Research Perspectives on the Role of Informatics in Health Policy and Management

Christo El Morr
York University, Canada

A volume in the Advances in Healthcare
Information Systems and Administration
(AHISA) Book Series

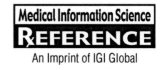

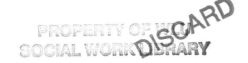

Managing Director: Lindsay Johnston
Editorial Director: Joel Gamon
Production Manager: Jennifer Yoder
Publishing Systems Analyst: Adrienne Freeland
Development Editor: Christine Smith
Assistant Acquisitions Editor: Kayla Wolfe
Typesetter: Lisandro Gonzalez
Cover Design: Jason Mull

Published in the United States of America by
    Medical Information Science Reference (an imprint of IGI Global)
    701 E. Chocolate Avenue
    Hershey PA 17033
    Tel: 717-533-8845
    Fax: 717-533-8661
    E-mail: cust@igi-global.com
    Web site: http://www.igi-global.com

Library of Congress Cataloging-in-Publication Data

Research perspectives on the role of informatics in health policy management / Christo El Morr, editor.
      pages cm
   Summary: "This book focuses on the advancements of Health Information Science in order to solve current and forthcoming problems in the health sector, helping to widen healthcare professionals' and researchers' perspectives on healthcare delivery"-- Provided by publisher.
   Includes bibliographical references and index.
   ISBN 978-1-4666-4321-5 (hardcover) -- ISBN 978-1-4666-4322-2 (ebook) -- ISBN 978-1-4666-4323-9 (print & perpetual access) 1. Health services administration--Data processing. 2. Information resources management. 3. Medical informatics--Research. 4. Management information systems. I. El Morr, Christo, 1966- editor of compilation.
   RA971.6.R47 2014
   610.285--dc23
                              2013011180

This book is published in the IGI Global book series Advances in Healthcare Information Systems and Administration (AHISA) (ISSN: 2328-1243; eISSN: 2328-126X)

British Cataloguing in Publication Data
A Cataloguing in Publication record for this book is available from the British Library.

All work contributed to this book is new, previously-unpublished material. The views expressed in this book are those of the authors, but not necessarily of the publisher.

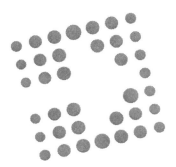

Advances in Healthcare Information Systems and Administration (AHISA) Book Series

Anastasius Moumtzoglou
Hellenic Society for Quality & Safety in Healthcare and P. & A. Kyriakou Children's Hospital, Greece
Anastasia N. Kastania
Athens University of Economics and Business, Greece

ISSN: 2328-1243
EISSN: 2328-126X

MISSION

The **Advances in Healthcare Information Systems and Administration (AHISA) Book Series** aims to provide a channel for international researchers to progress the field of study on technology and its implications on healthcare and health information systems. With the growing focus on healthcare and the importance of enhancing this industry to tend to the expanding population, the book series seeks to accelerate the awareness of technological advancements of health information systems and expand awareness and implementation.

Driven by advancing technologies and their clinical applications, the emerging field of health information systems and informatics is still searching for coherent directing frameworks to advance health care and clinical practices and research. Conducting research in these areas is both promising and challenging due to a host of factors, including rapidly evolving technologies and their application complexity. At the same time, organizational issues, including technology adoption, diffusion and acceptance as well as cost benefits and cost effectiveness of advancing health information systems and informatics applications as innovative forms of investment in healthcare are gaining attention as well. **AHISI** addresses these concepts and critical issues.

COVERAGE

- Clinical Decision Support Design, Development and Implementation
- E-Health and M-Health
- IT Applications in Physical Therapeutic Treatments
- IT Security and Privacy Issues
- Management of Emerging Health Care Technologies
- Pharmaceutical and Home Healthcare Informatics
- Rehabilitative Technologies
- Role of Informatics Specialists
- Telemedicine
- Virtual Health Technologies

IGI Global is currently accepting manuscripts for publication within this series. To submit a proposal for a volume in this series, please contact our Acquisition Editors at Acquisitions@igi-global.com or visit: http://www.igi-global.com/publish/.

Titles in this Series

For a list of additional titles in this series, please visit: www.igi-global.com

Advancing Medical Practice through Technology Applications for Healthcare Delivery, Management, and Quality
Joel J.P.C. Rodrigues (Instituto de Telecomunicações, University of Beira Interior, Portugal)
Medical Information Science Reference • copyright 2014 • 361pp • H/C (ISBN: 9781466646193) • US $245.00 (our price)

Patient Safety and Quality Care through Health Informatics
Vaughn Michell (University of Reading, UK) Deborah J. Rosenorn-Lanng (University of Reading, UK) Stephen R. Gulliver (Royal Berkshire Hospital Foundation Trust Reading, UK) and Wendy Currie (Audencia, Ecole de Management, Nantes, France)
Medical Information Science Reference • copyright 2014 • 357pp • H/C (ISBN: 9781466645462) • US $245.00 (our price)

Research Perspectives on the Role of Informatics in Health Policy and Management
Christo El Morr (York University, Canada)
Medical Information Science Reference • copyright 2014 • 351pp • H/C (ISBN: 9781466643215) • US $245.00 (our price)

Cross-Cultural Training and Teamwork in Healthcare
Simona Vasilache (Academy of Economic Studies, Romania)
Medical Information Science Reference • copyright 2014 • 326pp • H/C (ISBN: 9781466643253) • US $245.00 (our price)

Serious Games for Healthcare Applications and Implications
Sylvester Arnab (Coventry University, UK) Ian Dunwell (Coventry University, UK) and Kurt Debattista (University of Warwick, UK)
Medical Information Science Reference • copyright 2013 • 370pp • H/C (ISBN: 9781466619036) • US $245.00 (our price)

Telemedicine and E-Health Services, Policies, and Applications Advancements and Developments
Joel J. P. C. Rodrigues (Instituto de Telecomunicações, University of Beira Interior, Portugal) Isabel de la Torre Díez (University of Valladolid, Spain) and Beatriz Sainz de Abajo (University of Valladolid, Spain)
Medical Information Science Reference • copyright 2012 • 572pp • H/C (ISBN: 9781466608887) • US $245.00 (our price)

E-Healthcare Systems and Wireless Communications Current and Future Challenges
Mohamed K. Watfa (University of Wollongong, UAE)
Medical Information Science Reference • copyright 2012 • 462pp • H/C (ISBN: 9781613501238) • US $245.00 (our price)

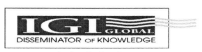

www.igi-global.com

701 E. Chocolate Ave., Hershey, PA 17033
Order online at www.igi-global.com or call 717-533-8845 x100
To place a standing order for titles released in this series, contact: cust@igi-global.com
Mon-Fri 8:00 am - 5:00 pm (est) or fax 24 hours a day 717-533-8661

Table of Contents

Section 1
Informatics and Health Management Perspectives

Detailed Table of Contents

Section 1
Informatics and Health Management Perspectives

The first section takes a look at innovative ways in using Health Informatics in health management to provide solutions for many of the field's challenges.

Through review of medical decision-decision making theories, this chapter identifies the elements affecting the nature of support that is required. These elements are demonstrated to be three: discipline, objective, and setting. Authors attempt to provide metrics that can be used to compare and evaluate the decision support systems.

Clinical decisions based on inaccurate sources of information can lead to medical errors. This chapter is a detailed discussion of the advantages of the PARIHS framework for implementing change in the decision-making process, in comparison to traditional models. It also summaries a knowledge translation attempt based on PARIHS framework, emphasizing the considerable need for health informatics in its context.

The chapter elucidates the use of a rehabilitation model to improve the decision-making processes in Long-Term Care (LTC) facilities in order to enhance the outcomes of seniors across the Ontario LTC continuum. It explains the effects of the model on quality of care and cost savings for the LTC industry and the health system. Finally, the chapter highlights the need to identify strategies for harnessing health informatics innovations to enable health system transformation.

Chapter 4

This chapter discusses the need to provide radiographers' performance appraisals in a continuous way, in order to enhance total quality in the radiology department. It provides the results of an empirical study that provided objective performance indicators derived from data stored in the PACS and RIS. The study indicates the ability to use informatics to enable PACS-RIS to act as a Decision Support System (DSS). Finally, the chapter outlines a model of a DSS that allows radiographers' continuous performance appraisals.

Chapter 5

The chapter discusses the shift in Ontario hospitals from global to activity-based funding and its impact on operational budget and cost management; it describes how case costing data and case mix information are collected and used for funding. It proposes a framework that connects input variables for determining resource utilization and long stays trim point. The author describes a clinical decision-making tool that supports hospital administrators in defining admission criteria and predicts length of stay. The chapter highlights the importance of informatics and data quality and concludes with 10 key success factors for better funding and benchmarking.

Chapter 6

This chapter describes the implementation of case costing using Ontario Case Costing Initiative (OCCI) as a guideline for a hospital. It addresses the implementation process and discusses ways for planning, implementing, transitioning, and evaluation of case costing. The chapter discusses the use of informatics to allow health care professionals to analyze integrated health information and enable evidence-based decision-making.

Chapter 7
Informatics and Health Services: The Potential Benefits and Challenges of Electronic Health
Records and Personal Electronic Health Records in Patient Care, Cost Control, and Health
Research – An Overview 89

This chapter focuses on the use of personal electronic health records as a key factor to improve health
care for patients, empower them by increasing their ability to self-manage their care, share decision
making. It discusses the utilizing information technology to moderate the cost of health care services,
improve clinical research, and determining best practices. Moreover, it reveals the many challenges to
implementation that must be addressed before these potential improvements in order to fully realize the
perceived benefits.

Section 2
Informatics and Health Policy Perspectives

*The second section of this book will take a look at innovative ways in using Health Informatics to provide
solutions in the Health Policy field.*

Chapter 8
The Administrative Policy Quandary in Canada's Health Service Organizations 116

This chapter analyzes the process for administrative health service policy development with respect to
information sharing and decision-making as well as the relationship of policy to decision making. It
identifies the challenges experienced by health service managers, and gives an example from a health
policy experience in Nova Scotia. By exploring the importance and nature of administrative policy as
a foundation for quality improvement in healthcare delivery, a case is made for greater use of health
informatics tools and processes.

Chapter 9
Towards Healthy Public Policy: GIS and Food Systems Analysis 135

This chapter makes the case for incorporating food systems analysis into public health practices. It addresses the challenges regarding food security, and investigates the ways health informatics can help in
establishing a Decision Making for food security taking into account production, processing, distribution, access, consumption, and waste management. It demonstrates how public health informatics can
offer potential answers to handling and using the large amount of information and geospatial data in a
food systems analysis approach. The author provides a scenario that envisions using a type of spatial
analytic tool, called Spatial On-Line Analytic Processing (spatial OLAP or SOLAP), for public health
decision-making.

Chapter 10

This chapter makes the case for the adoption of various healthcare technologies in order for the public sector to manage scarce resources and healthcare dollars to improve the health of seniors and the care available closer to home in Ontario, Canada. The Computerized Physician Order Entry (CPOE) Systems and Telehomecare are given as examples of health informatics solution working for attaining the policy concerns goal of caring for aging population in a manageable cost effective manner.

Section 3
Informatics Challenges

This section explores the information technology challenges and opportunities related to the use of health informatics in the health sector and particularly in health policy and management.

Chapter 11

This chapter analyzes the technological offerings and result of the epSOS (European Patient Smart Open Services) framework and how it has impacted strategic decisions in electronic prescription in Greece. It explores a new e-health national application and demonstrates that by rethinking healthcare, reusing established standards, it is conceivable to suggest new innovative systems.

Chapter 12

The chapter analyzes the reasons behind the little improvements witnessed in health, despite investments in health information technology. It examines the diverse priorities of stakeholders in the health system, particularly four stakeholder groups: patients, providers, pharmaceuticals, and payers. The chapter maps these priorities against the priorities of government and public health within the United States healthcare system. The authors find that these priorities are incongruent and in conflict, and suggest that policy makers and public health officials must understand these dichotomous priorities and work to bring them in line.

Chapter 13

This chapter explores the use of home telecare as an alternative medical approach to managing the increase in acute and long-term care admissions. The authors propose the use of a cardiac implant in conjunction with a mobile device to assist managing chronic heart failure. They discuss how this proposal helps in overcoming emergent limitations related to home telecare such as usability, self-management, and confinement to the home. Mobile wireless technology is suggested as an innovation that will drastically improve clinical decision-making and management of health services in the future.

Chapter 14

Chiara Libreri, Università Cattolica del Sacro Cuore, Italy
Guendalina Graffigna, Università Cattolica del Sacro Cuore, Italy

This chapter discusses how Web 2.0 has allowed knowledge sharing and construction between patients, in particular chronic patients. It also demonstrates that it is still unclear how patients use Web 2.0 for knowledge processes: what kind of knowledge processes happen in Web 2.0 between patients? How does Web 2.0 sustain or impede these processes? The authors develop a systematic exploration of the Web and analyze the diabetes sites in Italy. According to a psychosocial perspective, their findings highlight the main features of online knowledge processes among patients.

Foreword

Research Perspectives on the Role of Informatics in Health Policy and Management is an important new piece of work in the field that will be of interest and very useful for researchers, decision makers, and graduate students interested in the application of health informatics to a broad array of health system issues. The book's uniqueness and importance is evident in three respects.

First, this volume, which is divided into three sections, integrates work from a broad range of other disciplines. Research in health informatics, health policy, and healthcare organization and management is often discipline specific – an approach that is important for the deeper understanding of theory and practice it encourages in each of these areas. However, the current book, *Research Perspectives on the Role of Informatics in Health Policy and Management,* fills a gap that persists in the application of knowledge from other disciplines to existing and emerging health management and policy problems. As a field, healthcare practitioners and researchers would benefit tremendously from taking greater advantage of and integrating well-developed bodies of work that exist in the social sciences and other relevant fields such as engineering. *Research Perspectives on the Role of Informatics in Health Policy and Management* does an excellent job of integrating knowledge from a wide number of these disciplines and applying that knowledge to the study of pressing health care challenges. In doing so, the current work recognizes that the application of health informatics solutions is not a straightforward rational process in which new and superior technology is seamlessly applied to improve information and quality of care. Instead, many of the chapters recognize and make efforts to address the kind of non-rational barriers to the use of information technology that remain pervasive (e.g. competing stakeholder interests).

Second, there is a very broad micro to macro application approach that is evident when these 14 chapters are considered together. *Research Perspectives on the Role of Informatics in Health Policy and Management* brings a cross-disciplinary approach to applying health informatics to health management and health policy challenges. Inherent in this work is an underlying recognition that health informatics, as a field, provides more than technological solutions to small-scale practical problems. Instead, knowledge and applications from the field of health informatics can be applied to a broad range of significant health care, management, and policy issues that plague health systems at the most macro as well as the most micro levels.

Finally, the compilation of chapters found in this volume move beyond traditional settings and sectors. *Research Perspectives on the Role of Informatics in Health Policy and Management* is a must read for those interested in thinking about how health informatics can be applied beyond in-patient and out-patient settings to other sectors such as public health and health policy decision making.

Liane Ginsburg
York University, Canada

Liane Ginsburg *trained in healthcare organization and management at the University of Toronto where she received her PhD. She is an Associate Professor in the School of Health Policy and Management at York University and an Ontario Ministry of Health Career Scientist. Liane teaches Applied Research Methods in Health to 4th year undergraduate students in the Honors Bachelor of Health Studies Program at York. Her research interests focus on patient safety culture and learning from patient safety events. She has published several recent peer reviewed papers in these areas, most recently in Health Services Research, Social Science and Medicine, Quality and Safety in Health Care and Implementation Science. Liane is also interested in knowledge translation, specifically with respect to the utilization of research, data, and other information by health system managers, and she is the scientific officer of the Canadian Institutes for Health Research (CIHR) Knowledge Translation peer review committee. Liane is currently principal investigator on CIHR and CPSI funded studies.*

Preface

The discipline of health informatics is growing in importance and is attracting attention in both fields of health and information technology. Disciplines as varied as health management, health policy, psychology, kinesiology, nursing, information technology, computer science, software engineering, computer engineering, and telecommunication are taking advantage of health informatics and contributing to the evolution of the discipline.

The application area of health informatics is wide; it varies from Extra-Hospital applications (i.e., tele-medicine, tele-care, tele-monitoring), to Intra-Hospital application (e.g., Picture Archiving and Communication Systems, Hospital Information Systems, Radiologic Information System), as well as other more recent applications such as Health Virtual communities and Decision Support Systems. The aim of health informatics stays the same: offering support for health care delivery by providing the right information at the right time to the right people in the right cost.

While Health Informatics, Health Management, and Health Policy are well-established fields of research and teaching, rare are the books that intertwine these fields in order to explore innovative cross-disciplinary approaches to health management as well as to health policy, using health informatics.

This book is here to partially fill this gap; we hope it as a first step of a series of books investigating new innovative interdisciplinary approaches in healthcare. There is a lack of investigation of the potential advantages of health informatics, especially in the public policy sector; this book will provide an overview of important ways in which health informatics can contribute to finding solutions in health policy and management.

The unique perspective of this book is the integration of Health Informatics into health Management and health policy perspectives. The book includes analyses that show how Health Informatics can be used by Health Management and Health policy researchers in order to provide solutions to pending problems in the health sector. It sketches a vision for the coming and supplies it with practical research examples in both health management and health policy.

Many stakeholders can take advantage of this book. Masters and PhD students can use this book to widen their perspective in health management, health policy, and health informatics. The book can provide a textbook-like source for advanced health informatics, management, and policy courses. Researchers in the fields of management, policy, and informatics will profit from this book's holistic and integrative perspective. It will provide them with a rich pool of ideas in how to use informatics in their respective field of research. Managers in non-governmental organizations as well as governmental bodies can use the book to understand the new solutions that informatics can provide in their strategic planning.

Research Perspectives on the Role of Informatics in Health Policy and Management is divided into three sections.

Section 1 takes a look at innovative ways in using health informatics in health management to provide solutions for many of the field's challenges.

Chapter 1 identifies the elements affecting the nature of support that is required. These elements are demonstrated to be three: discipline, objective, and setting. The authors attempt to provide metrics that can be used to compare and evaluate the decision support systems.

In chapter 2, we encounter a detailed discussion the advantages the PARIHS framework for implementing change in the decision making process, in comparison to traditional models. The chapter also summaries a knowledge translation attempt based on PARIHS framework, emphasizing the considerable need for a health informatics in its context.

Chapter 3 elucidates the use of a rehabilitation model to improve the decision-making processes in Long-Term Care (LTC) facilities in order to enhance the outcomes of seniors across the Ontario LTC continuum. It explains the effects of the model on quality of care and cost savings for the LTC industry and the health system. Finally, the chapter highlights the need to identify strategies for harnessing health informatics innovations to enable health system transformation.

Chapter 4 discusses the need to provide radiographers' performance appraisal in a continuous way, in order to enhance total quality in the radiology department. It provides the results of an empirical study that provided objective performance indicators derived from data stored in the PACS and RIS. The study indicates the ability to use informatics to enable PACS-RIS to act as a Decision Support System (DSS). Finally, the chapter outlines a model of a DSS that allows radiographers' continuous performance appraisal.

Chapter 5 discusses the shift in Ontario hospitals from global to activity-based funding and its impact on operational budget and cost management; it describes how case costing data and case mix information are collected and used for funding. It proposes a framework that connects input variables for determining resource utilization and long stays trim point. The author describes a clinical decision-making tool that supports hospital administrators in defining admission criteria, and predicts length of stay. The chapter highlights the importance of informatics and data quality and concludes with 10 key success factors for better funding and benchmarking.

In chapter 6, we find a description about the implementation of case costing using Ontario Case Costing Initiative (OCCI) as a hospital guideline. The chapter addresses the implementation process and discusses ways for planning, implementing, transitioning, and evaluation of case costing. The chapter discusses the use of informatics to allow health care professionals to analyze integrated health information and enable evidence-based decision-making.

Chapter 7 focuses on the use of personal electronic health records as a key factor to improve health care for patients, empower them by increasing their ability to self-manage their care, and share decision-making. It discusses utilizing information technology to moderate the cost of health care services, improve clinical research, and determining best practices. Moreover, it reveals the many challenges to implementation that must be addressed before these potential improvements in order to fully realize the perceived benefits.

Section 2 investigates innovative health informatics applications in the health policy.

Chapter 8 analyzes the process for administrative health service policy development with respect to information sharing and decision-making as well as the relationship of policy to decision making. It identifies the challenges experienced by health service managers and gives an example from a health policy experience in Nova Scotia. By exploring the importance and nature of administrative policy as a foundation for quality improvement in healthcare delivery, a case is made for greater use of health informatics tools and processes.

Chapter 9 makes the case for incorporating food systems analysis into public health practices. It addresses the challenges regarding food security, and investigates the ways health informatics can help in establishing a decision making for food security taking into account production, processing, distribution, access, consumption, and waste management. It demonstrates how public health informatics can offer potential answers to handling and using the large amount of information and geospatial data in a food systems analysis approach. The author provides a scenario that envisions using a type of spatial analytic tool, called Spatial On-Line Analytic Processing (spatial OLAP or SOLAP), for public health decision-making.

Chapter 10 makes the case for the adoption of various healthcare technologies in order for the public sector to manage scarce resources and healthcare dollars to improve the health of seniors and the care available closer to home in Ontario, Canada. The Computerized Physician Order Entry (CPOE) Systems and Telehomecare are given as examples of health informatics solution working for attaining the policy concerns goal of caring for aging population in a manageable cost-effective manner.

Section 3 explores the information technology challenges and opportunities related to the use of health informatics in the health sector and particularly in health policy and management.

In chapter 11, we find an analysis of the technological offerings and result of the epSOS (European Patient Smart Open Services) framework and how it has impacted strategic decisions in electronic prescription in Greece. The chapter explores a new e-health national application and demonstrates that by rethinking healthcare, reusing established standards, it is conceivable to suggest new innovative systems.

Chapter 12 analyzes the reasons behind the little improvements witnessed in health despite investments in health information technology. It examines the diverse priorities of stakeholders in the health system, particularly four stakeholder groups: patients, providers, pharmaceuticals, and payers. The chapter maps these priorities against the priorities of government and public health within the United States healthcare system. The authors find that these priorities are incongruent and in conflict, and suggest that policy makers and public health officials must understand these dichotomous priorities and work to bring them in line.

Moreover, chapter 13 explores the use of home telecare as an alternative medical approach to managing the increase in acute and long-term care admissions. The authors propose the use of a cardiac implant in conjunction with a mobile device to assist managing chronic heart failure. They discuss how this proposal helps in overcoming emergent limitations related to home telecare such as usability, self-management, and confinement to the home. Mobile wireless technology is suggested as an innovation that will drastically improve clinical decision-making and management of health services in the future.

Finally, chapter 14 discusses how Web 2.0 has allowed knowledge sharing and construction between patients, in particular chronic patients. It also demonstrates that it is still unclear how patients use Web 2.0 for knowledge processes: what kind of knowledge processes happen in Web 2.0 between patients? How does Web 2.0 sustain or impede these processes? The authors develop a systematic exploration of the Web and analyze diabetes sites in Italy. According to a psychosocial perspective, their findings highlight the main features of online knowledge processes among patients.

Christo El Morr
York University, Canada

Section 1
Informatics and Health Management Perspectives

Chapter 1
Decision–Making and Decision Support in Acute Care

Brett W. Taylor
Dalhousie University, Canada

ABSTRACT

Clinical Decision Support Systems (CDSS) are information tools intended to optimize medical choice, promising better patient outcomes, faster care, reduced resource expenditure, or some combination of all three. Clinical trials of CDSS have provided only insipid evidence of benefit to date. This chapter reviews the theory of medical decision-decision making, identifying the different decision support needs of novices and experts, and demonstrates that discipline, objective and setting, and affect of the nature of support that is required. A discussion on categorization attempts to provide metrics by which systems can be compared and evaluated, in particular with regard to decision support mechanics and function. Throughout, the common theme is the placement of clinical decision makers at the center of the design or evaluation process.

BACKGROUND

Life is short, art long, opportunity fleeting, experience treacherous, judgment difficult. -Hippocrates Aphorisms, Section 1

Clinical decision support comes with an implicit promise: better patient outcomes, faster care, reduced resource expenditure or some combination of all three. There is no shortage of improvements to be had. In 2003, Bates and his coauthors lamented the issues found in a review of their own institution's practices: "... only 27% of antiepilep-

tic drug levels had an appropriate indication and, among these, half were drawn at an inappropriate time ... only 16% [of digoxin levels] were appropriate ... 28% [of lab tests] were ordered too early[to be useful]... the initial thyroid test performed was [inappropriate] in 52% ... Only 17% of diabetics who needed eye examinations had them ... guidelines for vancomycin use were not followed 68% of the time." (Bates, et al., 2003, p. 523) Brigham and Women's Hospital (Bates' home institution) is a well known center of excellence for medical care; the issues listed are indicative of an epidemic of medical error and inefficiency found in virtually every care setting. The scope of this problem was made clear three years earlier by the publication

DOI: 10.4018/978-1-4666-4321-5.ch001

of "To Err is Human" by the Committee on Quality of Health Care in America (Kohn, Corrigan, & Donaldson, 2000). Their review suggests that between 3% and 4% of all hospitalizations are associated with adverse events, over half of which result from medical error. Extrapolation suggests that "at least 44,000 Americans die each year as a result of medical errors." (Kohn, Corrigan, & Donaldson, 2000, p. 1) Many other publications have since expanded on this issue.

Clinical Decision Support Systems (CDSS) are tools intended to optimize medical choice such that error is minimized and efficiencies are found. Early versions of these products became available in the late 1950s (Miller, 2009); with the advent of cheap and widely available computing, interest in CDSS has exploded. Literally thousands of medical apps are now available for mobile devices, electronic health information systems generally come with the promise of decision support, and the concept is ubiquitous in modern culture.

Medical error is a huge problem, and one which decision support seems well suited to answer. It is a bit frustrating, then, to see that the evidence of benefit from CDSS is relatively insipid.

In 1998, a systematic review of CDSS revealed that while 60% of studies on drug dosing systems and 74% on preventative care systems showed positive effects on physician performance, only 42% of studies showed benefits to patient-oriented outcomes. Diagnostic support was particularly troubling; only 20% of these studies documented evidence of benefit (Hunt, Haynes, Hanna, & Smith, 1998). In 2012, Bright and her colleagues performed another systematic review (Bright, et al., 2012), revealing little evidence of benefit for length of stay, mortality, or risk of adverse event. Only modest impact on morbidity was found. CDSS did appear to be effective at improving the health care process; the delivery of recommended treatments, studies, and preventative care appeared better with the systems than without them. However, 14 years after Hunt's initial systematic review,

Bright and her colleagues found that there was still insufficient literature to assess the effect on user knowledge, clinician workload, physician efficiency, or patient satisfaction (Bright, et al., 2012). A review in 2010 by Lau, more generally aimed at health information systems, demonstrated that while medication errors were reduced and preventative care was somewhat improved, these systems did not lead to improvements in resource utilization, healthcare cost or patient oriented health care outcomes. Thirty percent of studies demonstrated a negative effect on provider time efficiency; that is, the use of the system actually slowed the clinician down (Lau, Kuziemsky, Price, & Gardner, 2010). A more recent review concluded that "the majority of CCDSSs demonstrated improvements in process of care, but patient outcomes were less likely to be evaluated and far less likely to show positive results" (Sahota, et al., 2011).

The evidence, in other words, that decision support improves the health of patients, efficiency of clinicians or the cost of health care is slim at best. "Better patient outcomes, faster care, reduced resource expenditure or some combination" does not seem to be a promise we are fulfilling.

Why is there so little consistent evidence of benefit for decision support systems?

One answer may lie in the quality and nature of the literature. Systematic reviews tend to lump together disparate systems (Berlin, Sorani, & Sim, 2006). Those that demonstrate excellence might be lost in the great mixing pots that reviews and broad based surveys become; any conclusions regarding efficacy from these reviews are dubious at best. As well, although things are improving, the quality of academic writing regarding benefits and risks of decision support has been notably poor. Descriptive articles or case studies are much more common than controlled clinical trials, and even these often suffer from inadequate statistical power (Lau, Kuziemsky, Price, & Gardner, 2010). Such studies do not offer much to a systematic review of the literature.

However, even given these concerns, the evidence strongly suggests issues with fundamental system design. In this area, there are reasons to be optimistic. Medical decision making theory is in the process of extensive renovation, and our interventions might improve once these advances have been incorporated into CDSS planning. The relatively new development of a hybrid worker, the "health informatician" who has an understanding of both medical care and information management, is encouraging. The opportunity for clinicians to actually have input into the key elements of their own decision support is only now gaining strength. It may be that after a few decades of inappropriately interrupting clinical workflow with inefficient methods of communication about data with little potential benefit to the decision-making process, we may finally be ready to start from a sound theoretical framework, with leaders who have been specifically trained and the right collection of people around the table.

This chapter will explore the key features of decision support as it applies to acute care. One key thesis of this text is the notion that to date modern theories of complex decision making have not been widely implemented in CDSS design; this text will open with an overview of this theory as it relates to acute care. A discussion on how the diversity of user and decision type affects CDSS design will follow. Finally, the chapter ends with thoughts on how best to categorize these products, based on the premise that methods of categorization inform key metrics important to designers, purchasers and end users.

Where available, relevant and provocative literature is referenced. The principle objective is to challenge the current process of CDSS design and implementation. Too often, these occur on the basis of poorly supported assumptions about decision making mechanics and a lack of understanding of the health care process at the provider level. Ultimately, this text argues that designers, administrators and academics should include real life decision making in design and evaluation.

AN OVERVIEW OF MEDICAL DECISION-MAKING

An understanding of the basics of medical decision-making is important in designing or evaluating decision support. This section of text will provide a brief review of decision-making theory, particularly as it applies to medical care. Prescriptive models of decision-making, which require logic and deductive reasoning, will be differentiated from naturalistic models, which are based on pattern recognition and heuristics. These will be discussed as separate entities, although in real clinical situations decision-making probably involves elements of each. The point will be made that providers of clinical decision support should be prepared for both strategies, and that naturalistic models have been relatively ignored.

The dominant theories of decision-making for much of the last two millenia have assumed the superiority of logic and reason over non-analytical approaches such as intuition, judgement and emotion (Lehrer, 2009; March & Olsen, 1986). In fact this view is still so widely held that "good decision-making" is often felt to be impossible without logic. Modern theory, however, casts doubt on this.

The classic model implies that good decision-making occurs when a cold, rational calculus informs the entire process. In this view, more data and processing time inevitably results in better decisions, while emotionality, hunch and intuition are viewed with suspicion. Short cuts through the logic process are seen as potential sources of error. This view has led to the "prescriptive approach", which attempts to describe an optimal decision process for a given set of circumstances. Choices are assumed to be made by a rational decision maker (Djulbegovic, Hozo, Beckstead, Tsalatsanis, & Pauker, 2012), whom is fully informed and able to compute with perfect accuracy.

Alternatively, the naturalistic approach attempts to describe "how humans actually make decisions in complex real-world settings", in circumstances characterised by "dynamic and continually changing conditions, real-time reactions to these changes, ill-defined tasks, time pressure, significant personal consequences for mistakes, and experienced decision makers" (Klein & Klinger, 1991, p. 16). Medicine in an acute care setting, such as the emergency department, clearly fits this description. In these decision spaces there is often inadequate data available and there is no fully rational, fully informed, computationally perfect decision maker. Interestingly, work from the real world suggests that the most successful actors in these complex decision spaces use many logic short cuts, and routinely rely on emotionality, hunch, and intuition. Naturalistic models try to describe decision making as it actually happens, rather than prescribing perfection.

In naturalistic models, experience is seen as a critical enabler. Decision makers engage in very rapid, experientially informed pattern recognition (Klein & Klinger, 1991; Norman, Young, & Brooks, 2007), mediated at least in part by tacit, emotion based processes (Lehrer, 2009). Players see "themselves as acting and reacting on the basis of prior experience ... generating, monitoring and modifying plans to meet the needs of the situation" (Klein & Klinger, 1991, p. 17). Evidence of extensive, rational option generation is not found; that is, there is little indication that a logic based, optimal choice model is being followed. Indeed, under these circumstances, decision makers "rarely use analytical methods and nonanalytical methods can be identified that are flexible, efficient, and effective" (Klein & Klinger, 1991, p. 17).

This is a problem for decision support designers, because it is much easier to provide knowledge, which supports prescriptive decision making, than it is to augment experience.

One example of real world non-analytical methods are heuristics, or rules of thumb (this text will use the word "heuristic" and "algorithm" interchangeably). These are sets of easily followed instructions that can be used to short cut more lengthy reasoning techniques. Heuristics are used in decision theory to explain how remarkable decisions are made when the resources required for a full logical appraisal are lacking.

Consider, for example, the now classic case of catching a baseball. When an outfielder catches a baseball in the air, he acts as though he had solved, in the time between the crack of the bat and the catch, a set of differential equations involving the mass of the ball, the impact of the bat, the effect of wind and gravity, the exact distance between the batter and himself, and many other parameters. Unfortunately for those who might be tempted to model this with a fully informed, perfectly rational baseball player, our meager computational capabilities are clearly inadequate to the task. So how do we do it?

The answer appears to be the application of the "gaze heuristic", which can be simply stated: "Fixate your gaze on the ball, start running, and adjust [direction and] speed so that the angle of the gaze remains constant" (Gigerenzer, 2008). A catcher following this rule has no need to calculate or even know the parameters involved in Newton's laws of motion. He also has no way to predict where the ball will land; rather, by following the heuristic, he will be there when it does.

The best heuristics appear to be those that Gerd Gigerenzer describes as both "fast and frugal" (Gigerenzer, 2008). That is, the algorithm should provide a solution quickly enough to work in real world settings, and should do so without requiring a large computational resource. Explicit heuristics are those that are consciously created, modified and used; one medical example is the rapid decision rule which allows bedside screening for certain types of stroke (Gigerenzer & Gaissmaier, 2011, p. 469) and which, in a few minutes at the bedside, outperforms an MRI scan which costs hours of wait time and thousands of dollars. In contrast, tacit heuristics represent "understanding without rationale" (Bond & Cooper, 2006). Baseball players, for example, typically cannot describe the gaze heursitic; they have no conscious understanding of the decision mechanics involved. Through practice and experience, they simply catch the ball. Gigerenzer theorizes that some of our decision heuristics are hard wired into our biology, modeled by evolutionary pressures (Gigerenzer, 2008).

Tacit decision-making is probably best modeled as a self correcting neural network, in which experience (or perhaps, as above, evolution) plays a substantial role in establishing net architecture. Recognition and to some extent response are informed by a pre-cognitive process, one that does not require an internal dialogue or a chain of reason (Lehrer, 2009). In such cases, it is relatively pointless to ask physicians, for example, to describe their internal logic because, literally, there is no logic to describe (Norman, Young, & Brooks, 2007).

Pattern recognition is an essential component of complex naturalistic decision making, an example of tacit heuristics that are very difficult to distil and teach. A child presenting with difficulty breathing, for example, can be safely and rapidly identified as a "wheezer," judged as being low to moderate risk, and placed on an asthma protocol within minutes of arrival, in spite of the wide range of other possible etiologies, such as inhaled foreign body, pneumonia, cardiac problems, etc. Experienced clinicians do not appear to spend much time assessing this decision space during their initial examination; rather, they appear to very rapidly categorize the presentation into a "type" of patient, then unpack the appropriate intervention algorithm for that group. Then, like decision makers in other domains, they seek feedback about the accuracy of the initial classification, and adjust responses accordingly (Klein & Klinger, 1991). This rapid categorization occurs to some extent across all levels of expertise, but more experienced clinicians perform more accurately (Elstein, Shulman, & Sprafka, 1978; Bordage & Lemieux, 1991).

Pattern recognition, then, is an early component of naturalistic decision making in acute care, and appears to be largely tacit. Further, the pattern recognized clearly determines subsequent decision-making; researchers have found that decision makers in complex settings "... relied on their ability to recognize and appropriately classify a situation. Once they knew it was 'that' type of case, they usually also knew the typical way of reacting to it" (Klein & Klinger, 1991). In other words, it was the initial pattern recognition that selected the subsequent intervention.

There are clear risks here. The clinician might anchor inappropriately on first impressions, or be swayed by the experience that asthma is common and inhaled foreign bodies are not, and so might err on the basis of a decision making process that, because it is tacit and not accessible to consciousness, is not auditable for critical review later. Collectively these and other similar mistakes are labelled "cognitive error", and will be discussed a bit later in the text.

Because of the implicit reliance on experience, it is perhaps not surprising that novices tend to more explicit data analysis and logic, while experts rely increasingly on pattern recognition and heuristics (Elstein, Shulman, & Sprafka, 1978). The impact of environment, the decision mechanics, and subsequently the decision support required differ depending upon the decision mechanics involved.

Consider the decisions involved in working through the large cohort of toddlers who present each winter with an unfocused fevers to emergency care. By "unfocused" we mean that no obvious cause will be found on examination; there is, in other words, no red throat, no easily identified viral rash, no obvious skin infection, etc. In this group, bacterial infections like pneumonia, sepsis or meningitis are rare, comprising perhaps one to two percent of the group at most (Trainor & Stamos, 2011). The vast majority have illnesses that, however uncomfortable, are managed principally with fluids, over the counter medications and time.

Investigating an individual patient for the rare bacterial causes is painful, involves exposure to x-rays, affects patient flow in the department, and is expensive. It is simply not justifiable in most such children. However, missing a patient with meningitis, for example, can be devastating. Some children from this group must be selected for further investigation, while in others the decision must be made to watch and wait. This is, simply, a categorization decision, in which the decision maker must choose what "type" of patient (in this case, low versus high risk) is presenting.

The prescriptive decision-making model is rational, stepwise and logical. The clinician should begin with an unbiased mind, thoroughly interrogate the parent and child, and perform a complete physical exam. Information gained is then used to construct a series of theories that might explain the clinical findings. These are ranked both according to likelihood and risk, and specific investigations and treatment, if needed, are then provided.

Those who are new to clinical medicine often appear to behave in precisely this fashion. The process is laborious and time consuming; it requires immense amounts of acquired data and laboratory work and therefore is quite interventionist ... more pokes and cost per child. Abnormality in medicine is often a statistical definition, in which "low" values are defined as being below the 5th percentile, for example. Natural biological variation is also an issue. Consequently, the more tests performed, the greater the risk that false "abnormalities" will be detected merely by chance. The consequence is that ambiguous or even conflicting data is often obtained.

Nonetheless the prescriptive model is logical, results in a reconstructable decision-making process that is clearly understood and articulated by the decision maker when presenting later to a supervisor.

Experienced clinicians, however, simply don't work this way. Experts will pluck one child out of their febrile population on the basis of a history and exam that takes seconds to minutes to perform. They will then "unpack" a previously constructed treatment algorithm, and initiate an immediate action plan. Investigations and therapy are characteristically conducted simultaneously; by the time confirmatory blood work returns, specific treatment has often already been given. Conversely, other (low risk) children will be directed, equally rapidly, into less aggressive pathways. Even in cases where more traditional logic style decision models are evident, where more extensive history, physical and laboratory parameters are sought, the initial data collection process is very truncated. The decision tree is aggressively pruned prior to being used, on the basis of very little explicit data (Elstein, Shulman, & Sprafka, 1978; Bond & Cooper, 2006).

In experienced hands, this process is pre-cognitive, alingual, and *fast*, one that communicates with the decision maker through emotions rather than internal dialogue. When asked by students later to explain their decision-making process, how one child was chosen over another, why this hot tachycardic toddler was given antipyretics and left to be re-assessed later while his apparent peer was subjected to costly and often painful intervention, most physicians will not be able to clearly articulate their reasons. Indeed, the experienced clinician in a rapidly evolving situation such as the one above will often simply (and honestly) reply "the child frightened me".

We can oversimplify by saying that while medical trainees may think their way through problems, medical experts recognize them. A more accurate statement, though, would be that in the absence of experience, trainees may be forced to rely on logic and the sort of generic information conveyed by textbooks and lectures, while their more senior colleagues can utilize pattern recognition borne of years of practice, and fed by the sort of patient-specific information conveyed by context and circumstance.

Designing decision support for the expert in this setting is clearly much more challenging than it is for the novice. The student merely requires access to knowledge in a user-friendly, just-in-time fashion. Expert users already have well developed knowledge structures (Bordage & Lemieux, 1991; Schmidt & Boshuizen, 1993); augmenting these seems to provide little additional benefit to the decision making process.

Support structures that allow rational short cuts to these decision makers, such as pre-existing assessment algorithms in flow-chart format, for example, may be useful. Unfortunately, this hypothesis is not borne out by the limited literature available. For example, the only publication found on CDSS for unfocused fever involved a prescriptive model that provided a risk score on the basis of user-entered data. Compliance was low at 49%, and compared to controls who were not exposed to the CDSS, no benefit in care was observed. In fact there was a non-significant trend to increased time in the department for those using the tool, and more tests were ordered for the CDSS cohort than the control group. Use of the CDSS was subsequently discontinued (Roukema, Steyerberg, van der Lei, & Moll, 2008).

It seems that where prescriptive decision making requires rapid access to knowledge and machine generated heuristics, pattern recognition benefits from data which challenges the selected practice plan. Pattern recognizers are eager consumers of data, so long as it is appropriately presented, easily visualized, and contextual. They are poor consumers of instruction, preferring in study after study to trust their (pattern based, customized, contextual) assessment of the individual patient, or a similar assessment performed by their peers (Tamber, 2012; Lin, Lin, & Roan, 2011), than the (non-contextual, generic, literature based) advice of anonymous "experts".

In other settings, where the task is managing a wide range of chronic illnesses following guidelines that are constantly updated, prescriptive CDSS has been shown to decrease laboratory testing and therefore the costs of providing health care (Poley, et al., 2007). In this instance, acquir-

ing and maintaining expertise in optimal care is difficult, and prescriptive methods are shown to be valuable. Clearly, decision support designers need to be aware of, and provide for, both contexts.

Naturalistic decision-making represents distinct risks. Pattern recognition represents an opportunity to anchor inappropriately, to explain away important discrepancies in data in favor of the pattern that has been imposed (Bond & Cooper, 2006). Naturalistic decision-making may be more prone to other cognitive errors as well; a number of these have been described (Norman, 2009). Humans are very good at imposing a pattern on streaming data, even when one doesn't exist (a process known as "pattern forcing"). Combined with the "availability error" (a tendency to judge diagnoses as more likely if they are more easily retrievable from memory) this means that in the absence of a clear emergent pattern the clinician is likely to impose one, very often based on recent, rather than extended experience. Once a false pattern has been identified, it is often difficult to see others in an even handed fashion ("anchoring error"). Clinicians are prone to stop searching when the first abnormality or explanation is detected ("premature closure") and there is a great tendency to seek data to confirm, not refute the initial hypothesis ("confirmation bias"). Finally, tacit processes are confounded by emotional bias; the clinician may be more likely to be frightened by a given patient if recent clinical experience has been harrowing, or to be overly cavalier if coming off a long run of therapeutic success.

Recognition of these and other cognitive errors has led some to rate heuristic, intuitive decision-making as relatively unreliable, error prone, and associated with low scientific rigor (Croskerry, 2009), yet this appears to be based on previous information theory, and not on empirical (scientifically rigorous) data. Conversely, "there is very little evidence to associate diagnostic errors with ... [non-analytical reasoning] ... experts are as likely to commit errors when they are attempting to be systematic and analytical." (Norman & Eva, 2010). Indeed, it is tempting to say that non-analytical methods are better, if they provide greater speed and lower resource utilization, yet with comparable error rates. Clearly this issue needs further investigation.

Decision-making in medicine is not as dichotomous as has been presented in this text. Rather, choice is probably made using a two system process or perhaps a spectrum of strategies, with more experienced decision makers selecting the method that works best for any given presentation (Norman, 2009; Croskerry, 2009; Osman, 2004). All clinicians, regardless of experience, routinely see patient presentations that are new to them. Pattern recognition may still play a role with regard to the initial triage and stabilization of such patients, but it is hard to see how intuitive data processing can provide a diagnosis in the absence of experience. Prescriptive methods, logic and deductive reasoning are crucial. Similarly, even the greenest novice brings experiential knowledge to a clinician / patient interaction, and is clearly guided by this in the weighing of clinical data.

Croskerry has noted that the research community is uncomfortable with naturalistic theory, in particular with the difficulties in studying its mechanism, and producing testable predictions. As a result " an important feature of clinicians' decision-making is apparently disqualified from study by those who research the field of medical decision-making" (Croskerry, 2009). This is no less true for clinicians, managers, and informaticians. While designing CDSS for naturalistic models is admittedly difficult, and requires a re-thinking of both architecture and output, examples such as the febrile child suggest that the current prescriptive approaches may not be particularly ef-

fective. Discomfort with non-analytical decision-making seems to be a poor reason to exclude it from decision support.

In summary, then, our overview of medical decision-making theory:

- Modern decision-making theory can be divided into:
  - Prescriptive models of decision-making, which require fully informed, computationally accurate and wholly rational clinicians.
  - Naturalistic models, which are based on pattern recognition and heuristics.
  - In real clinical situations, this probably reflects a spectrum of strategies which are deployed depending on circumstance and experience.
- Prescriptive strategies are characterised by logic and deductive reasoning. Although superior in the theoretical setting of infinite knowledge, resources and rationality, these suffer in the face of limited knowledge, limited (human) computational resources, and time pressures.
- Naturalistic reasoning, characterised by pattern recognition and heuristics, is extremely prevalent, and extraordinarily functional in the face of limited resources and time pressures. However, these processes are prone to early anchoring and pattern forcing, cannot be dissected, audited or rationally confirmed, and are prone to be affected adversely by recent (negative) experience.
- While debate continues about which of these two models represent optimal decision-making strategy, data would indicate that sophisticated decision makers use both, depending on patient circumstance

and setting. Clearly, optimal decision support should provide for both types of decision mechanics, if it hopes to be relevant to acute care clinicians.

POPULATIONS OF USERS, AND THEIR DECISION SUPPORT NEEDS

CDSS is best evaluated on the basis of how well it meets the needs of its users. These can be clustered according to domain (e.g. nursing, medicine, pharmacy), by experience (learner versus expert), and by administrative level (front line worker, area manager, institutional manager, etc.) as well as any number of other site specific dimensions. Designing and evaluating decision support requires that the needs of these various users be taken into account. It is therefore essential to understand which population (or populations) will be using the technology involved.

Support required will also vary according to the nature of the decision the system is asked to augment. For example, if the intent is to encourage compliance with practice guidelines for a given diagnosis, the task is directing the caregiver along a defined path. Asthma maps in emergency care frequently consist of simple pathways with a number of optional branch points (Figure 1).

If a CDSS were designed to support such a path, the task might be reduced to reminding caregivers about the guideline, and providing a template with automatic drug calculation. Note that even in this simple example, the need (encouraging compliance with the pathway, and avoiding calculation error) can result in a powerful emergent consequence

Figure 1. Medication orders from an asthma care map used in a pediatric emergency department

Medication Orders	
Start Date: Time:	
■ Supplemental oxygen to keep oxygen saturation > 91%	
■ Corticosteroid (choose ONE option): ❑ predniSONE/prednisoLONE ______mg PO x 1 dose (Dose = 1 mg/kg/dose rounded up to nearest 5 mg, max. 50 mg/dose) ❑ dexamethasone ________ mg PO x 1 dose (Dose 0.3 mg/kg/dose rounded up to nearest 1 mg, max. 12 mg/dose) ❑ methylPREDNISolone ________ mg IV x 1 dose) (Dose = 2 mg/kg/dose, max. 125 mg/dose)	
❑ MDI / SPACER:	❑ WET NEBULIZATION
Ipratropium - given to all Level 2 patients and at the discretion of physician for Level 3-5 patients.	
■ First Dose: salbutamol 100 micrograms/puff 10 puffs > 5 yr; 5 puffs < 5 yr ❑ ipratropium bromide 20 micrograms/puff -8 puffs > 5 yr; 4 puffs < 5 yr	■ First mask: salbutamol (5 mg by inhalation) (2.5 mg < 5 yr) ❑ ipratropium bromide 250 micrograms < 5 yr; 500 micrograms > 5 yr
■ Second Dose (5-10 minutes following first MDI/Spacer): salbutamol -10 puffs > 5 yr; 5 puffs < 5 yr) ❑ ipratropium bromide 20 micrograms/puff - 8 puffs > 5 yr; 4 puffs < 5 yr	■ Second mask (immediately following above steroid administration) salbutamol 5 mg (2.5 mg < 5 yr old) ❑ ipratropium bromide 250 micrograms < 5 yr; 500 micrograms > 5 yr
■ Third dose (5-10 minutes following second MID/Spacer): salbutamol - 10 puffs > 5 yr; 5 puffs < 5 yr ❑ ipratropium bromide - 8 puffs > 5 yr; 4 puffs < 5 yr	■ Third mask: salbutamol 5 mg (2.5 mg < 5 yr) ❑ ipratropium bromide 250 micrograms < 5 yr; 500 micrograms > 5 yr
■ Room air saturation level 10 minutes following third MDI/spacer or mask	
■ Resume oxygen therapy if oxygen saturation level < 91% on room air	
■ Use salbutamol - 5 or 10 puffs for subsequent doses	■ Use salbutamol 5 mg (2.5 mg< 5 yrs old) (standard dose) for subsequent masks
Other Orders	**Disposition from ED**
❑ NPO ❑ CBC Done @ hours ❑ Capillary Blood Gas Done @ hours ❑ PA and Lateral Chest X-ray Done @ hours ❑ Lytes Done @ hours	• Saturation on room air while awake > 92% • Respiratory, neurological & cardiovascular stable 2 hour post therapy • Written Discharge Home Instructions

(knowledge translation about the pathway itself, and therefore optimal asthma care). Also note that this support mechanism is prescriptive, and is to some extent self terminating; after a very brief exposure, presumably, the map would be memorized, limiting the value of the intervention to the (nonetheless important) role of automating drug dosage calculation.

Frequently, both the task and the optimal user base are more complex. Consider, for example, providing decision support for the triage process in an emergency department. The primary purpose of triage is to ensure that care is delivered first to those who need it most. A head to head comparison of CDSS for triage (eTriage) versus standard practice has been published (Dong, et al., 2005), as has an evaluation of its reliability (Dong, et al., 2006). eTriage provided lists of patient parameters to triage nurses and automated scoring for their patients in an attempt to improve recognition of higher needs individuals. Again, this was a prescriptive approach, in this instance directed at triage nurses who are, by selection, expert in their craft. The performance of the system was relatively lukewarm. It appeared to be less specific in identifying individuals in the "Emergent" (Canadian Triage and Acuity Scale - CTAS - 2) category, placing far more individuals into this category than standard triage. Further, the correlation between triage level and admission rate for CTAS 2 patients seemed better for the unsupported nurse. Agreement between triage nurses and the CDSS was moderate.

Clearly, when first transitioning into the triage role, there is a learning curve. Everyone is a novice at some point. Further, presentations to the emergency department are intrinsically varied; while many patients will have conditions and complaints that are common, each shift provides an opportunity for even an experienced triage nurse to see a patient presentation that is entirely new to her. Some role exists for a prescriptive approach, perhaps available through user-customization. However, rather than attempting to augment the well developed knowledge structures of expert tri-

age nurses, eTriage might have been more effective if it supported and expanded clinical experience, perhaps by highlighting patient presentations that are statistically likely to be mis-triaged, or by identifying patient presentations that the individual triage nurse has problems with.

In any case, the triage process also provides critical direction to other health care workers in the department. When the waiting room contains less urgent patients, more time can be spent providing complete care. However, as the acuity in the waiting room rises, so does the pressure on acute care staff to provide the essentials only. For unit managers, funders and policy makers, triage is one of several metrics used to evaluate the overall needs of the patient population served. Collated triage data is a valid predictor of resource utilization (Chang, Ng, Wu, Chen, Chen, & Hsu, 2012). Optimal design of triage decision support might logically expand, therefore, beyond the initial task of triage to include these secondary needs. A holistic approach to this problem might also include a dashboard reflecting the triage status of the waiting room to the rest of the acute care staff, an alert system to let more senior administrators know when the ED is experiencing a crisis of patient flow, and a data cube that could be accessed by management and policy makers to help support higher level analyses and decisions. Privacy concerns and use would dictate a different granularity of information for each user group; the ability to "drill down" into more personal information would be more important to the triage nurse, for example, while the ability to "roll up" (collate) would be utilized primarily by those involved in planning.

So in summary, we can say the following about decision maker populations and the decision support needs they represent:

- Different decision support is needed depending upon the complexity of the decision task. We showed the differences between very narrow, simple applications of CDSS (e.g. the asthma care map example) versus more broad based, complex implementations (e.g. triage support). A determination of the decision support needs of the population must be based upon a clear understanding of the intended data use and clinical outcome of the support application. This should be assessed on a case by case basis.

- Different decision support is needed for different health care actors based on their training and fundamental roles. Front line clinicians need access to high granularity patient specific information (e.g. the triage nurse who needs access to the patient's past medical visits). Their colleagues, at different points in the care path for the same patient population, need access to real time information with immediate resource implications (e.g. the acute care nurses and physicians in the ED, who need to prepare for the patients in the waiting room). Administrators, funders and policy makers need increasingly high level population data that represent longer term population need and cost. Again, the use and clinical impact of the data will guide those needs, generally on a case by case basis.

- Support needs are also different depending on decision-making strategy employed, supporting learners and novices with more prescriptive methods, and experts with more experiential information.

- Each of these factors inter-relate; the final assessment of needs for any decision support population will be based on the sum of these effects.

CATEGORIZING CLINICAL DECISION SUPPORT SYSTEMS

The term CDSS references a large and diverse group of systems with a variety of intended uses. Any discussion of CDSS is facilitated by a clear categorization of the many different types available. While a variety of classification schemas are available, none have been validated against efficacy (as measured by changes in resource, efficiency or patient oriented outcomes), and few are designed to provide an easy set of metrics for system selection by either clinicians or administrators. As with so much associated with decision support, an ideal classification scheme seems to still be on the "to-do" list.

Commonly in medical (as opposed to informatics) literature, systems are categorized by setting. References such as "decision support in the emergency department" (Graber & VanScoy, 2003; Kulkarni, 2005) or "pediatric clinical decision support" (Ramnarayan & Britto, 2002) are readily found. This classification is useful for the end user who wishes to peruse the systems available for a particular domain, but is not particularly helpful to those who would design or evaluate such systems. It is clear that there are distinct similarities in both decision-making structure and strategy across clinical settings (i.e. the logic of an "Emergency Department" CDSS might work very well in a family medicine clinic), and also that there are distinct differences within each setting (decisions regarding the elderly with chest pain are quite different than those involving pre-school children, regardless as to whether they both present to an Emergency Department). A grouping of the varied types of CDSS by disease or clinical setting therefore should be seen as a useful search strategy for perusing options, but is otherwise rather limited as a classification schema.

Another approach is to lump applications together on the basis of the platform upon which they are based. Members of the American Academy of Pediatrics Steering Committee on Clinical Information Technology, for example, separated CDSS into those based on mobile devices ("handheld computers"), those housed on the Internet, and those intimately linked to an electronic medical record system (Longhurst & Hahn, 2005). This classification had the advantage of recognizing the differences implied by the immediately local (to the decision maker) nature of information on mobile devices, the much greater computational capacity of Web based services and the value of a direct link with patient data. The problem is that this technological context is becoming increasingly dated; the line between systems residing on mobile devices and those housed online has been blurred by increasing connectivity and the increasing power of mobile. It is unlikely that any platform based categorization schema will age well in the future. Aside from the obvious implementation issues in which available technology places a limit on the choice of system, this schema has limited value.

Yet another approach describes systems on the basis of the decision support mechanics involved. "Mechanics" here means the details involving the timing and nature of the information delivered, the delivery process itself, and the intended impact of the decision support intervention. In other words, the classification of the CDSS in this model is based on the way in which it manages (queries, customizes, creates) knowledge, and how it inserts the resulting output into the decision-making process. Concerns such as the timing of support (before, during or after the clinical encounter / decision), passivity versus activity of the user ("pull" versus "push" of information) are examples, as well as the reasoning method used (Berner & La Lande; Berlin, Sorani, & Sim, 2006). Each of these has distinct advantages; however, in general none are sufficient in isolation.

A taxonomic classification has been published by Berlin and colleagues (Berlin, Sorani, & Sim, 2006). In this schema, CDSS is classified according to several axes:

- **Context:** Including clinical setting, clinical task, anticipated outcome, relation to point of care, institutional buy in and change management, and potential barriers.

- **Knowledge and Data Sources:** Including the source for clinical knowledge such as guidelines, etc; sources for patient data such as EMR, paper chart, data coding, degree of customization and update mechanism.

- **Decision Support:** Including reasoning method, clinical urgency, recommendation explicitness, logistical complexity and response requirement.

- **Information Delivery:** Including the format, mode, integration and usability of the information provided.

- **Workflow:** Including the identity of the user, the target decision maker, the need for data input or output intermediaries, and the degree of workflow integration.

As a metric for funders or clinicians looking to purchase decision support this classification system conceptually addresses the critical points of having a clear objective ("context") for the system, and makes explicit the communication and workflow issues that arise. This schema or something like it seems very well suited to be part of any formal assessment process for CDSS. However, a critical player, the end user, is not specifically represented. Consequently there is little understanding of user type (novice or expert) and therefore what type of support (prescriptive or naturalistic) is required.

In our institution, we have experimented with a "clinician centered" approach to decision support categorization that recognizes that the contribution of the system lies not just with its internal logic, platform or setting, but also on the basis of the decision-making function provided, the manner in which the decision support adds value to a decision making process.

Using this approach, it is possible to identify a number of functions that are provided by decision support systems:

- **Knowledge Base Enhancement:** Knowledge base enhancers range in simplicity from products like Isabel (Isabel Health Care, 2012) which are simply electronic textbooks, to systems with more sophisticated logic attached. Since expert decision makers already have sophisticated knowledge structures, knowledge enhancement is more useful to learners, or to clinicians who are otherwise expert but approaching a novel clinical situation.

- **Information Visualization:** The field of computer assisted visualization is based on recognition that for humans, the visual information channel has a very large capacity, and very fast processing speeds, resulting in nearly immediate (so-called "pre-cognitive") recognition of data anomalies (Ware, 2004). As noted, experienced naturalistic decision makers are challenged by discerning an appropriate signal (important information) in a sea of noise (irrelevant information). Techniques which report some data dimensions visually can markedly enhance the signal in such settings. Some of these can be quite simple, even paper based. For example, highlighting abnormal lab values with a distinctive color or changing their placement on the page allows for the transfer of data in a "glancable" fashion; a quick look can confirm that all is normal, or that a particular part of the information needs to be more carefully scrutinized. Visualization can also allow for the immediate recognition of possible patterns in the data, as in the clustering of data points on a screen showing infectious disease surveillance information. Critically, information visualization

helps both the expert and the learner, since appropriate visualization helps to frame and re-frame the clinical problem.

- **Patient Care Heuristics / Clinical Care Guidelines:** A paper copy of a clinical guideline is abstract and general, while the electronic copy can be as complicated and specific as required, taking into account the patient's age, gender, risk factors, etc, effectively piloting the caregiver through the process of planning a truly customized treatment regimen. The asthma care map example given previously in this chapter is a simple example of this type of support mechanics. Often, encapsulated within this support type is automatic calculation, knowledge translation about appropriate care, and integrated monitoring of those aspects of patient outcomes that determine care farther down the pathway. This sort of support offers something for most decision makers, however it should be recognized that the expert decision maker will likely come to rely only on the automated features, having internalized the knowledge implicit in the pathway over time. This knowledge translation is very functional, particularly when this sort of decision support is applied to self guided care.

- **Error Detection and Reduction:** This function can be seen in the automation of clinical pathways and as an aspect of visualization; however the importance of this function suggests that it should be provided its own category. Drug dosage calculators, automated pre-op checklists, automatic alerts and other functions that are intended to draw the often limited attention of a busy practitioner to a common source of error, or to avoid error prone processes entirely (e.g. calculation) are included in this functionality. Many of these utilize "push" technology, since by definition they are required to insert information into the decision-making process that is not being specifically sought.

We relate these four basic decision-making functions to the costs, usability, system and workload implications when evaluating decision support structures. It must be emphasized that this is a localistic approach, not validated against patient or user outcomes, and that it is a relatively new approach for our institution. Clearly more research is required, both regarding this "clinician-centered" approach and other categorization schemas.

Categorization does not judge quality of product directly, yet it is clear that low quality products will not be used, or worse, will contribute to a deterioration in care. Bates lists "10 Commandments" of decision support design (Bates, et al., 2003). Amongst these is recognition that systems must not delay care, and that the fit with workflow must be carefully considered. System usability and the delivery of the right information at the right time are also highlighted. Bates states that the requirement for user input should be minimized in the sense that information from clinicians should be sought only when absolutely necessary. User satisfaction is sometimes seen as a sales pitch rather than a measure of system competence, but this is not so. "The advice that a CDDSS offers to highly trained, knowledgeable clinicians must be of sufficient quality to merit the clinicians' trust and respect" (Miller, 2009). To be effective, a system must be used, and irritating, slow systems that give advice that is either obvious or not credible will simply be discarded. Key features involve the inclusion of clinicians in the development cycle and the emphasis of speed

and work flow issues. Feedback from users and evidence of benefit during the iterative development cycle is vital. Maintaining these knowledge systems once produced is also crucial to success.

In summary, some combination of Berlin's taxonomic categorization method, and perhaps our decision-maker centered approach seems to answer most of the needs of those who would select, evaluate and use decision support systems. It must be emphasized again that this is an emerging discussion, and that more work sophisticated and holistic metrics are badly needed. Regardless of the categorization schema involved, a separate assessment of quality, including impact on workflow, usability, and credibility / usefulness of support provided is necessary.

CONCLUSION

Those of us who work in the front lines of medical care routinely see amazing things. Remarkable decisions and sound judgement are the norm in our care systems, and the sophistication with which complex clinical issues are recognized, stabilized and definitively managed is, at times, simply breathtaking.

Yet, that remarkable system is under threat. The costs involved with providing care are unsustainably rising in every constituency, to the point where the future of service delivery is being seriously questioned. The explosion in medical knowledge has not been matched by a knowledge translation process that reliably converts understanding into more effective care. Although outcomes are generally good, error is pervasive; we cannot deny that we are systematically harming an unconscionable number of patients through mistakes, inconsistency, misunderstanding and shear medical ignorance. The waste in medicine through inappropriate investigations, useless or even harmful interventions, and error in diagnosis and management represents huge potential revenues. The quality of life, and in a distressing number of cases life itself, is at stake for our patients.

The discipline of decision support has been invigorated by technological advances and an increased appreciation for the mechanics of decision-making. In the area of preventative health, drug prescribing and compliance with recommendations, CDSS appears to facilitate distinct improvements in the delivery of care. In acute care, the challenges of supporting diagnosis, improving efficiencies and demonstrably altering patient outcomes remain at this point works in process.

There is an ongoing need to continue to improve the scientific rigor with which we approach the assessment of decision support. We are well past the point where simple proof of concept or demonstration work should engender much buzz; the onus must be on developers and marketers to prove that costs, efficiencies, or patient outcomes are positively affected by their systems. We need study data on both successful and unsuccessful design and delivery. Implementation at the institutional level should, simply, be considered incomplete until such evaluations are made; these should be in the budget from the beginning, enclosed within the development cycle and widely distributed through publication and presentation. The expectation should be an openness about the bang for any bucks spent. Otherwise knowledge is held in institutional silos, and further progress is inhibited.

This chapter has reviewed the nature of medical decision-making, identifying the different decision support needs of novices and experts. It has discussed the various players and sampled clinical contexts to show that discipline, objective and setting each affect the nature of support that is required. An attempt has been made, through the

discussion on categorization, to provide metrics by which systems can be compared and evaluated, in particular with regard to decision support mechanics and function. Throughout, the common theme was the placement of clinical decision makers at the center of the design or evaluation process, so that systems that are built or purchased can be clearly seen to work with the users for whom they are notionally intended.

The question is not whether we take steps to support the decision-making of health care workers, it is, rather, how we will do so. Regardless of background, each of us is a patient, and each a medical decision maker. The challenge we face is significant, to be bombarded by data, yet to find wisdom within it.

ACKNOWLEDGMENT

The author would like to acknowledge Dr. Katrina Hurley for her discussions and proofing related to this chapter.

REFERENCES

Bates, D., Kuperman, G., Wang, S., Gandhi, T., Kittler, A., & Volk, L. et al. (2003). Ten commandments for effective clinical decision support: Making the practice of evidence-based medicine a reality. *Journal of the American Medical Informatics Association*, 10(6), 523–530. doi:10.1197/jamia.M1370 PMID:12925543.

Berlin, A., Sorani, M., & Sim, I. (2006). A taxonomic description of computer-based clinical decision support systems. *Journal of Biomedical Informatics*, 39(6), 565–667. doi:10.1016/j.jbi.2005.12.003 PMID:16442854.

Berner, E., & La Lande, T. (n.d.). Overview of clinical decision support systems. In Berner, E. (Ed.), *Clinical Decision Support Systems Theory and Practice*. Academic Press.

Bond, S., & Cooper, S. (2006). Modelling emergency decisions: Recognition-primed decision making: The literature in relation to an opthalmic critical incident. *Journal of Clinical Nursing*, *15*(8), 1023–1032. doi:10.1111/j.1365-2702.2006.01399.x PMID:16879547.

Bordage, G., & Lemieux, M. (1991). Semantic structures and diagnostic thinking of experts and novices. *Academic Medicine*, *66*(Suppl), 70–72. doi:10.1097/00001888-199109000-00045 PMID:1930535.

Bright, T., Wong, A., Dhurjati, R., Bristow, E., Bastian, L., & Coeytaux, R. et al. (2012). Effect of clinical decision-support systems a systematic review. *Annals of Internal Medicine*, *157*(1), 29–43. doi:10.7326/0003-4819-157-1-201207030-00450 PMID:22751758.

Chang, Y., Ng, C., Wu, C., Li-Chin, C., Chen, C., & Kuang-Hung, H. (2012). Effectiveness of a five-level pediatric triage system: an analysis of resource utilization in the emergency department in Tawaan. *Emergency Medicine Journal*. doi:10.1136/emermed-2012-201362 PMID:22983978.

Croskerry, P. (2009). A universal model of diagnostic reasoning. *Academic Medicine*, *84*(8), 1022–1028. doi:10.1097/ACM.0b013e3181ace703 PMID:19638766.

Djulbegovic, B., Hozo, I., Beckstead, J., Tsalatsanis, A., & Pauker, S. (2012). Dual processing model of medical decision-making. *BMC Medical Informatics and Decision Making*, *12*(1), 94. doi:10.1186/1472-6947-12-94 PMID:22943520.

Dong, S., Bullard, M., Blitz, S., Ohinmaa, A., & Holroyd, B. et al. (2006). Reliability of computerized emergency triage. *Academic Emergency Medicine*, *13*(3). doi:10.1111/j.1553-2712.2006.tb01691.x PMID:16495428.

Dong, S., Bullard, M., Meurer, D., Colman, I., Blitz, S., & Holroyd, B. et al. (2005). Emergency triage: comparing a novel computer triage program with standard triage. *Academic Emergency Medicine*, *12*(6), 502–507. doi:10.1111/j.1553-2712.2005.tb00889.x PMID:15930400.

Elstein, A., Shulman, L., & Sprafka, S. (1978). *Medical problem solving: An analysis of clinical reasoning*. Cambridge, MA: Harvard University Press.

Gigerenzer, G. (2008). Fast and frugal heuristics. In *Rationality for Mortals: How People Cope with Uncertainty*. New York: Oxford University Press.

Gigerenzer, G., & Gaissmaier, W. (2011). Heuristic decision making. *Annual Review of Psychology*, *62*, 451–482. doi:10.1146/annurev-psych-120709-145346 PMID:21126183.

Graber, M., & VanScoy, D. (2003). How well does decision support software perform in the emergency department? *Emergency Medicine Journal*, *20*(5), 426–428. doi:10.1136/emj.20.5.426 PMID:12954680.

Hunt, D., Haynes, R., Hanna, S., & Smith, K. (1998). Effects of computer-based clinical decision support systems on physician performance and patient outcome. *Journal of the American Medical Association, 280*(15), 1339–1346. doi:10.1001/jama.280.15.1339 PMID:9794315.

Isabel Health Care. (2012). *Home*. Retrieved 07 05, 2012, from www.isabelhealthcare.com/home/default

Klein, G., & Klinger, D. (1991). Naturalistic decision making. *Human Systems IAC Gateway, 11*(3), 16–19.

Kohn, L., Corrigan, J., & Donaldson, M. (2000). *To err is human: Building a safer health system*. Washington, DC: The National Academioes Press.

Kulkarni, G. (2005). Diagnostic decision support in the ED: Practical considerations. *Emergency Medicine Journal, 22*(6), 462. PMID:15911967.

Lau, F., Kuziemsky, C., Price, M., & Gardner, J. (2010). A review on systematic reviews of health information system studies. *Journal of the American Medical Informatics Association, 17*(6), 637–645. doi:10.1136/jamia.2010.004838 PMID:20962125.

Lehrer, J. (2009). The Predictions of Dopamine. In *How We Decide* (pp. 28–56). New York: Houghton Mifflin Harcourt Publishing Co..

Lin, C., Lin, I., & Roan, J. (2012). Barriers to physicians' adoption of healthcare information technology: An empirical study on multiple hospitals. *Journal of Medical Systems, 36*(3), 1965–1977. doi:10.1007/s10916-011-9656-7 PMID:21336605.

Longhurst, C., & Hahn, J. (2005). Clinical decision-support systems in pediatrics. *COCIT Newsletter, 10*.

March, J., & Olsen, J. (1986). Garbage can models of decision making in organizations. In March, K., & Weissinger-Baylon, R. (Eds.), *Ambiguity and Command* (pp. 11–35). New York: Longman Inc..

Miller, R. (2009). Computer-assisted diagnostic decision support: History, challenges and possible paths forward. *Advances in Health Science Education, 14*(Suppl 1), 89–106. doi:10.1007/s10459-009-9186-y PMID:19672686.

Norman, G. (2009). Dual processing and diagnostic error. *Advances in Health Science Education, 14*(Suppl 1), 37–39. doi:10.1007/s10459-009-9179-x.

Norman, G., & Eva, K. (2010). Diagnostic error and reasoning. *Medical Education, 44*(1), 94–100. doi:10.1111/j.1365-2923.2009.03507.x PMID:20078760.

Norman, G., Young, M., & Brooks, L. (2007). Non-analytical models of clinical reasoning: The role of experience. *Medical Education, 41*(12), 1140–1145. doi: doi:10.1111/j.1365-2923.2007.02914.x PMID:18004990.

Osman, M. (2004). An evaluation of the dual-process theories of reasoning. *Psychonomic Bulletin & Review, 11*(6), 988–1010. doi:10.3758/BF03196730 PMID:15875969.

Poley, M., Edelenbos, K., Mosseveld, M., van Wijk, M., Bakker, D., & van der Lei, J. et al. (2007). Cost consequences of implementing an electronic decision support system for ordering laboratory tests in primary care: Evidence from a controlled prospective study in The Netherlands. *Clinical Chemistry, 53*(2), 213–219. doi:10.1373/clinchem.2006.073908 PMID:17185371.

Ramnarayan, P., & Britto, J. (2002). Pediatric decision support systems. *Archives of Disease in Childhood, 87*(5), 361–362. doi:10.1136/adc.87.5.361 PMID:12390900.

Roukema, J., Steyerberg, E., van der Lei, J., & Moll, H. (2008). Randomized trial of a clinical decision support system: Impact on the management of children with fever without apparent source. *Journal of the American Medical Informatics Association*, 15(1), 107–113. doi:10.1197/jamia.M2164 PMID:17947627.

Sahota, N., Lloyd, R., Ramakrishna, A., Mackay, J., Prorok, J., & Weise-Kelly, L. et al. (2011). Computerized clinical decision support systems for acute care management: A decision-maker-researcher partnership systematic review of effects on process of care and patient outcomes. *Implementation Science; IS*, 6(91). PMID:21824385.

Schmidt, H., & Boshuizen, H. (1993). On the origin of intermediate effects in clinical case recall. *Memory & Cognition*, 21(3), 338–351. doi:10.3758/BF03208266 PMID:8316096.

Tamber, P. (2012). *Doctors only trust doctors*. Retrieved 09 01, 2012, from http://blogs.bmj.com/bmj/2012/07/09/pritpal-s-tambar-doctors-only-trust-doctors/

Trainor, J., & Stamos, J. (2011). Fever without a localizing source. *Pediatric Annals*, 40(1), 21–25. doi:10.3928/00904481-20101214-06 PMID:21210596.

Ware, C. (2004). Foundation for a Science of data visualization. In Ware, C. (Ed.), *Information Visualization Perception for Design* (pp. 1–27). San Francisco, CA: Morgan Kaufman Publishers. doi:10.1016/B978-155860819-1/50004-2.

KEY TERMS AND DEFINITIONS

Acute Medical Care: Health care provided without substantial a priori planning on the part of the patient, in response to rapidly developing circumstances, generally provided in ambulatory clinics, emergency departments, and intensive care wards.

Clinical Decision Support Systems: Those systems which "link health observations with health knowledge to influence health choices by clinicians" Robert Hayward's definition.

Cognitive Errors: Common biases which potentially confound clinical and other decision making, identified by studying real life decision making.

Health Information Systems: The hardware and software required to store, search, view and use information regarding the care of patients, including patient, caregiver, and system data.

Medical Heuristics: Rule sets that provide rapid method of proceeding from data to decision without the expenditure of extensive overt logical processing. These can be considered to be decision making strategies, rather than decision making methods.

Naturalistic Decision theory: An alternative approach to the study of decision making that attempts to identify the steps taken by decision makers in real world settings.

Prescriptive Decision Theory: An approach to the understanding of decision making that attempts to identify the best process for arriving at the optimal outcome, and further supports the implementation of this identified best practice.

Chapter 2
Implementation of Evidence-Based Practice and the PARIHS Framework

Shahram Zaheer
York University, Canada

ABSTRACT

Patients receiving healthcare are commonly exposed to harm that is systematic and often severe. Clinical decisions based on inaccurate sources of information can lead to medical errors, high treatment costs, and poor patient outcomes. Evidence-based practice has the potential to overcome these problems by improving clinical decision-making processes. The PARIHS framework was developed to address the inability of traditional unidimensional models to successfully implement evidence-based practice. The PARIHS framework proposes that successful implementation of evidence into practice is a function of evidence, culture, and facilitation. The PARIHS framework can be used to design, implement, and evaluate knowledge translation projects at both acute and chronic care facilities. This chapter discusses the PARIHS framework as well as its advantages for implementing change at a healthcare setting compared to traditional models. The chapter also outlines a feasible knowledge translation project based on the principles of the PARIHS framework while highlighting health informatics and availability of easily accessible high quality patient outcome data as key enablers in designing and successfully implementing such a project at a healthcare setting.

MEDICAL ERRORS AND EVIDENCE-BASED MEDICINE

In modern health care stakes are high as a medical error can potentially have fatal consequences. The cost to health care system due to medical errors is enormous both in terms of finance and patient

well-being. It is estimated that 44,000 to 98,000 Americans die annually due to medical errors and that the annual costs for adverse events are between $38 billion to $50 billion (Institute of Medicine, 2000). An adverse event is defined as, "an unintended injury or complication that results in disability at the time of discharge, death or prolonged hospital stay and that is caused by health care management rather than the patient's

DOI: 10.4018/978-1-4666-4321-5.ch002

underlying disease process" (Baker et. al, 2004, p. 1679). A recent Canadian study found adverse event rate of 7.5 per 100 hospital admissions in participating Canadian hospitals after adjustment for sampling strategy. The same study associated approximately 1521 additional hospital days with adverse events (Baker et. al, 2004). It is quite evident that lowering the occurrence of medical errors in health care will not only lower financial costs but will also improve patient safety outcomes.

Research has shown that clinical decisions based on inaccurate sources of information can lead to medical errors, high treatment costs, and poor patient outcomes. Evidence based medicine has the potential to overcome these problems by enhancing healthcare staff clinical decision making processes. The term evidence based medicine, coined in the early 1990s, is defined as "the process of systematically finding, appraising and using contemporaneous research findings as the basis for clinical decisions" (Straus & McAlister, 2000, p. 837). It is a multistep process that takes into consideration not only the current best evidence from research but also the clinical expertise and patient values during clinical decision making (Haynes & Haines, 1998; Straus & McAlister, 2000). However, development and introduction of policies or guidelines based on current best evidence alone is not sufficient to change or modify clinical practice. For example, Rosser (1993) found that only 5% of surveyed Ontario family physicians followed the lipid lowering guidelines. Implementation of evidence often fail to change practice as policy makers, researchers, and managers frequently rely on unidimensional change models that are incapable to take into consideration all the complexities associated with the change process (Davis & Taylor-Vaisey, 1997; Kitson, Harvey, & McCormack, 1998). Healthcare organizations are living systems that are influenced by a large number of interdependent agents (such as patients, healthcare staff, hospital administration, accreditation and licensing bodies etc.) and external forces (such as political ideologies, provincial laws and regulations etc.)

in a nonlinear and discontinuous manner (Begun, Zimmerman, & Dooley, 2003). As a consequence, successful adoption of current best evidence into practice will necessitate the utilization of a holistic or a multidimensional framework that takes into consideration various contextual factors such as culture and leadership while implementing the change process.

In 1998, a team of researchers at Royal College of Nursing Institute developed a multidimensional framework, Promoting Action on Research Implementation in Health Services (PARIHS), that proposes that the successful implementation of evidence based practice is a function of evidence, context, and facilitation (Estabrooks et al., 2009b). A salient advantage of the PARIHS framework over the traditional implementation models is that it can allow health informatics to be integrated seamlessly within the change process during the implementation of evidence based practice. For example, it can be used to design a decision support tool that can suggest appropriate facilitating strategies such as leadership retreat, academic detailing, audit and feedback, and computer based reminders depending on the needs of a particular situation. The aim of this chapter will be to discuss in detail the advantages, challenges, and limitations of the PARIHS framework for implementing change at a healthcare setting. The chapter will also outline a feasible project to improve the uptake of clinical practice guidelines for prevention of pressure ulcers at a nursing care setting while highlighting the role of health informatics and availability of easily accessible high quality patient outcome data as key enablers in designing a project that can benefit from the comprehensive nature of the PARIHS implementation model without being limited by financial and logistical constraints.

THE PARIHS FRAMEWORK

The implementation of evidence into practice (also referred as knowledge translation or transfer) is a complex and challenging task as the process is influenced by a variety of factors simultaneously. However, most of the conceptual models or frameworks describing the implementation process are often linear and unidimensional in nature. For example, the Department of Health in England followed a framework for implementation of evidence into practice that consisted of three linear steps of "informing, monitoring, and changing practice" (Kitson, Harvey, & McCormack, 1998, p. 149). Implementation of evidence based on such frameworks often fails to change practice as they are incapable to take into consideration all the complexities associated with the change process.

In 1998, a team of researchers at Royal College of Nursing Institute identified a number of key variables that appear to influence the implementation of evidence into practice (Kitson, Harvey, & McCormack, 1998). The research team developed a multidimensional framework based on research evidence and on experience gained through working closely with clinicians directly involved in knowledge translation activities. This conceptual framework, Promoting Action on Research Implementation in Health Services (PARIHS), took into consideration the relationships and interdependence of key factors influencing simultaneously the implementation of evidence into practice (Kitson, Harvey, & McCormack, 1998; Rycroft-Malone, 2004).

The PARIHS framework proposes that the successful implementation of evidence based practice is a function of evidence, context, and facilitation (Estabrooks et al., 2009b). More specifically, the framework states that there must be clarity about "the nature of evidence being used, the quality of context, and the type of facilitation" required to ensure successful implementation of current best evidence into practice (Rycroft-Malone, 2004, p. 298). The framework envisions each of these three elements on a high to low continuum and having a simultaneous dynamic relationship with each other (Rycroft-Malone, 2004). The importance of these three elements to knowledge translation is discussed in detail below.

Evidence

The PARIHS framework defines evidence as "knowledge derived from a variety of sources that has been subjected to testing and has found to be credible" (Rycroft-Malone, 2004, p. 298). The framework identify three important components of evidence that are essential for clinical decision making: research, clinical experience, and patient experience (Rycroft-Malone et al., 2002). These three components of evidence are located on high to low continuum. For example, patient experience is high when patient narratives are considered a valid source of evidence and patient preferences are included in clinical decision making process (See Rycroft-Malone et al., 2004 for an in-depth concept analysis of the evidence dimension in the PARIHS framework).

The PARIHS framework suggests that to maximize the uptake of evidence into practice these three components should be located towards high on the continuum. However, the framework acknowledges that different components of evidence will be valued in different situations (Rycroft-Malone et al., 2002). For example, a treatment based on current best evidence offering long term benefits might not be appropriate in a given situation where a patient prefer an alternative treatment with less immediate risk. In other words, a clinician needs to balance research, clinical expertise, and patient preferences while making a clinical decision, a conclusion that is supported by other research studies (e.g., Haynes & Haines, 1998; Straus & McAlister, 2000) (see Figure 1).

Context

The PARIHS framework define context as "the environment or setting in which the proposed change is to be implemented" (Kitson, Harvey, & McCormack, 1998, p. 150). Research has shown that contextual factors can play an important mediator role during the implementation of evidence into practice (Davis & Taylor-Vaisey, 1997;

Figure 1. Components of evidence in the PARIHS framework (adapted from Rycroft-Malone, et al., 2002)

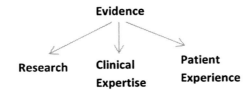

Evidence

Research   **Clinical Expertise**   **Patient Experience**

- Research is well conceived, designed, and conducted.
- Clinical experience tested and reflected upon.
- Patients are treated as partners and their experiences are valued.
- Research, clinical expertise, and patient experience are all considered during clinical decision making.

Rycroft-Malone, 2004, Estabrooks et al., 2009b). In the PARIHS framework, context is subdivided into three core components: culture, leadership, and evaluation.

To lower medical errors and improve patient safety outcomes, health care organizations need to change or modify their organizational culture in order to maximize the uptake of evidence into daily practice. Research in healthcare has primarily focused on addressing micro issues such as minimizing medication errors, improving anaesthesia care, and reducing diagnostic and treatment errors. However, for these efforts to bear fruit, attention also needs to be paid to the macro issue of organizational culture (Ruchlin, Dubbs, Callahan, & Fosina, 2004). Organizational culture "is the basic pattern of shared assumptions, values, and beliefs considered to be the correct way of thinking about and acting on problems and opportunities facing the organization" (McShane, 2006, p. 442). The PARIHS framework emphasizes the need to understand the dominant cultural values and beliefs at an organization before trying to implement current best evidence into practice (Rycroft-Malone et al., 2002). For example, the implementation process

might fail because clinicians are reluctant to accept new evidence in an environment that is task driven and places low value to the contributions of individual staff members. On the other hand, an organizational culture that values healthcare staff, promotes organizational learning, and facilitates teamwork is more likely to maximize the uptake of new evidence into daily practice (Kitson, Harvey, & McCormack, 1998; Rycroft-Malone et al., 2002).

Evidence based practice cannot be implemented without the help and guidance of visionary leadership figures. The PARIHS framework suggest that transformational leaders create a culture conducive to the uptake of evidence into practice by encouraging teamwork and inclusive decision making, and by teaching and empowering individual staff members (Rycroft-Malone et al., 2002). McClure and Hinshaw (2002) have shown that feelings of empowerment and autonomy in a hospital setting are associated with improved patient outcomes. Leadership that stresses the participation of all layers of staff in decision making leads to better outcomes in patient care and contributes to a cultural shift at a healthcare organization (Sherer, 1994). The degree of participation of employees in decision making is important since participativeness as a leadership dimension may interact with cultural variables (Fisher & Bibo, 2000). Participative leaders exhibit coaching behaviours that encourage unit members to speak openly and share their concerns (Chuang, Ginsburg, & Berta, 2007). It is important to note here that at a generic level "transformative leadership can be characterized as participative" leadership (Castellese, 2006, p. 39).

Evaluation is another component of the context that plays an important role in translating evidence into practice. Measurement is not only an integral part of research process for generating evidence but it is also an important feedback and evaluation mechanism for an organization to test the suitability, effectiveness, and efficacy of proposed changes to practice (Rycroft-Malone et al., 2002; Rycroft-Malone, 2004). An organization looking to implement evidence into practice must provide different sources of information/feedback (at indi-

vidual, team, and system levels) and rely on multiple methods (clinical, performance, economic, and experience) of evaluation (Rycroft-Malone et al., 2002). The physical environments in which healthcare services are delivered are complex and dynamic. The PARIHS framework acknowledges this fact by recognizing the importance of culture, leadership, and evaluation to the successful implementation of evidence into practice (See McCormack et al., 2002 for an in-depth concept analysis of the context dimension in the PARIHS framework) (see Figure 2).

Facilitation

The PARIHS framework defines facilitation as "the process of enabling (making easier) the implementation of evidence into practice" (Rycroft-Malone, 2004, p. 300). The task of facilitation is carried out by an individual (facilitator) that is specifically appointed to the task of translating evidence into practice at an organization/facil-

Figure 2. Components of context in the PARIHS framework (adapted from Rycroft-Malone, et al., 2002)

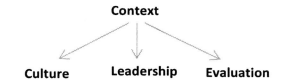

Context

Culture **Leadership** **Evaluation**

- Organizational culture and subcultures promotes learning, teamwork, and values individual staff.
- Leaders rely on transformational leadership approaches & democratic decision making processes.
- Reliance on multiple evaluation methods (clinical, economic, and performance etc.) and feedback is provided at individual, team, and system levels.

ity. It is important for the facilitator to possess appropriate knowledge, skills and attributes to successfully guide the implementation of evidence based practice. The facilitator play a key role in the implementation process by 1) helping clinicians make sense of the current best evidence and by 2) helping to modify the context (practice setting) where the change process in taking place (Rycroft-Malone et al., 2002).

The PARIHS framework stresses the importance of using "appropriate" mechanisms of facilitation for the implementation of evidence based practice "depending on the needs of the situation" (Rycroft-Malone et al., 2002, p. 177). In other words, a facilitator needs to take into consideration the purpose of the implementation process (i.e., to facilitate completion of a specific task or a complex holistic change) before selecting appropriate roles, skills and attributes that can be utilized to successfully implement

evidence into practice. Moreover, the facilitator can employ a range of strategies such as leadership retreat, academic detailing, audit and feedback, and computer based reminders depending on the needs of the situation to enable individuals, teams, and organizations to implement evidence into practice (See Harvey et al., 2002 for an in-depth concept analysis of the facilitation dimension in the PARIHS framework) (see Figure 3).

BENEFITS OF THE PARIHS FRAMEWORK TO THE HEALTH SYSTEM

During the last few decades, healthcare expenditure in Canada has grown at a significantly higher rate than the growth in economy and the government tax revenues (Ontario Hospital Association, 2010; Mawani, 2011). Due to current

Figure 3. Components of facilitation in the PARIHS framework (adapted from Rycroft-Malone, et al., 2002)

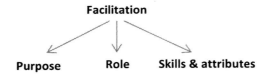

- Appropriate mechanisms for facilitation needs to be selected based on the needs of a given practice setting.

- Purpose can range from task specific facilitation requiring episodic contact to holistic facilitation requiring sustained partnerships.

- Role of the facilitator can range from completing specific tasks to enabling others to carry out large scale change at a practice setting.

- A facilitator would require a variety of skills and attributes based on the needs of a given situation such as project management, technical, marketing, co-counselling, and critical reflection skills.

economic realities, healthcare delivery organizations such as hospitals and nursing homes are coming under increasing government pressure to invest in sustainability efforts, that is, to deliver more care and ensure better outcomes at a lower financial cost (Ontario Hospital Association, 2010; Mawani, 2011). Canada is ranked fifth on healthcare spending on a per capita basis among industrialized countries; however, it is ranked last out of 30 countries in terms of value for money spent on healthcare (Mawani, 2011). A recent report by OECD emphasized that the Canadian healthcare system can achieve efficiency improvements at all levels with the implementation of appropriate strategies and interventions (Mawani, 2011). Governments are attracted to the concept of evidence based practice as it has the potential to reduce health expenditures while at the same time improve quality of care by reducing medical errors and redundant or harmful treatments. The PARIHS Framework can help administrators, clinicians, and researchers to employ appropriate strategies for successful knowledge translation projects based on the characteristics of a particular practice setting, thereby providing value for money to the healthcare sector, where money is often allocated to programs that yield subpar results.

Healthcare organizations such as hospitals and nursing homes are Complex Adaptive Systems (CASs) that are influenced by a large number of interdependent agents (such as patients, healthcare staff, hospital administration, accreditation and licensing bodies etc.) and external forces (such as political ideologies, provincial laws and regulations etc.) in a nonlinear and discontinuous manner (Begun, Zimmerman, & Dooley, 2003). Each CAS is context dependent and unique as it undergoes constant change from complicated interactions among a large number of interdependent agents and forces (Begun, Zimmerman, & Dooley, 2003). As a consequence, a knowledge translation strategy that was successful at one practice setting might not work at another practice setting. Most conceptual frameworks describing the implementation of evidence into practice are linear and unidimensional. Research has shown that reliance on such models for implementing evidence based practice often encounter resistance and the implementation process might even fail all together (Davis & Taylor-Vaisey, 1997; Kitson, Harvey, & McCormack, 1998). The PARIHS framework was developed based on research evidence and on experience gained through working directly with clinicians in order to address the apparent shortcomings of traditional models. The PARIHS framework takes into consideration the dynamic multidimensional nature of the change process that involves the interplay and interdependence of a variety of factors unique to a given CAS. As a consequence, the PARIHS framework can help clinicians and researchers in the planning, implementation, and evaluation of evidence based practice much more effectively compared to the traditional unidimensional models. Study protocols based on the PARIHS framework are being developed and refined to help improve the knowledge translation process (e.g., Estabrooks et al., 2009a).

The PARIHS framework is a comprehensive knowledge translation model that takes into consideration the dynamic interdependence and interplay of evidence, context, and facilitation. As a consequence, clinicians and researchers can not only use it to implement evidence based practice but can also utilize the model to identify potential new avenues of research, generate hypotheses that are grounded in research and practice, test these hypotheses in a systematic way by utilizing a variety of research methodologies, and finally suggest innovative strategies to maximize the uptake of evidence into practice. Translating Research in Elder Care (TREC) project is an excellent example that demonstrates the ability of the PARIHS framework to generate new research, develop new measurement tools such as the Alberta Context Tool (ACT), and guide knowledge translation at the same time (TREC and ACT are discussed in detail later in this chapter). The

PARIHS framework can also serve as a simple checklist for clinicians and managers to see what steps they need to take at their organization to successfully implement best current evidence into practice (Kitson, Harvey, & McCormack, 1998). Moreover, the framework can be used as a guideline to design a decision support tool that can suggest what type or kind of facilitation steps a manager, an organizational leader, or a research team could undertake to improve the uptake of evidence into practice (see Table 1).

KEY ENABLERS FOR THE APPLICATION OF THE PARIHS FRAMEWORK

The PARIHS framework can help an organization implement evidence into practice with a higher success rate compared to traditional models. Successful implementation of evidence based practice would lead to lower medical errors, better clinical decision making and improved patient outcomes. The challenge is to design a feasible project that is able to benefit from the comprehensive nature of

Table 1. Benefits to the health system

PARIHS Framework	Traditional Models
Improves clinical decision making	Fails to improve clinical decision making
Increases acceptance of EBP by frontline staff	Fails to overcome staff reluctance to adopt EBP
Change in practice is often permanent	Change in practice is often temporary
Helps improve patient outcomes	Fails to improve patient outcomes
Lowers healthcare costs through reduction in medical errors & harmful treatments	Financial/human resources are often wasted due to unsuccessful change process
Enables integration of health informatics in the change process	Use of health informatics is minimal
Can generate new avenues for research	Linear mode of implementation is not conducive to generating new research

the PARIHS implementation model without being limited by financial and logistical constraints. This section will briefly discuss the emergence of health informatics and the availability of easily accessible high quality outcome data as two key factors that can facilitate the successful application of the PARIHS framework for the implementation of evidence based practice.

Health Informatics

The cost of delivering healthcare has steadily increased in almost all developed economies as a consequence of a number of factors including expensive medical technologies, aging population, inflation, and citizens' expectations etc. (TD Economics, 2010; Norris, 2002). In response to the emerging challenges facing the healthcare sector, a number of prominent reports have called for a greater investment in health informatics to curve expenditures while at the same time improve patient safety, quality of care, accessibility to services, and to provide better value for money (e.g., Institute of Medicine, 2000; Institute of Medicine, 2001; TD Economics, 2010) Health informatics (HI) is defined as "the systematic application of information management and technology (IM&T) to the planning and delivery of high quality and cost-effective healthcare" (Norris, 2002, p. 205). Health informatics facilitates the collection, storage, communication, and interpretation of medical information to enhance the delivery of healthcare services. HI add value to patients, clinicians, and managers interactions with the system by providing access to relevant information leading to improved convenience and decision making (Norris, 2002). For example, clinical decision support systems can enhance a physicians' ability to select the most appropriate treatment regimen for a particular patient while simultaneously taking into consideration a number of important variables such as patient medical history, drug interactions, drug cost and availability etc. Similarly, online triage services and workflow planning systems provide convenience and improve decision making for patients and managers respectively (Norris, 2002). There are number of other applications of HI that have transformed the face of healthcare delivery system including electronic health records, telecare, telemedicine, robotic surgery, online prescribing, clinical information systems, and tools to facilitate the practice of evidence based medicine etc. (Norris, 2002; Imhoff, Webb, & Goldschmidt, 2000).

Developments in health informatics during the past few decades have fueled the acceptance and utilization of evidence based medicine by the healthcare sector and the research community (Georgiou, 2002). The emergence of clinical search engines, evidence based medicine reviews such as the Cochrane library, clinical decision support tools, and accessible online databases are some of the key driving forces behind the implementation of evidence-based practice. Furthermore, the emergence of evidence-based practice in parallel to the technological advancements in health informatics can be explained by the synergy among the goals of evidence based medicine and health informatics, that is, the creation and utilization of knowledge derived from health data and information (Georgiou, 2002).

High Quality Outcome Data

Most of the past research studies in the acute, ambulatory, and nursing home settings were only able to infer a link between evidence based medicine and actual clinical outcomes primarily due to the lack of availability of high quality databases on health outcomes. However, accreditation and other safety agencies in Canada have now started to regularly report health outcome data collected from medical facilities. For example, the Ministry of Health and Long-Term Care in Ontario has started to report patient safety outcome data on variables such as Clostridium Difficile Infection (reported monthly as of September 2008) and Ventilator Associated Pneumonia (reported quar-

terly as of April 2009) from all eligible Ontario hospitals. Similarly, new regulations now require nursing homes in Canada to collect outcome data on resident health and well-being such as Pressure Ulcer Prevalence and Restraint Use on a regular basis (quarterly) through the Resident Assessment Instrument-Minimum Data Set version 2 (RAI-MDS 2.0). The provincial, regional, and/or facility custodians are responsible for maintaining RAI-MDS 2.0 databases (Estabrooks et al., 2009b). As a consequence, it is now possible for research teams to design, implement, and evaluate a knowledge translation project to examine whether successful implementation of evidence into practice actually translated to improved health/safety outcomes.

The PARIHS framework is a comprehensive and multidimensional conceptual model of implementing evidence into practice. However, this strength of the framework can also prove to be a limitation for designing and implementing a project due to the financial and logistical constraints. A project trying to implement evidence into practice by relying on the PARIHS framework would need to measure contextual variables at regular intervals (for example, quarterly), frequently access information located in a variety of databases, and design appropriate facilitation strategies to help modify the context so as to maximize the uptake of evidence. As a consequence, integration of health informatics and availability of high quality outcome data are two essential ingredients for designing and successfully implementing a feasible knowledge translation project that is based on the principles of PARIHS framework.

PUTTING IT ALL TOGETHER: A RESEARCH PROJECT

This section will outline a study project to evaluate the effectiveness of the PARIHS framework to improve the uptake of clinical practice guidelines for prevention of pressure ulcers at a nursing care setting compared to a traditional implementation model. It is not feasible to use an experimental design to investigate the role of modifiable factors such as leadership and culture on patient outcomes at residential long term care facilities. It is not possible to randomly assign study participants such as health care providers and long term care residents to different groups (nursing care units) and treatments (for example, varying level of safety culture) as it is neither practical nor ethical. As a consequence, a multiple time series study (quasi-experiment) will be designed to investigate the implementation of clinical practice guidelines to reduce prevalence of pressure ulcers at a long term care setting. An advantage of multiple time series design is that it can better control for alternative explanations by eliminating reactive and history effects compared to basic quasi-experimental design.

A knowledge translation project with a multiple time series design will require access to longitudinal data on context (culture, leadership, evaluation) and prevalence of pressure ulcers at resident care facilities. This will necessitate the project investigator to forge partnerships with other research teams and medical facilities. For example, the project investigator can seek collaboration with the research team involved in Translating Research in Elder Care (TREC) program. The TREC team is studying the role of modifiable factors of organizational context (i.e., leadership, culture, and human, material, and structural resources etc.) on resident and provider outcomes in long term care settings (*Translating Research in Elder Care*, 2012). TREC is collecting data from providers, managers, and residents at nearly 100 nursing care units in Alberta, Saskatchewan, and Manitoba by using the TREC survey (Estabrooks et al., 2009b). The TREC survey is composed of a number of survey instruments such as the Alberta Context Tool (ACT). The ACT is a survey designed to measure "organizational context as conceptualized in the PARIHS framework" (Estabrooks et al., 2009b, p. 5). The TREC team also collects resident outcome data quarterly from all participating long term care facilities by using an electronic version of RAI-MDS 2.0. As a consequence, the project investigator will use the longitudinal data obtained through TREC to choose two resident care units that are as closely matched as possible by examining their base line scores on appropriate characteristics (unit demographics, culture, leadership, evaluation, and prevalence of pressure ulcers). The researcher can than introduce clinical practice guidelines to reduce pressure ulcers (Registered Nurses' Association of Ontario, 2005) at the two nursing care units. The PARIHS framework will be used at one of these two nursing care units while a traditional model (i.e., introduce guidelines and monitor practice change) will be applied at the other care unit (See Figure 4). This will enable the researcher to investigate whether or not the PARIHS framework is better suited to implement evidence into practice at a long term care setting compared to a traditional model.

The project investigator will collect contextual data (culture, leadership, and evaluation) by using the ACT questionnaire at a fixed interval (e.g., every month) from the nursing care unit where evidence is being implemented through the PARIHS framework. This context data directly obtained by the researcher will be used to decide what type of facilitation strategies are needed to maximize the uptake of the clinical practice guidelines to reduce pressure ulcers (See Figure 4). For example, the researcher can employ an academic detailing strategy to convey the importance of transformational leadership style to improved resident outcomes if the ACT data indicate that the nursing care unit is led by a manager who primarily rely on traditional command and control

Figure 4. Project design

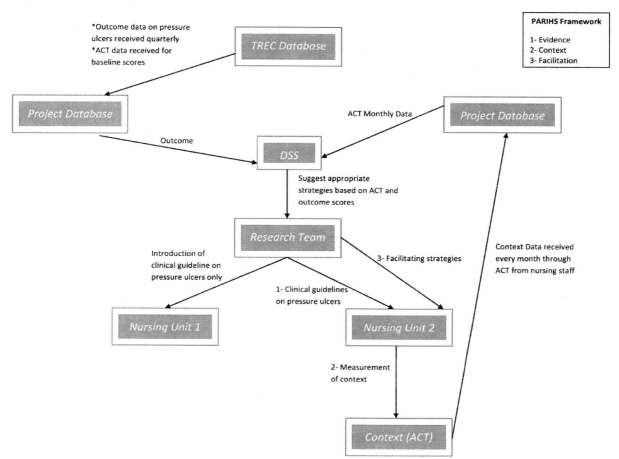

leadership style. In most instances, the researcher will need to rely on multiple facilitating strategies to help modify the context of the nursing home where the PARIHS framework is being applied.

Moreover, the project investigator can design a decision support tool to streamline the facilitation process. The raw data from ACT that is being obtained directly by the researcher on a monthly basis can be converted into separate scores for culture, leadership, and evaluation. These scores can then be uploaded to a database server containing the decision support tool. The decision support tool can be programmed by the IT experts to consider these scores before it can suggest

facilitation strategies that are most appropriate to maximize the uptake of evidence into practice (See Figure 4). The researcher will continue to monitor the outcome data on the prevalence of pressure ulcers being send by the TREC team on a quarterly basis to observe if any differences over the baseline scores have emerged between the two participating nursing care units employing two different implementation models. After a predetermined time period, the researcher will be able to conclude whether or not the prevalence of pressure ulcers decreased significantly at the nursing care unit where the PARIHS framework was applied compared to the nursing care unit where a traditional model was used.

It is important to note here that confidentiality and usability issues must be considered while designing and implementing a project that involves collection and analysis of confidential data. The researcher of the project will ensure that the data being obtained from TREC team (to set the initial baseline scores and quarterly updates on prevalence of pressure ulcers) is stored on a secure database. Furthermore, the ACT data collected on a monthly basis from the care unit where the PARIHS framework is being applied will be stored on a separate secure database. The proposed decision support tool will access these databases through a server that will require insertion of a smart card and entry of an encrypted password. Furthermore, this server will be designed to automatically log off the researcher from the system when the smart card is removed.

FUTURE RESEARCH DIRECTIONS

Critics have questioned whether the use of evidence-based practice actually translates into improved patient outcomes (Straus & McAlister, 2000). There is a need to conduct empirical studies to examine whether or not evidence-based practice translates into improved patient outcomes. Research community has only recently started to turn their attention to using the PARIHS framework for designing empirical research projects to investigate the link between evidence based practice and improved health outcomes (e.g., Estabrooks et al., 2009b; Rycroft-Malone et al., 2009; Perry et al., 2011).

Moreover, research on medical errors and factors influencing health outcomes has primarily been carried out in acute care settings such as hospitals. Medical and scientific community also needs to focus on investigating factors influencing knowledge translation and health outcomes in long term care facilities and nursing homes.

It is expected that nearly 23.4% of the Canadian population will be over 65 years of age by 2031 (Estabrooks et al., 2009b). As a consequence, this issue is of particular significance for health professionals, researchers, and policy makers as the Canadian population will continue to age over the next several decades.

CONCLUSION

System and human medical errors can lead to substantial treatment and patient well-being costs. Evidence based practice has the potential to reduce errors by improving healthcare staff decision making and subsequently improving patient outcomes. However, the implementation of evidence into practice often faces resistance and is not always successful in changing practice behaviours. Research has suggested that the inability of traditional implementation models to consider the dynamic nature and the simultaneous interaction of a variety of variables such as culture and leadership during the change process might be responsible for the failure to translate evidence into practice. The PARIHS framework was developed to address the shortcomings in the traditional implementation models and to maximize the uptake of evidence into practice. The PARIHS framework proposes that the implementation of evidence into practice is a function of research evidence, context, and facilitation. In the past, it was not feasible to design empirical studies under the PARIHS framework. However, it is now possible to design such studies primarily due to advancements in health informatics and availability of easily accessible high quality outcome data both at acute care and long term care settings. This chapter has suggested a feasible research project to evaluate the effectiveness of the PARIHS framework to improve the uptake of clinical practice guidelines for prevalence of pressure ulcers at a nursing care setting compared to a traditional implementation model. Hence, the PARIHS framework can be used to design effective knowledge translation projects as well as innovative decision support tools to maximize the uptake of evidence into practice.

REFERENCES

Baker, G. R., Norton, P. G., Flintoft, V., Blais, R., Brown, A., & Cox, J. et al. (2004). The Canadian adverse event study: The incidence of adverse events among hospital patients in Canada. *Canadian Medical Association Journal*, *170*(11), 1678–1686. doi:10.1503/cmaj.1040498 PMID:15159366.

Begun, J. W., Zimmerman, B., & Dooley, K. (2003). Health care organizations as complex adaptive systems. In Mick, S. M., & Wyttenbach, M. (Eds.), *Advances in health care organization theory* (pp. 253–288). San Francisco, CA: Jossey-Bass.

Castellese, S. R. (2006). *Guatemala health care practitioners' leadership styles: Medical worker perception versus leader self-perception.* (Unpublished doctoral dissertation). Capella University, Minneapolis, MN.

Chuang, Y., Ginsburg, L., & Berta, W. B. (2007). Learning from preventable adverse events in health care organizations: Development of a multilevel model of learning and propositions. *Health Care Management Review*, *32*(4), 330–340. doi:10.1097/01.HMR.0000296790.39128.20 PMID:18075442.

Davis, D. A., & Taylor-Vaisey, A. (1997). Translating guidelines into practice: A systematic review of theoretic concepts, practical experience, and research evidence in the adoption of clinical practice guidelines. *Canadian Medical Association Journal*, *157*, 408–416. PMID:9275952.

Economics, T. D. (2010). *Charting a path to sustainable healthcare in Ontario: 10 proposals to restrain cost growth without compromising quality of care.* Retrieved January 20, 2012, from http://www.td.com/document/PDF/economics/special/td-economics-special-db0510-health-care.pdf

Estabrooks, C. A., Hutchinson, A. M., Squires, J. E., Birdsell, J., Cummings, G. G., & Degner, L. et al. (2009a). Translating research in elder care: An introduction to a study protocol series. *Implementation Science; IS*, *4*(51). PMID:19664285.

Estabrooks, C. A., Squires, J. E., Cummings, G. G., Teare, G. F., & Norton, P. G. (2009b). Study protocol for the translating research in elder care (TREC), building context - An organizational monitoring program in long-term care project (project one). *Implementation Science; IS*, *4*(52). PMID:19671166.

Fisher, G., & Bibo, M. (2000). No leadership without representation. *International Journal of Organisational Behaviour*, *6*(2), 307–319.

Georgiou, A. (2002). Data, information and knowledge: The health informatics model and its role in evidence-based medicine. *Journal of Evaluation in Clinical Practice*, *8*(2), 127–130. doi:10.1046/j.1365-2753.2002.00345.x PMID:12180361.

Harvey, G., Loftus-Hills, A., Rycroft-Malone, J., Titchen, A., Kitson, A., McCormack, B., & Seers, K. (2002). Getting evidence into practice: The role and function of facilitation. *Journal of Advanced Nursing*, *37*(6), 577–588. doi:10.1046/j.1365-2648.2002.02126.x PMID:11879422.

Haynes, B., & Haines, A. (1998). Barriers and bridges to evidence based clinical practice. *British Medical Journal*, *317*, 273. doi:10.1136/bmj.317.7153.273 PMID:9677226.

Imhoff, M., Webb, A., & Goldschmidt, A. (2001). Health informatics. *Intensive Care Medicine*, *27*, 179–186. PMID:11280631.

Institute of Medicine. (2000). *To err is human: Building a safer health system*. Washington, DC: National Academy Press.

Institute of Medicine. (2001). *Crossing the quality chasm: A new health system for the 21st century*. Washington, DC: National Academy Press.

Kitson, A., Harvey, G., & McCormack, B. (1998). Enabling the implementation of evidence based practice: A conceptual framework. *Quality in Health Care, 7*, 149–158. doi:10.1136/qshc.7.3.149 PMID:10185141.

Mawani, A. (2011). *Can we get better for less: Value for money in Canadian health care*. Retrieved December 2, 2011 from http://www.cga-canada.org/en-ca/ResearchReports/ca_rep_2011-04_healthcare.pdf

McClure, M., & Hinshaw, A. S. (Eds.). (2002). *Magnet hospitals revisited: Attraction and retention of professional nurses*. Washington, DC: American Nurses Publishing.

McCormack, B., Kitson, A., Harvey, G., Rycroft-Malone, J., Titchen, A., & Seers, K. (2002). Getting evidence into practice: The meaning of 'context'. *Journal of Advanced Nursing, 38*(1), 94–104. doi:10.1046/j.1365-2648.2002.02150.x PMID:11895535.

McShane, S. L. (2006). *Canadian organizational behaviour* (6th ed.). New York: McGraw-Hill Ryerson.

Norris, A. C. (2002). Current trends and challenges in health informatics. *Health Informatics Journal, 8*, 205–213. doi:10.1177/146045820200800407.

Ontario Hospital Association (OHA). (2010). *Ideas and opportunities for bending the health care cost curve: Advice for the government of Ontario*. Retrieved December 2, 2011 from http://www.ccac-ont.ca/Upload/on/General/Bending%20the%20Health%20Care%20Cost%20Curve%20(Final%20Report%20-%20April%2013,%202010).pdf

Perry, L., Bellchambers, H., Howie, A., Moxey, A., Parkinson, L., Capra, S., & Byles, J. (2011). Examination of the utility of the promoting action on research in health services framework for implementation of evidence based practice in residential aged care setting. *Journal of Advanced Nursing, 67*(10), 2139–2150. doi:10.1111/j.1365-2648.2011.05655.x PMID:21535089.

Registered Nurses' Association of Ontario. (2005). *Risk assessment and prevention of pressure ulcers (revised)*. Toronto, Canada: Registered Nurses' Association of Ontario.

Rosser, W. W. (1993). Dissemination of guidelines on cholesterol: Effects on patterns of practice of general practitioners and family physicians in Ontario. *Canadian Family Physician Medecin de Famille Canadien, 39*, 280–284. PMID:8495119.

Ruchlin, H. S., Dubbs, N. L., Callahan, M. A., & Fosina, M. J. (2004). The role of leadership in instilling a culture of safety: Lessons from literature. *Journal of Healthcare Management, 49*(1), 47–59. PMID:14768428.

Rycroft-Malone, J. (2004). The PARIHS framework - A framework for guiding the implementation of evidence-based practice. *Journal of Nursing Care Quality, 19*(4), 297–304. doi:10.1097/00001786-200410000-00002 PMID:15535533.

Rycroft-Malone, J., Dopson, S., Degner, L., Hutchinson, A. M., Morgan, D., Stewart, N., & Estabrooks, C. A. (2009). Study protocol for the translating research in elder care (TREC), building context through case studies in long-term care project (project two). *Implementation Science; IS, 4*, 53. doi:10.1186/1748-5908-4-53 PMID:19671167.

Rycroft-Malone, J., Kitson, A., Harvey, G., McCormack, B., Seers, K., Titchen, C., & Estabrooks, C. (2002). Ingredients for change: Revisiting a conceptual framework. *Quality & Safety in Health Care, 11*, 174–180. doi:10.1136/qhc.11.2.174 PMID:12448812.

Rycroft-Malone, J., Seers, K., Titchen, A., Harvey, G., Kitson, A., & McCormack, B. (2004). What counts as evidence in evidence-based practice. *Journal of Advanced Nursing, 47*(1), 81–90. doi:10.1111/j.1365-2648.2004.03068.x PMID:15186471.

Sherer, J. L. (1994). Retooling leaders: Facilitative leadership helps clarify process and underpin culture change. *Hospitals & Health Networks, 68*(1), 42–44. PMID:8269006.

Straus, S. E., & McAlister, F. A. (2000). Evidence-based medicine: A commentary on common criticisms. *Canadian Medical Association Journal, 163*(7), 837–841. PMID:11033714.

Translating Research in Elder Care: TREC Overview. (2012). Retrieved March 18, 2012, from http://www.trec.ualberta.ca/TRECOverview.aspx

ADDITIONAL READING

Anderson, J. G., & Aydin, C. E. (2005). *Evaluating the organizational impact of healthcare information systems* (2nd ed.). New York, NY: Springer. doi:10.1007/0-387-30329-4.

Baumbusch, J. L., Kirkham, S. R., Khan, K. B., McDonald, H., Semeniuk, P., Tan, E., & Anderson, J. M. (2008). Pursuing common agendas: A collaborative model for knowledge translation between research and practice in clinical settings. *Research in Nursing & Health, 31*(2), 130–140. doi:10.1002/nur.20242 PMID:18213622.

Bullard, M. J., Emond, S. D., Graham, T. A. D., Ho, K., & Holroyd, B. R. (2007). Informatics and knowledge translation. *Academic Emergency Medicine, 14*(11), 996–1002. PMID:17967961.

Davis, D., Evans, M., Jadad, A., Perrier, L., Rath, D., & Ryan, D. et al. (2003). The case for knowledge translation: Shortening the journey from evidence to effect. *British Medical Journal, 327*(7405), 33–35. doi:10.1136/bmj.327.7405.33 PMID:12842955.

Degner, L. F. (2005). Knowledge translation in palliative care: Can theory help? *Canadian Journal of Nursing Research, 37*(2), 105–113. PMID:16092783.

Doebbeling, B. N., Chou, A. F., & Tierney, W. M. (2006). Priorities and strategies for the implementation of integrated informatics and communication technology to improve evidence-based practice. *Journal of General Internal Medicine, 21*, S50–S57. doi:10.1007/s11606-006-0275-9 PMID:16637961.

Doran, D., Paterson, J., Clark, C., Srivastava, R., Goering, P. N., & Kushniruk, A. et al. (2010). A pilot study of an electronic interprofessional evidence-based care planning tool for clients with mental health problems and addictions. *Worldviews on Evidence-Based Nursing, 7*(3), 174–184. doi:10.1111/j.1741-6787.2010.00191.x PMID:20367805.

Doran, D. M., Mylopoulos, J., Kushniruk, A., Nagle, L., Laurie-Shaw, B., & Sidani, S. et al. (2007). Evidence in the palm of your hand: Development of an outcome-focused knowledge translation intervention. *Worldviews on Evidence-Based Nursing, 4*(2), 69–77. doi:10.1111/j.1741-6787.2007.00084.x PMID:17553107.

Doran, D. M., & Sidani, S. (2007). Outcomes-focused knowledge translation: A framework for knowledge translation and patient outcomes improvement. *Worldviews on Evidence-Based Nursing, 4*(1), 3–13. doi:10.1111/j.1741-6787.2007.00073.x PMID:17355405.

Drenning, C. (2006). Collaboration among nurses, advanced practice nurses, and nurse researchers to achieve evidence-based practice change. *Journal of Nursing Care Quality, 21*(4), 298–301. doi:10.1097/00001786-200610000-00004 PMID:16985397.

Englebardt, S. P., & Nelson, R. (2002). *Health care informatics: An interdisciplinary approach.* St. Louis, MO: Mosby.

Haines, T. P., & Waldron, N. G. (2011). Translation of falls prevention knowledge into action in hospitals: What should be translated and how should it be done? *Journal of Safety Research, 42*(6), 431–442. doi:10.1016/j.jsr.2011.10.003 PMID:22152261.

Ho, K., Novak, L. H., Best, A., Walsh, G., Jarvis-Selinger, S., Fedeles, M., & Chockalingam, A. (2004). Dissecting technology-enabled knowledge translation: Essential challenges, unprecedented opportunities. *Clinical and Investigative Medicine. Medecine Clinique et Experimentale, 27*(2), 70–78. PMID:15202826.

Holroyd, B. R., Bullard, M. J., Graham, T. A. D., & Rowe, B. H. (2007). Decision support technology in knowledge translation. *Academic Emergency Medicine, 14*(11), 942–948. PMID:17766733.

Kitson, A. (2011). Mechanics of knowledge translation. *International Journal of Evidence-Based Healthcare, 9*(2), 79–80. doi:10.1111/j.1744-1609.2011.00181.x PMID:21599839.

Kitson, A. L. (2009). The need for systems change: Reflections on knowledge translation and organizational change. *Journal of Advanced Nursing, 65*(1), 217–228. doi:10.1111/j.1365-2648.2008.04864.x PMID:19032518.

Kosel, K. C., Clark, T., Haywood, T. T., & Lonappan, M. (2012). VHA blueprints: Redefining the way clinical knowledge is transferred. *American Journal of Medical Quality, 27*(3), 226–232. doi:10.1177/1062860611422270 PMID:22114153.

Kudyba, S. (2010). *Healthcare informatics: Improving efficiency and productivity.* Boca Raton, FL: CRC Press. doi:10.1201/9781439809792.

Leahey, M., & Svavarsdottir, E. (2009). Implementing family nursing: How do we translate knowledge into clinical practice? *Journal of Family Nursing, 15*(4), 445–460. doi:10.1177/1074840709349070 PMID:19783792.

Lemieux-Charles, L., McGuire, W., & Blidner, I. (2002). Building interorganizational knowledge for evidence-based health system change. *Health Care Management Review, 27*(3), 48–59. doi:10.1097/00004010-200207000-00006 PMID:12146783.

Lin, C., Tan, B., & Chang, S. (2008). An exploratory model of knowledge flow barriers within healthcare organizations. *Information & Management, 45*(5), 331–339. doi:10.1016/j.im.2008.03.003.

Lin, S. H., Murphy, S. L., & Robinson, J. C. (2010). Facilitating evidence-based practice: Process, strategies, and resources. *The American Journal of Occupational Therapy., 64*, 164–171. doi:10.5014/ajot.64.1.164 PMID:20131576.

Lyons, J. S. (2009). Knowledge creation through total clinical outcomes management: A practice-based evidence solution to address some of the challenges of knowledge translation. *Journal of the Canadian Academy of Child and Adolescent Psychiatry, 18*(1), 38–45. PMID:19270847.

Palinkas, L. A., & Soydan, H. (2012). *Translation and implementation of evidence-based practice.* New York: Oxford University Press.

Petr, C. G. (2009). *Multidimensional evidence-based practice: Synthesizing knowledge, research and values.* New York: Routledge.

Proctor, E. K. (2004). Leverage points for the implementation of evidence-based practice. *Brief Treatment and Crisis Intervention, 4*(3), 227–242. doi:10.1093/brief-treatment/mhh020.

Reason, J. (1990). *Human error.* New York: Cambridge University Press. doi:10.1017/CBO9781139062367.

Reason, J. (1995). Understanding adverse events: Human factors. *Quality in Health Care, 4,* 80–89. doi:10.1136/qshc.4.2.80 PMID:10151618.

Reason, J. (1997). *Managing the risks of organizational accidents.* Burlington, UK: Ashgate Publishing Limited.

Rundall, T. G., Martelli, P. F., Arroyo, L., Mc-Curdy, R., Graetz, I., & Neuwirth, E. B. et al. (2007). The informed decisions toolbox: Tools for knowledge transfer and performance improvement. *Journal of Healthcare Management, 52*(5), 325–341. PMID:17933188.

Rycroft-Malone, J. (2007). Theory and knowledge translation: Setting some coordinates. *Nursing Research, 56*(4), S78–S85. doi:10.1097/01.NNR.0000280631.48407.9b PMID:17625479.

Rycroft-Malone, J., & Bucknall, T. (2010). *Models and frameworks for implementing evidence-based practice: Linking evidence to action.* Chichester, UK: Wiley-Blackwell.

Shortliffe, E. H., & Perreault, L. E. (2001). *Medical informatics: Computer applications in health care and biomedicine* (2nd ed.). New York: Springer.

Smith, M. L., & Raab, S. S. (2011). Assessment of latent factors contributing to error: Addressing surgical pathology error wisely. *Archives of Pathology & Laboratory Medicine, 135*(11), 1436–1440. doi:10.5858/arpa.2011-0334-OA PMID:22032570.

Spath, P. L. (2011). *Error reduction in health care: A systems approach to improving patient safety* (2nd ed.). San Francisco, CA: Jossey-Bass.

Springer, P. J., Corbett, C., & Davis, N. (2006). Enhancing evidence-based practice through collaboration. *The Journal of Nursing Administration, 36*(11), 534–537. doi:10.1097/00005110-200611000-00009 PMID:17099439.

Tan, J. K. H. (2008). *Healthcare information systems and informatics: Research and practices.* Hershey, PA: IGI Global. doi:10.4018/978-1-59904-690-7.

Thompson, C., McCaughan, D., Cullum, N., Sheldon, T., & Raynor, P. (2005). Barriers to evidence-based practice in primary care nursing – Why viewing decision-making as context is helpful. *Journal of Advanced Nursing, 52*(4), 432–444. doi:10.1111/j.1365-2648.2005.03609.x PMID:16268847.

Thompson, G. N., Estabrooks, C. A., & Degner, L. F. (2006). Clarifying the concepts in knowledge transfer: A literature review. *Journal of Advanced Nursing, 53*(6), 691–701. doi:10.1111/j.1365-2648.2006.03775.x PMID:16553677.

Trinder, L., & Reynolds, S. (2000). *Evidence-based practice: A critical appraisal.* Oxford, UK: Blackwell Science. doi:10.1002/9780470699003.

Veluswamy, R. (2008). Golden nuggets: Clinical quality data mining in acute care. *Physician Executive, 34*(3), 48–53. PMID:18605272.

KEY TERMS AND DEFINITIONS

Context: It is the environment/setting where healthcare is being delivered. Culture, leadership, and evaluation are core components of a given practice setting.

Evidence: In clinical decision-making, evidence consists of credible knowledge derived from research, clinical expertise, and patient experience.

Evidence-Based Medicine or Evidence-Based Practice: The judicious use of current best evidence, clinical expertise, and patient preferences during diagnosis, treatment, and other clinical decision making processes.

Facilitation: The process of helping or enabling others to successfully implement change.

Health Informatics: HI is the systematic accumulation, storage, retrieval, analyses, and interpretation of health data to facilitate healthcare policy, management, and delivery.

Knowledge Translation: The process of implementing current best evidence into practice.

The PARIHS Framework: A multidimensional conceptual model that stipulates that successful implementation of evidence into practice requires simultaneously considering evidence, context, and facilitation.

Chapter 3
Investing in a "Rehabilitation Model" to Improve the Decision–Making Process in Long–Term Care

Connie D'Astolfo
SPINEgroup®, Canada & York University, Canada

ABSTRACT

An aging population is a primary factor associated with escalating healthcare costs due to increased drug spending, chronic diseases and co-morbidities, physician visits, and hospital costs (TD Report, 2010). There has already been a marked increase in the number of Long-Term Care (LTC) residents with co-morbidities, and chronic diseases will be more prevalent in future years (Conference Board of Canada, 2011). The chapter explores the use of a rehabilitation model to improve the current decision-making processes that impact the health outcomes of seniors across the Ontario LTC continuum. Improved clinical management of this population through rehabilitation could result in not only enhanced quality of care but also significant cost savings for both the Long-Term Care (LTC) industry and the health system at large. The chapter highlights the need for the LTC sector to identify strategies for harnessing innovation to improve its own activities and outcomes and become a leader in health system transformation.

INTRODUCTION

The sustainability of our healthcare system (due to rising costs and quality challenges) is the most pressing policy issue facing Canada and the provinces in this decade (TD Report, 2010). In 2010,

DOI: 10.4018/978-1-4666-4321-5.ch003

Canada's health-care system is forecast to consume 11.9 percent of Gross Domestic Product (GDP) as the costs of health-care continue to rise. By 2025, healthcare is projected to consume 15 percent of GDP (Conference Board of Canada, 2011). The TD Economic Report and the Conference Board of Canada report that "innovation" while reducing the rate of health-care costs and improving health outcomes is the best option for keeping Canada's health-care system sustainable (Conference Board of Canada, 2011; TD Report, 2010). In Ontario, healthcare costs currently make up 46% of total program spending and is expected to continue to rise in the future due to increasing utilization of services, our aging population, and the prevalence of chronic disease (MOHLTC, 2010).

The number and proportion of seniors in the population is growing and chronic diseases are increasingly prevalent; impairing the ability of many Ontarians to live independently. In this decade, the number of people aged 65 and older is expected to rise to over 1.9 million. By 2035—when boomers are 71 to 89 years old—there will be nearly 238,000 Ontarians in need of long-term care, versus about 98,000 today (StatsCan, 2006; Government of Ontario, 2009). Long term care homes provide care for people who are not able to live independently in their own homes and who require 24-hour nursing or personal care support.

In 2006, Canada's expenditure on Long-Term Care (LTC) alone was equivalent to about 1.5% of its Gross Domestic Product (GDP). More than 80% of these expenditures were targeted to institutional care (OECD Health Data, 2010). Given the continued rise in our aging population as well as high costs associated with LTC, re-engineering health care delivery through improved decision-making processes in this sector may be an effective strategy in reducing expenditures.

There are currently 625 long-term care homes in Ontario with approximately 76,904 residents who are unable to live independently in the community (Conference Board of Canada, 2011). Hospitalization of LTC residents is highly prevalent and contributes to clogging of emergency rooms and hospital bed shortages (Conference Board of Canada, 2011). The nursing home literature reports estimated rates of hospitalization averaging approximately 35% per year, most of which were classified as Ambulatory Care Sensitive Conditions which are typically considered as unnecessary hospital transfers (Hutt et al., 2002;

Coburn et al., 2002). In Ontario, between 7 and 17 percent of all hospitalizations are Alternate Level of Care (ALC) related—that is, where the healthcare needs of the patient are such that they do not require hospitalization, and could be managed in another setting, provided that other setting is available (Conference Board of Canada, 2011). There are multiple risk factors and predictors of hospitalization for the LTC population including cognitive and functional decline (Hutt et al., 2002; Coburn et al., 2002; Conference Board of Canada, 2011). Numerous studies report that these conditions also contribute to rising costs associated with hospitalization (Cornette, 2005; Intrator et al., 2004; Carter, 2003).

The Canadian healthcare system is effectively designed for reactive, episodic care making it an ideal system for acute disease management but under performs in the prevention and management of chronic diseases. This system has significant shortcomings for improving and maintaining the health of an aging population with multiple co-morbidities, as found in the LTC population (Conference Board of Canada, 2011; TD Economic Report, 2010). See Table 1 for list of current and estimated future percentages and rates of co-morbidities among LTC residents.

The health-care system is not alone in under-performance on new initiatives. In the Conference Board's 2010 report, How Canada Performs: A Report Card on Canada, Canada received a grade of——D grade on innovation performance, ranking 14th out of 17 peer countries (Conference Board of Canada, 2011). Although lack of innovation is yet to be a priority of the government, the Ontario Ministry of Health and Long-Term Care (MOHLTC) is currently concerned with the impact of population aging on the costs of healthcare. The MOHLTC is focusing on quality to drive value in healthcare: "Excellent Care for All Act, 2010" provides a foundation to reform the health system around the client. This focus promotes innovation while creating incentives for quality, value and evidenced-based care for patients. Both

Table 1. Rates of selected co-morbidities in long-term care residents

Co-Morbidity	Percentage of Residents with Co-Morbidity	Estimated Number of Residents with each Co-Morbidity		
		2015	2025	2035
Alzheimer's Disease	19.0	21,776	29,593	45,176
Dementia Other Than Alzheimer's Disease	42.4	48,665	66,134	100,960
Anxiety Disorder	6.5	7,496	10,187	15,551
Depression	27.4	31,406	42,680	65,155
Hypertension	50.0	57,376	77,971	119,031
Osteoporosis	25.0	28,685	38,982	59,509
Diabetes Mellitus	24.0	27,516	37,394	57,085
Arthritis	34.5	39,572	53,776	82,095
(The Conference Board of Canada, 2011)				

hospitals and LTC homes, for example, agree that lack of access to community resources results in higher rates of avoidable ER admissions, contributing to the Alternative Level of Care (ALC) problem. Stakeholders also agree that efficient healthcare delivery is dependent on the availability and use of information effective management technology (Conference Board of Canada, 2011; TD Economics, 2010).

Overlooked in the healthcare system is the importance of rehabilitation through the long term care continuum (Conference Board of Canada, 2011). A case study will be presented to illustrate the challenges and opportunities in long-term care and the importance of investing in "rehabilitation" supported by new decision making processes to increase patient health outcomes and revenue opportunities. It is important to note that hospitals, drug costs, and physician compensation currently absorb 60% of healthcare spending and a significant portion of public spending (TD Economic Report, 2010). There is an urgent need to exploit opportunities to increase "value for money" in the current system that would free up resources to be invested in other activities that would restore the social gradient in health outcomes.

BACKGROUND

Clinical decision-making processes address the quality, integration, analysis and use of information for evidence-based decision making for screening, diagnosis, treatment, monitoring and follow-up; aimed at enhancing health outcomes (Osheroff et al., 2006; Garg et al., 2005; O'Connor et al., 2011). Health outcomes are generally understood in the context of population and individual health including mortality, morbidity, self-reported health status, and prevalence/incidence rates of diseases; or as process indicators, including responsiveness of the system, namely, access, wait times, patient satisfaction, safety and rates of medical errors (Knaus et al., 1986). The most common use of clinical decision support is for addressing clinical needs, such as ensuring accurate diagnoses, screening in a timely manner for preventable diseases, or averting adverse drug events. The healthcare industry, one of the most information intensive industries has been extremely slow in the uptake and efficient use of information systems to assist in healthcare delivery (TD Economic Report, 2010). The LTC sector, due to budget constraints, is even further behind (California Healthcare Foundation,

2008). Researchers described a system approach to the care of populations with chronic disease that is built around two essential elements: (1) educating and preparing clinical practice teams and (2) activating and educating individuals with chronic disease (Hatzakis et al, 2006). Essential to this model is the use of tools such as evidence-based guidelines, data repositories, and an Electronic Medical Record (EMR) to manage high-risk groups with specific conditions (Wagner, 1999).

Arthritic Disorders and Back Pain

Arthritic disorders have reached epidemic proportions across all industrialized nations. Canada faces a significant challenge with the costs associated with arthritic pain. In Canada, arthritis was associated with 5.9% (129,205) of the total hospitalizations, and accounted for 12.7% (91,556) in surgical hospitalizations in 2005-6 (Public Health Agency, 2010). The economic burden of arthritis in Canada was estimated to be $6.4 billion in 2005-6 (Public Health Agency, 2010). In 2008, hospital costs attributable to arthritis totaled $1.2 billion for patients under 65 years and $1.7 billion for seniors (Public Health Agency, 2010).

Back pain is the most common arthritic complaint and ranks first as a cause of disability and inability to work, a top reason for physician visits, with a significant impact on quality of life (Public Health Agency, 2010; Health Canada, 2003). In Ontario, spinal pain currently affects 1.6 million people and by 2026, an estimated 2.8 million Ontarians aged 15 and over will be suffering with the condition (Public Health Agency, 2010). With the aging population, the prevalence of back pain is expected to rise to 20% of the Canadian population, resulting in approximately 7 million or 1 in 5 Canadians by 2031 (Public Health Agency, 2010). A U.S. national survey of patients aged 75 and older demonstrated that back pain is the third most frequently reported symptom and reason for physician visit. In another study, 17.3% of total back pain visits occurred in the 65 years and

older age group (Cypress et al, 1983; Hart et al, 1995). Goel et al, suggests that back pain is the 3rd leading cause of chronic health problems in the over 65 year old category for women and the fourth leading cause of chronic health problems for men in the same age group (Goel et al, 1996). Although back pain is one of the most common health problems seen in primary care; because of its benign nature, back pain is often seen as a trivial problem compared to other afflictions that generate a high mortality i.e. cancer, heart disease or infectious diseases (Coyte et al, 1998).

Results from an Ontario study of LTC seniors (average age 84 years) identified a 40% prevalence rate for reported back pain, which is more than other conditions prevalent in seniors i.e. diabetes (8%), atherosclerotic heart disease (6%), depression (13%) and hypertension (36%) (D'Astolfo et al., 2008). The study reported that back pain in this population was also under-reported and inadequately managed. Chronic non-malignant spinal pain management in older vulnerable patients is inadequate and improvement is needed in screening, clinical evaluation, follow up and attention to potential toxicities of drug therapy (D'Astolfo et al., 2008). There is a significant correlation found between back pain and various chronic diseases including cognitive impairment, dementia, hypertension, diabetes and depression (D'Astolfo et al., 2008).

Long-Term Care Funding and Challenges

Long Term Care is funded per diem primarily through the Ministry envelopes with the addition of a resident co-payment for accommodation. As of October 2010, LTC facilities receive $147.77 per resident per day, of which residents pay $53.23 per day for basic accommodation—a level set not by the market, but by the province. Adjustments are also made to LTC funding to reflect the acuity levels of residents. Additionally, LTC operators are eligible for a variety of other specialized funding programs for such things as the construction of new beds and replacement beds, capital funding for new construction and retrofits, premiums to meet structural compliance classification standards, and dialysis funding among many other things (Conference Board of Canada, 2011).

In April 2010, the Ministry moved to adopt a new classification system for LTC called Resource Utilization Groups (RUGs) for the purposes of adjusting the base per diem funding of the Nursing and Personal Care Envelope. Also, the calculation of Case Mixed Index (CMI) using RUGs is a result of the move to integrate RAI-MDS across the LTC sector (MOHLTC, 2010). The RUG-III 34-group model uses over 100 MDS items to determine the appropriate RUG III category. Membership in a RUG category is based on how much care a resident needs, types of treatments received, and whether or not the resident has certain conditions or diagnoses. See Table 2 (MOHLTC, 2010).

It is increasingly clear that Ontario's capacity to provide accessible, and high quality care in healthcare settings will not meet future needs without significant innovation and transformation (Conference Board of Canada, 2011). Patients who enter LTC homes in the future are expected to have higher and more complex health care needs than previous generations of residents, adding stress to staff and facilities. There will be higher expectations of baby boomers for enhanced accommodation and choice in quality health services, thus requiring different service models from LTC providers and operators (Conference Board of Canada, 2011). While the pressures faced by the LTC sector in Ontario may not be characterized as competitive pressures, the pressures the sector does face in Ontario include increasing demand from individuals with higher expectations, preferences for home care and reputational pressures from increased public reporting of outcomes (Conference Board of Canada, 2011).

Current emphasis on compliance with regulations rather than accountability for outcomes is driving new ways of complying/reporting rather than strategies to improve outcomes through real innovation. It has been recommended that a government-directed shift away from the regulatory compliance towards accountability for outcomes is worth exploring. (Conference Board of Canada, 2011) As an example, LTC operators are currently faced with multiple costly challenges which burden the health system, i.e. cost of care, assessment and documentation associated with high prevalence of falls, use of restraints (including psychotropic drugs) for cognitively impaired residents and skin breakdown. With the new RUGs III classification system, they also face the prospect of reduced funding for nursing care services due to lower CMI scores for the treatment of less complex residents. This may, in all likelihood, translate to significant loss in profits for a LTC corporation. Since the implementation of the RUGs, the LTC industry has struggled with ways to increase their CMI scores. To date, strategies have centred on training of staff and/or use of software on how to effectively document and capture additional points to increase the overall score. Improving documentation has demonstrated some positive results, but most homes are still struggling. It is crucial for both government and LTC operators to recognize that the new RUGS III classification has the potential to be an incentive for innovation in the area of rehabilitation which can potentially unleash a cascade of health improvements for the LTC residents as well as the health system.

The long-term care sector in Ontario continues to face significant challenges related to shortage of human health resources, technology, funding and regulations. Ministry regulations, policies, and funding are viewed as restrictive and serve as a disincentive for homes to design and implement creative solutions to effectively administer quality cost effective care (Conference Board of Canada, 2011). The ratio of persons aged 20-64 (i.e., the working age population) to the number of people aged 85 or older (i.e., those most likely to need LTC) is diminishing. In 2009, the ratio was 19 to 1; in 2035 the expected ratio will be 10

Table 2. Current funding and outcomes evaluation for long-term care

Resident Assessment Instrument-Minimum Data Set (RAI-MDS)	The RAI-MDS is an example of a widely adopted technology that has great promise to improve efficiency and care outcomes in Ontario's LTC facilities. The RAI-MDS assessment instrument for Skilled Nursing Facilities (SNFs) and Ontario CCC facilities was originally developed by InterRAI between 1988 and 1990. InterRAI is a collaborative network of researchers in over 30 countries committed to improving healthcare for persons who are elderly, frail, or disabled. Their goal is to promote evidence-based clinical practice and policy decisions through the collection and interpretation of high quality data about the characteristics and outcomes of persons served across a variety of health and social services settings. RAI-MDS was designed for use in U.S. nursing homes in response to a contract offered by the U.S. Healthcare Financing Administration (now the Centres Centersfor Medicare and Medicaid Services). The tool was first used by U.S. nursing homes in 1990 and was subsequently updated in 1994-1995. The MDS data is derived from comprehensive and standardized assessments that are mandated for all skilled nursing facilities across Canada and the US. The assessment data is used as a care planning tool in clinical management and to determine facility payment for residents. It provides information on residents' socio-demographic characteristics, physical and cognitive status, psychological and health conditions, behavioural problems, service use, and medication use. Trained staff members in LTC facilities complete the full MDS 2.0 assessments 7-13 days after admission and then annually thereafter, with quarterly assessments completed every 90 days. The time period of interest for each assessment is the previous seven days. Resident-level assessments and facility information are collected and entered in the LTC facilities. Data are submitted to the Ontario MOHLTC by the LTC facilities on a quarterly basis. At the end of each fiscal year, the database for the year is released to ICES (CIHI, 2006). According to the Ontario Family Councils Program, the RAI-MDS has many benefits, including: improved ease in sharing information among care workers in LTC facilities, due to the use of a common "language" and metrics; improved efficiency and accuracy of assessments; enhanced information for decision-making regarding quality improvement, assessment, and planning; and a greater capacity to sharing information across the health system as a whole, due to the transmission opportunities provided by digital records (Conference Board of Canada, 2012).
Case Mix Index (CMI)	Case mix index, which is a measure of the relative cost or resources needed to treat the mix of patients or residents. The system comprises seven main clinical groups devised as a hierarchy, ranked by cost. These groups are rehabilitation, extensive services, special care, clinically complex, impaired cognition, behavioural problems and reduced physical function. These main groups are further divided into subgroups on the basis of an Activity of Daily Living (ADL) score that reflects the intensity of ADL dependency, receipt of certain types of care (including rehabilitation input from nurses) and the presence or absence of depression. The groups at the top of the hierarchy represent clinical characteristics that were found to be associated with increased care costs. The ADL subdivisions within the hierarchy reflect the importance of physical function as a driver of cost. The contribution of cognitive function in the absence of other clinical characteristics is recognized in the impaired cognition group. Case mix is by definition a system that classifies people into groups that are homogeneous in their use of resources. A good case-mix system also gives meaningful clinical descriptions of these individuals. The application of case mix is broad; it provides the basis, not only for reimbursement, but also for comparing facilities or programs, practice patterns, as an adjunct to quality of care and efficiency measurement, a staff planning tool, etc. (MOHLTC, 2012).
Resource Utilization Groups (RUG)	The best known of the interRAI case-mix systems is the Resource Utilization Groups (RUG-III) used in institutional long term care settings. Resource Utilization Groups (RUGs) is a case mix grouping methodology that can be calculated using data from the RAI-MDS. Compared to ARCS, RUGs provides a more comprehensive view of residents based on diagnosis and informs which services residents receive with a focus on activities of daily living and measurable outcomes. In partnership with the LTC sector, the MOHLTC adopted the RUG III 34 group model as the case mix grouping methodology to adjust the NPC envelope for LTC homes in Ontario. The 34-group model includes 4 groups for residents that receive rehabilitation services. The 34-group model is more suitable for long-term care programs where nursing care is the primary cost driver. Membership in a RUG category is based on how much care a resident needs, types of treatments received, and whether or not the resident has certain conditions or diagnoses. These could include: • Assistance with Activities of Daily Living (ADLs) – bed mobility, transferring from one position to another, eating, and toilet use. A total ADL score of 4 – 18 is possible. The ADL score is a main part of determining case mix classification. The more assistance that is need, the higher the ADL score will be; • Treatments such as Intravenous (IV) medication, fluids, or nutrition; • Depression or behavioural symptoms; • Decreased ability to communicate or make decisions; • Therapy needs: Speech, Occupational, and/or Physical therapy (Canadian RAI Conference, 2008).

to 1. This will make it difficult to recruit future LTC clinical staff. (Conference Board of Canada, 2011) Regulatory and funding barriers limit the sector's adoption of technologies that can help provide high quality, efficiently and cost-effective care. LTC providers also lack sufficient resources in light of current and future demand, acuity levels, and resident preferences. The LTC sector is highly regulated making it difficult for LTC providers to innovate (Conference Board of Canada, 2011).

Investing in an Innovative Rehabilitation Strategy

In their report to the Ontario Long Term Care Association, the Conference Board of Canada recommended that the sector seek innovative strategies to better integrate LTC into the overall health system and to identify new services and products for their changing environment (Conference Board of Canada, 2011). An investment in a rehabilitation strategy for LTC would arguably impact the main drivers for CMI funding as well as significantly reduce hospital costs. Physical and cognitive function, mobility and pain are significant health outcomes for the LTC senior population (D'Astolfo, 2008; Coburn et al, 2002; Burton et al, 2001). An emerging trend in healthcare is the efficient use of human health resources, as seen in the rise of family health teams in Ontario. (MOHLTC, 2010) Interdisciplinary teams and healthcare integration have for some time been widely considered as essential to the delivery of rehabilitation (Rubin et al., 1972).

Many studies have demonstrated significant reductions in hospital readmission rates and numbers of office visits; increases in social activities, improvements in depression scores, functional status, and perceived well-being with interdisciplinary patient management (Sommers et al, 2009). Inter-professional collaboration or "teamwork" has also demonstrated improvement in patient outcomes (Newhouse et al, 2012). The APACHE II study involving over 5000 patients in thirteen intensive

care settings found significant patient mortality reductions in hospitals where physicians and nurses collaborated clinically (Sommers et al, 2009). Five fundamental variables to effective clinical collaborative teamwork have been identified in the literature. These include goal definition, role expectations, a flexible decision-making process, open communication and leadership. The use of an information system or decision tool to increase efficiencies in clinical teamwork may further enhance and improve patient outcomes (Newhouse et al, 2012). Essential to the advancement of rehabilitation is the development of new models of care, i.e. use of interdisciplinary, collaborative teams and non-OHIP funded health professionals, i.e. psychologists, chiropractors, etc., for re-defined roles in the management of multiple chronic diseases for LTC residents (Conference Board of Canada, 2011).

In addition to interdisciplinary teams, a Clinical Decision Support (CDS) tool could assist in the coordination of care of each individual patient based on specific rehabilitation needs (Conference Board of Canada, 2011). The tool could integrate the use of electronic medical records as they have the potential to properly document CMI scores associated with rehabilitation. Information technology is also essential for planning, horizontal management (collaboration among cross-sectoral partners), and the tracking of patient outcomes. Its use may help ensure coordinated planning, development, and implementation of innovative programs.

FUTURE RESEARCH DIRECTIONS

There is a trend for healthcare services to be downloaded to the community as opposed to the more costly hospital setting (Conference Board of Canada, 2011). Investing in innovative strategies to enhance integrated delivery of care for rehabilitation in long term care homes will enable a more coordinated approach to managing healthcare cost drivers (Conference Board of Canada, 2011). At the same time this will have significant pay off for the home operator as well as the broader system including increased CMI scores for LTC homes, time savings for nurses and broader healthcare savings in terms of cost avoidance for hospital emergency rooms, reduction in wait times, and lessening of Alternate Levels of Care (ALC) days (Conference Board of Canada, 2011). Further research is recommended in the development of decision tools aimed at detection and coordinated management of disorders responsive to rehabilitation, including back pain. New funding models are also needed to support this new initiative.

CONCLUSION

The healthcare needs of our aging population is a primary factor associated with escalating costs due to increased drug spending, physician visits, chronic diseases, co-morbidities, emergency visits and hospital costs. Back pain is highly prevalent in the long term care senior population and is a significant health care cost driver (Bressler et al., 1999; Coyte, 1998). A case study in support of "investing in a LTC rehabilitation strategy" illustrated the importance of improved decision making processes to support patient health outcomes and increase funding opportunities in the long term care continuum.

REFERENCES

Bressler, H., Keyes, J., Rochon, P., & Badley, E. (1999). The prevalence of low back pain in the elderly. *Spine*, *24*, 1813–1819. doi:10.1097/00007632-199909010-00011 PMID:10488512.

Burton, L. C., German, P., Gruber-Baldini, A., Hebel, R., Zimmerman, S., & Magaziner, J. (2001). Medical care for nursing home residents: Differences by dementia status. *Journal of the American Geriatrics Society*, *49*, 142–147. doi:10.1046/j.1532-5415.2001.49034.x PMID:11207867.

California Healthcare Foundation. (2008). *Report: Improving decision support tools for long term care*. Sacramento, CA: California Healthcare Foundation.

Canadian, R. A. I. Conference. (2008). *Making the quality connection*. Slide presentation. Canadian RAI Conference.

Canadian Institute for Health Information. (2006). *Discharge abstracts database 2005-2006: Executive summary: Data quality documentation*. Ottawa, Canada: Canadian Institute for Health Information.

Canadian Institute for Health Information. (2010). *Healthcare in Canada 2010*. Ottawa, Canada: Canadian Institute for Health Information.

Carter, M. (2003). Factors associated with ambulatory care-sensitive hospitalizations among nursing home residents. *Journal of Aging and Health*, *15*(2), 295–329. doi:10.1177/0898264303015002001 PMID:12795274.

Coburn, A., Keith, R., & Bolda, E. (2002). The impact of rural residence on multiple hospitalizations in nursing facility residents. *The Gerontologist*, *42*(5), 661–666. doi:10.1093/geront/42.5.661 PMID:12351801.

Conference Board of Canada. (2011). *Elements of an effective innovation strategy for long term care in Ontario*. Ontario, Canada: Ontario Long Term Care Association.

Cornette, P., Swine, C., Malhomme, B., Gillet, J., Meert, P., & D'Hoore, W. (2005). Early evaluation of the risk of functional decline following hospitalization of older patients: Development of a predictive tool. *European Journal of Public Health*, *16*(2), 203–208. doi:10.1093/eurpub/cki054 PMID:16076854.

Coyte, P. C. (1998). The economic cost of musculoskeletal disorders in Canada. *Arthritis Care and Research*, *5*, 315–335. doi:10.1002/art.1790110503 PMID:9830876.

Cypress, B. (1983). Characteristics of physician visits for back symptoms: A national perspective. *American Journal of Public Health*, *73*, 389–395. doi:10.2105/AJPH.73.4.389 PMID:6219588.

D'Astolfo, C., & Humphreys, B. K. (2006). *A record review of reported musculoskeletal pain in an Ontario long term care facility*. BMJ Geriatrics.

Economics, T. D. (2010). *Charting a path to sustainable healthcare in Ontario*. TD Bank Financial Group.

Garg, A. X., Adhikari, N. K. J., & McDonald, H. et al. (2005). *Effects of computerized clinical decision support systems on practitioner performance and patient outcomes*. Academic Press. doi:10.1001/jama.293.10.1223.

Goel, V. (1996). Indicators of health determinants and health status. In *Patterns of HealthCare in Ontario: The ICES Practice Atlas* (2nd ed., pp. 5–26). Ottawa, Canada: CMA.

Government of Ontario. (2009). *Ontario population projections update 2009-2036*. Ontario, Canada: Government of Ontario.

Hart, L., Deyo, R., & Cherkin, D. (1995). Physician office visits for low back pain: frequency, clinical evaluation and treatment patterns from a US National survey. *Spine*, *20*, 11–19. doi:10.1097/00007632-199501000-00003 PMID:7709270.

Hatzakis, M., Allen, C., Haselkorn, M., Anderson, S., Nichol, P., Lai, C., & Haselkorn, J. (2006). Use of medical informatics for management of multiple sclerosis using a chronic-care model. *Journal of Rehabilitation Research and Development*, *43*(1), 1–16. doi:10.1682/JRRD.2004.10.0135 PMID:16847767.

Hutt, E., Ecord, M., Eilertsen, T., Fredrickson, E., & Kramer, A. (2002). Precipitants of emergency room visits and acute hospitalization in short-stay medicare nursing home residents. *Journal of the American Geriatrics Society*, *50*, 223–229. doi:10.1046/j.1532-5415.2002.50052.x PMID:12028202.

Intrator, O., Castle, N., & Mor, V. (1999). Facility characteristics associated with hospitalization of nursing home residents: Results of a national study. *Medical Care*, *37*(3), 228–237. doi:10.1097/00005650-199903000-00003 PMID:10098567.

Intrator, O., Zinn, J., & Mor, V. (2004). Nursing home characteristics and potentially preventable hospitalizations of long-stay residents. *Journal of the American Geriatrics Society*, *52*(10), 1–7. doi:10.1111/j.1532-5415.2004.52469.x PMID:14687307.

Knaus, W., & Draper, E. D. (1986). An evaluation of outcome from intensive care in major medical centers. *Annals of Internal Medicine*, *104*, 410–418. doi:10.7326/0003-4819-104-3-410 PMID:3946981.

Ministry of Health and Long Term Care. (2010, July 1). *LTCH level-of-care per diem funding policy*. Ottawa, Canada: Ministry of Health and Long Term Care.

Ministry of Health and Long Term Care. (2012, March). *Long term care home financial policy*. Ottawa, Canada: Ministry of Health and Long Term Care.

MOHLTC. (2010). *Externally-informed annual health systems trends report* (3rd ed.). Academic Press.

Newhouse, I., Heckman, G., Harrison, D., D'Elia, T., Kaasalainen, S., Strachan, P., & Demers, C. (2012). Barriers to the management of heart failure in Ontario long term care homes: An interprofessional perspective. *Journal of Research in Interprofessional Practice and Education, 2*(3).

O'Connor, A. M., Stacey, D., & Jacobsen, M. J. (2011). *Ottawa decision support tutorial: Improving practitioners' decision support skills Ottawa hospital research institute: Patient decision aids.* Academic Press.

OECD. (2011). *Help wanted? Providing and paying for long-term care.* Paris, France: OECD. Retrieved from www.oecd.org/health/longtermcare

OECD Health Data. (2010). Retrieved from www.oecd.org/health/healthdata

Osheroff, J. A., Teich, J. M., & Middleton, B. F. et al. (2006). *A roadmap for national action on clinical decision support.* Washington, DC: American Medical Informatics Association.

PointClickCare. (2011). Retrieved from http://www.pointclickcare.com/solutions/solutions.php

Raphael, D. (2007a). Canadian public policy and poverty in international perspective. In Raphael, D. (Ed.), *Poverty and Policy in Canada: Implications for Health and Quality of Life* (pp. 335–364). Toronto, Canada: Canadian Scholars' Press.

Rubin, I., & Beckhard, R. (1972). Factors influencing the effectiveness of health teams. *The Milbank Memorial Fund Quarterly, 50*(3), 317–335. doi:10.2307/3349352 PMID:5043085.

Sommers, L., Marton, K., & Barbaccia, J. C. (2000). Physician, nurse, and social worker collaboration in primary care for chronically ill seniors. *Archives of Internal Medicine, 160,* 1825–1833. doi:10.1001/archinte.160.12.1825 PMID:10871977.

StatsCan. (2007). *Residential care facilities (2006/2007).* StatsCan.

Wagner, E. H. (1998). Chronic disease management: What will it take to improve care for chronic illness? *Efficient Clinical Practice, 1*(1), 2–4. PMID:10345255.

ADDITIONAL READING

Billings, J. (1990). *Consideration of the use of small area analysis as a tool to evaluate barriers to access.* Washington, DC: US Dept of Health and Human Resources.

Canadian Institute for Health Information. (2009). *Health care in Canada 2009: A decade in review.* Ottawa, Canada: CIHI. Retrieved from http://www.cihiconferences.ca/HCIC2009/index.html

Canadian Institute for Health Information. (2010)... *Health Care in Canada, 2010.* Retrieved from https://secure.cihi.ca/estore/productFamily.htm?locale=en&pf=PFC1568&lang=en&media=0.

Christensen, C., & Bohmer, J. (2000, September-October). Kenagy will disruptive innovations cure health care? *Harvard Business Review,* 102–112. PMID:11143147.

Dycke, M. (2002). Nursing informatics: Applications for long-term care. *Journal of Gerontological Nursing, 28*(10), 30. PMID:12382458.

Eng, C., Pedulla, J., & Eleazer, G. (1997). Program of all-inclusive care for the elderly (PACE): An innovative model of integrated geriatric care and financing. *Journal of the American Geriatrics Society, 45*(2), 223–232. PMID:9033525.

Extendicare Canada. (2011). Retrieved from http://www.extendicare.com

Healthcare 2015. (n.d.). *Win-win or lose-lose?* Retrieved from http://www-05.ibm.com/de/healthcare/downloads/healthcare_2015.pdf

Raphael, D. (2006). Social determinants of health: Present status, unresolved questions, and future directions. *International Journal of Health Services, 36*, 651–677. doi:10.2190/3MW4-1EK3-DGRQ-2CRF PMID:17175840.

Wagner, E. H., Austin, B. T., & Von Korff, M. (1996). Organizing care for patients with chronic illness. *The Milbank Quarterly, 74*(4), 511–544. doi:10.2307/3350391 PMID:8941260.

KEY TERMS AND DEFINITIONS

Ambulatory Care Sensitive Conditions: Classification of conditions that can be managed effectively in a community setting (Carter, 2003).

Arthritis: Arthritis is a chronic condition characterized by the breakdown of the joint's cartilage causing stiffness, pain, and loss of movement. Arthritis is a common cause of back pain (Coyte, 1998).

Back Pain: Back pain originates from injury to muscles, nerves, bones, joints or other structures in the spine. Back pain can present as acute or chronic and is classified as a significant cause of disability (Coyte, 1998).

Case Mix Index: Case mix index is a measure of the relative cost or resources needed to treat the mix of patients or residents in long term care and is used as a measure of the average care requirements of the home (CIHI, 2012; MOHLTC, 2012).

Chronic Disease: Chronic diseases are persistent or otherwise long-lasting in its effects (more than three months). Common chronic diseases include arthritis, asthma, cancer, COPD, diabetes/back pain. Chronic diseases share common modifiable risk factors (Wagner, 1998).

Long Term Care: Long-term care involves providing medical care that requires the expertise of skilled practitioners to address chronic conditions associated with older populations. Long-term care can be provided at home, in assisted living facilities or in nursing homes (MOHLTC, 2008).

RAI-MDS: The Resident Assessment Instrument-Minimum Data Set (RAI-MDS) is an assessment data tool used for care planning in clinical management and to determine facility payment for residents. It provides information on residents' socio-demographic characteristics, physical and cognitive status, psychological and health conditions, behavioural problems, service use, and medication use (Canadian RAI Conference, 2008).

Rehabilitation: To restore to good health or pre-injury status, with physical and psychological therapy and patient education (D'Astolfo, 2006).

Resource Utilization Groups (RUGS): Resource Utilization Groups is a case mix grouping funding methodology that can be calculated using data from the RAI-MDS. RUGS are used in LTC institutional settings (Canadian RAI Conference, 2008).

Value for Money: Cost efficient use of resources and investments in our healthcare system (TD Economics, 2010).

Chapter 4

Making Quality Control Decisions in Radiology Department:
A Decision Support System for Radiographers' Performance Appraisal Using PACS

Valentina Al Hamouche
The Michener Institute for Applied Health Sciences, Canada

ABSTRACT

In the radiology department, radiographers' performance appraisal cannot be performed continuously due to time pressure and the lack of objective performance indicators. The authors conducted an empirical study where they assessed radiographers' performance based on objective performance indicators derived from data stored in the PACS and RIS. The study indicated that one is able to use the PACS-RIS environment as a Decision Support System (DSS) that delivers promptly objective indicators for performance appraisal purposes. Besides, the model of a DSS allows radiographers' continuous performance appraisal.

INTRODUCTION

Diagnostic imaging departments are becoming filmless; integrating Picture Archiving Communication System (PACS), Radiology Information System (RIS), Computed Radiography (CR), and many other digital imaging techniques are

DOI: 10.4018/978-1-4666-4321-5.ch004

currently common practice in medical imaging due to the adoption of Health Level 7 (HL7) standard (Health Level 7, 2006). Despite its high cost, medical imaging digitization provides many advantages, such as improved productivity, better efficiency, and reduced radiation dose to patient (Crowe & Sim, 2005; Kimura, 1991; Lawrence, 2005; Mulvaney, 2002; Rogoski, 2003; Worthy, Rounds, & Soloway, 2003). The integrated

PACS-RIS environment generates a vast amount of valuable data related to patients and users (e.g. radiographers, radiologists). Nevertheless, the capacity of this digital environment is not fully exploited yet; particularly in the domain of performance appraisal (Coates, 1996; Edmonstone, 1996; Fletcher, 1993; Gellerman & Hodgson, 1988; Grote, 2000; Johnson, 1991; Man, 2005; McGregor, 1972; Meyer, Kay, & French, 1989; Palmer, McElearney, & Harrington, 2004; Ryan, 2003; Wilson & Cole, 1990; Winstanley, 1980). Even though some propositions were made to enhance the quality in the radiology department, attempts were made to establish department wide quality indicators and dashboards (Abujudeh, Kaewlai, Asfaw, & Thrall, 2010; Kruskal, Anderson, Yam, & Sosna, 2009; Nagy et al., 2009) or scoreboards(Donnelly et al., 2010), or to measure the productivity of the imaging devices(Hu et al., 2011) or radiologists (Rubin, 2011); none has looked into the radiographers performance measurement and appraisal, and its relation to patient safety.

Appraising and providing feedback regularly is an advised practice (Boswell & Boudreau, 2000; Daft & Marcic, 2001) that aims to detect performance weaknesses as early as possible and to take corresponding corrective actions. However, two factors are hindering the establishment of policies enforcing frequent and ongoing appraisal: time and automation. Performance appraisal can be conducted under two modes one is evaluative and the other is developmental (Boswell & Boudreau, 2000). The evaluative approach is concerned with management problems, such as salary administration, promotion decision, and retention-termination decisions; therefore, it can be a source of anxiety and resistance of staff. On the other hand, the developmental approach is concerned with identifying individual training needs, providing performance feedback, determining transfers and assignments and identifying individual strength and weaknesses; and these aims are usually positively perceived by staff (Boswell

& Boudreau, 2000). We take developmental and participative approaches in our performance appraisal project. We build on Handy's (Handy, 1993) argumentation for a developmental approach in performance appraisal, particularly staff needs of encouragement, direction and freedom. These needs fit well the leader managerial participative role suggested by Mintzberg (Huczynski & Buchanan, 2001). We believe that a developmental approach to performance appraisal is characterized by fairness, and leads to job satisfaction and help personal career development.

Currently, there is no computerized tool that allows calculating objective radiographers' performance indicators. The objective of our study we present in this chapter, were to investigate the ability of PACS-RIS to serve as a basis to develop decision support model for a continuous radiographers' performance appraisal, using objective performance indicators derived from PACS-RIS databases. We will show the results of a qualitative flexible design study that includes six interviews with PACS administrators and radiology departments' managers, and a case study of performance appraisal in a hospital in Toronto. We will then draw a model for a developmental performance appraisal module that can be added to PACS-RIS and serve managers and radiographers as a Decision Support System (DSS), in a Total Quality Management (TQM) perspective (Dowd & Tilson, 1996; Edwards, 1986; Hackman & Wageman, 1995). We suggest that this model adds a managerial functionality, particularly a decision support one, to the PACS-RIS environment; thus, expanding PACS-RIS use to the field of human resource management.

METHODS

In order to investigate the ability to use of PACS-RIS for human resource management; we have used a qualitative flexible design approach including (1) six individual semi structured interviews with PACS administrators and radiology departments' managers, and (2) a case study of performance appraisal for 5 radiographers in a hospital in Toronto.

Interviews

We have chosen a convenience sample of three radiology managers and three PACS administrators at three different hospitals, in the city of Toronto, Ontario, Canada. One administrator and one manager were interviewed in each hospital. The interviewees were chosen based on their extensive experience in PACS and RIS. The interviews were semi-structured, organized in an open ended series of questions. All interviewees were asked the same questions; the interviews were conducted in depth, probes were used when necessary. All aspects of data collection and analysis concerning PACS and RIS were discussed in details. Two areas were investigated (1) the method and frequency in which radiographers' performance appraisal is performed and (2) the data that exist in the department and that can support objective performance appraisal.

Case Study

Two steps were involved in the case study: calculating performance indicators and conducting performance analysis for each radiographer.

We have calculated the performance indicators of five radiographers for four months in a hospital that has an integrated PACS-RIS. The radiology department manager selected five out of ten radiographers working in CR, and we collected the following data related to their performance:

- Years of experience
- Monthly schedule and assignment
- Number of hours worked per month
- Number of cases performed per month
- Number of images produced per month

- Number of repeat per month
- Number of rejected images by the radiologist per month
- Reasons of repeat

The RIS and CR allowed us to collect the following "Reasons of repeat":

- Clipped anatomy
- Inadequate X ray Exposure
- Positioning error
- Patient motion
- Technique
- Test image
- Other reasons (This category can include scatter radiation, artifact, double exposure, wrong marker, wrong examination, and equipment malfunction).

Besides, the total number of cases done, the total number of images produced, the total repeat of the whole department, as well as the number of repeats per "reason of repeat" category were collected on a monthly basis. We collected data related to the cases and images processed on three CR units.

As a result, the following performance indicators were calculated:

- Productivity (cases and images performed in a certain period of time).
- Number of hours worked.
- Number of images rejected by radiographers and repeated, and the reasons of repeat.
- Number of images rejected by radiologist (after they have been sent to PACS).

We analyzed each radiographer's performance using spreadsheets. In the absence of dedicated software developed for such purpose, the processing took extensive effort and substantial number of hours.

Analysis

The main objective for the three managers' interviews was to reveal the method used for radiographers' performance appraisal, the appraisal frequency, as well as the data present in the PACS-RIS. Therefore, we did not conduct a formal thematic analysis for the interviews.

We used spreadsheets to code and analyze the data collected for the five radiographers. Given that he sample size was small, we used simple statistical analysis of the case study, using percentages and averages, and we generated bar charts to illustrate the analysis results.

FINDINGS

Interviews' Results

The interviews showed that the three interviewed managers were conducting performance appraisal sessions once a year, or once every two years, using performance appraisal forms set by the human resources departments; besides, they revealed that the managers assess the performance subjectively by observation; the only objective,

tangible and quantifiable factors they relied on was the radiographers' attendance. Moreover, we have discovered that data needed to calculate performance indicators were scattered on different information systems and that they were not always stored in an electronic format. Table 1 summarizes the interview findings in relation to data availability and their format.

Case Study Results

The collected indicators reflected each radiographer's performance and allowed the manager to advise each one accordingly. For the first time, details about each radiographer's performance were visible in a quantified way, which gave the manager an objective insight into the radiographers' performance and enabled her to analyze their performance (Figures 1, 2, and 3). The manager was able to find out what factors are influencing performance, and supplied her observations with objective performance measurement. She then used the indicators to conduct the annual performance appraisal interview with radiographers. Finally, she provided a written qualitative feedback expressing satisfaction, of both radiographers and herself, during the appraisal sessions. The manager

Table 1. Data collected or calculated by PACS administrators in the hospitals A, B, and C

Data	Data Format		
	Hospital A	**Hospital B**	**Hospital C**
Imaging Modalities	Electronic on PACS except mammography	Electronic on PACS except mammography and Nuclear Medicine	Electronic on PACS except mammography
Radiographer's schedule	Electronic on RIS	Manually/Paper	Manually/Paper
Workload	Electronic on PACS/RIS	Electronic on PACS/RIS	Electronic on PACS/RIS
Acquisition repeat count and reasons of repeat	Electronic on CR	Electronic on CR	Electronic on CR
Radiologist rejection count (hence repeated) and reasons of rejection	Absent: Not stored on PACS	Absent: Not stored on PACS	Absent: Not stored on PACS
Number of images rejected by radiologists	Manual calculation	Manual calculation	Manual calculation
Patient complaints	Manual calculation	Manual calculation	Manual calculation

Figure 1. Workload per month

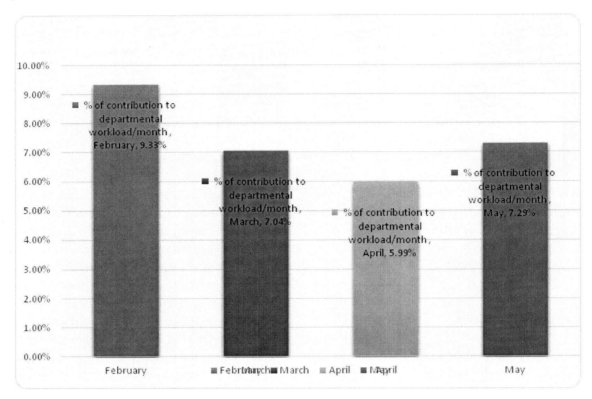

Figure 2. Radiographer A repeat rate (Radiographer A repeats/department total repeats)

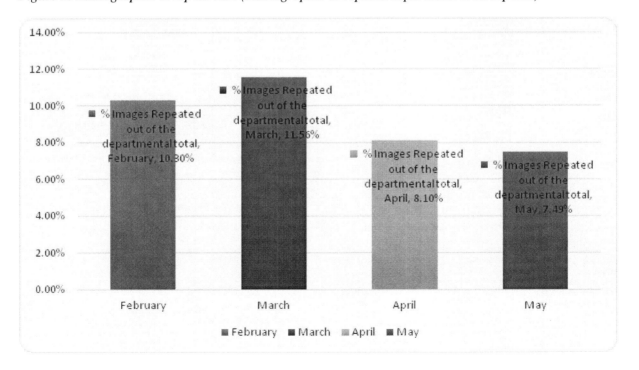

Figure 3. Individual repeat analysis

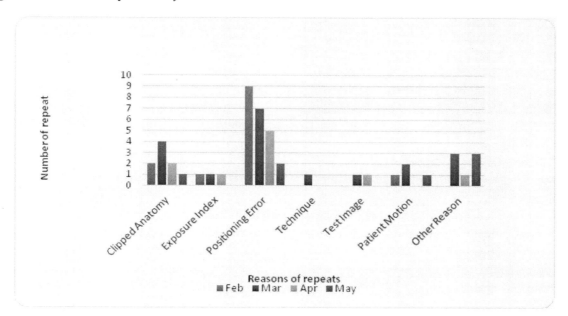

could discuss with the radiographers and advise them on specific performance issues that were imperceptible without the indicators.

A summary of the five radiographer's main deficiencies is shown in Table 2.

In the absence of an automated system, an objective and continuous performance appraisal is time consuming and impractical since managers are already overwhelmed in conducting day-to-day activities and solving emergent problems. Therefore, an automated developmental performance appraisal module needs to be developed and get integrated in the current PACS-RIS environment.

Figures 1, 2, and 3 illustrate the results of one of the radiographers: Radiographer A.

DISCUSSION

We could draw several lessons from the interviews as well as from the case study.

Interviews

Based on the interviews, we could draw two kind of conclusions one in relation to the *appraisal process* and the other in relation to the *data* available.

Table 2. Summary of the radiographer's main problems

Radiographer	Main Problems
Radiographer A	No indication of the specific reasons of repeat. Not helpful for him and his manager to evaluate the problem
Radiographer B	Positioning errors
Radiographer C	Clipped anatomy
Radiographer D	Exposure index
Radiographer E	Clipped anatomy, positioning error and "other reason." The other reasons are not specified while it should have been so.

On the process level, the performance appraisal was conducted subjectively based on observation and the attendance was only objective data used. Due to time pressure the appraisal frequency was once a year or once every two years. Besides, the managers judged the appraisal process to be time consuming, which prohibited them from doing a more frequent (and eventually continuous) performance appraisal. Our conclusion is that automation is an important and advantageous factor that can enable a desirable more frequent/continuous performance appraisal.

On the data level, not all available data were stored electronically. Some data, such as the radiographer schedule, were available on paper; some other data, such as acquisition repeat, were electronic and available on the CR but not captured in PACS. Finally, some data were absent and never captured, that was the case of the radiologist image rejection. Moreover, electronically stored data were scattered, and there were no software available to enable managers to query the available data. Our conclusion is that any attempt to automate the performance appraisal process should take into account (1) making all data related to performance appraisal electronically available in the PACS-RIS environment, (2) and integrating these data in order to allow one point of access to performance indicators.

Case Study

We analyzed the indicators of the five radiographers. Indicators of Radiographer D, showed that his repeats were due mainly to "exposure index." These repeats were related to Radiographer D having moved to a new rotation; we discovered that this situation is due to the fact that each X-ray equipment has different output exposure, so when a rotation is changed it took Radiographer D some time to get used to the new X-ray exposure settings. The manager advised Radiographer D to make use of the exposure charts available in each X-ray room. Radiographer A, had majority of her/his repeats due to "other reasons" with no further details. In this case, it was not possible for the manager and for the concerned radiographer to identify the exact reasons of repeat, hindering the possibility of identifying her weak areas. During the appraisal process, the manager advised Radiographer A as well as other radiographers, to enter data explaining the "other reasons' for repeat in the proper field available on the screen.

Future Perspectives

The individual measurements that we have used were mainly the workload, the repeat rate and the reasons of repeat. Compared to subjective assessment, the indicators were able to give a clearer and objective measurement of the productivity, and the quality of the radiographers' work.

Concerning radiographers' productivity, we were able to express it in terms of the number of cases performed per hour or the number of images performed per hour. It is the manager's choice to decide which numbers she wants to use to assess productivity. Nevertheless, it is worth mentioning that the time required to perform a case varies widely between cases, thus, it seems that using the number of images produced per hour can provide a better estimate of the work performed per hour. The number of hours spent on repeating images can be calculated by relying on the number of images performed per hour. This can help in calculating the cost incurred by repeating image acquisition, as a function of radiographer's rate per hour; besides, we can calculate the service cost reduction related to any improvement in skill that produces a reduction in repeat rate.

Since the radiographers are responsible of producing images of diagnostic quality, the quality that we have measured was the quality of the images produced expressed in terms of image acquisition repeat analysis and image rejection analysis. Repeat analysis can determine to a certain extent the quality of images produced, and the factors affecting the repeat rate.

Communication skills are also part of the radiographer's quality of work. They can be assessed partly by the "patient motion" factor. Since patient cooperation and immobilization depends on clear instructions provided by radiographer patient (Torres, Dutton, & Norcutt, 2003). However, we can determine better this factor if we add a patient feedback factor; we suggest to add a patient satisfaction input module to the system. A touch screen based system can enable patients to give their feedback in an easy to use way after the imaging procedure; this feedback can be useful in assessing performance of the whole service as suggested by Papp (2006).

The manager and the radiographers that used the performance indicators data in hospital A showed satisfaction and described the experience to be "very positive", and the tool to be "successful"; besides, the radiologists "appreciated" the indicators presented to them.

We could attribute the manager satisfaction to the fact that the generated spreadsheets were efficient and helped her to conduct an effective performance appraisal session. While we could relate the radiographers' satisfaction to the objectivity induced by the objective indicators, and the empowerment they would have experienced due to their ability to rely on based on sound data to take personal decisions related to their continuous education.

The study showed that objective performance indicators can be extracted from PACS-RIS environment and provide support for managers. The proposed Decision Support System could save time and allow the implementation of a continuous performance appraisal, allowing the managers to be proactive and to act on the fly when they notice a performance disturbance and before the service degrades.

Modeling

In order to summarize our view of the new role of PACS-RIS as a decision support system, we have developed an information flow model for a developmental performance appraisal module that would automate the indicators' collection and chart drawing. We also developed, another model that represents the way the PACS-RIS integrated system will behave when adapted to Performance appraisal of radiographers. The two proposed models are two high level designs of a decision support system following a developmental approach, and show that the proposed decision support system can be implemented with minimal changes to the PACS information system.

Developmental Performance Appraisal Model

Most of the data related to the indicators we have proposed were already present in the PACS-RIS. The data that was not present (acquisition repeat count, rejection repeat count) can easily be stored in the system; for instance, the information related to radiographers' schedule, rotation and workload can be gathered from RIS; while the information related to technical factors and repeat can be gathered from the digital modality (the CR in our case). Information related to the workload, rejected images by the radiologists can be collected from the PACS (after minor database schema modifications).

All these information can then constitute an input to a Developmental Performance Appraisal decision support system, allowing the radiographers' performance indicators to be computed in an automated manner and performance reports to be generated instantaneously in a systematic way. Such module would enable radiographers and managers to be aware of performance and quality problems whenever they take place.

We have built an information flow model (Figure 4) that summarizes the internal processing in the proposed module. The model shows the flow of data from the time a patient is scheduled for an appointment with a doctor, to the time a radiologist diagnose the medical images and a report is written.

Information System Model

We believe that the development of the proposed module is feasible and incurs minimal changes in the currently available systems, and consequently minimal cost. To be sure, the changes that we suggest implementing involve the following data:

1. Radiographer schedules
2. Acquisition repeat count
3. Rejection count

Figure 5 represents two Data Flow Diagrams that illustrate the changes in the internal information systems processes as well as in the data flows needed between these processes.

Study Limitation

The fact that the manager has selected the five radiographers in the Case Study is a methodological limitation since it could indicate some bias in the selection process. Another limitation to the study is the small number of radiographers (five) which limits the study generalizability; besides, the fact that the 'observed' radiographers knew that their performance will be evaluated may have caused some degree of bias. Further research could include more staff and be conducted in a blinded way using a random method to select the participants.

We conducted the empirical fieldwork in spring 2006, though the model was not implemented electronically for an on an ongoing decision support.

The implementation needed an involvement of a Vendor and we were not successful in reaching an implementation agreement with the vendor in the corresponding hospital. However, between 2006 and 2012, and to the best of our knowledge, no research has been conducted to address this burning issue in radiology department; we believe that our model is still valid and replies to a sure void in the radiology department.

CONCLUSION

We have showed the ability of PACS-RIS to serve as a managerial tool, and we have developed a decision support model for a continuous radiographers' performance appraisal using objective performance indicators derived from PACS-RIS.

Our empirical study shows that we can use an integrated PACS-RIS environment to support objective radiographer's performance appraisal sessions. The study showed that objective indicators gives insights to the actual capabilities of individual radiographers in relation to productivity and quality of work. Our approach relieves both managers and radiographers from a stressful and sensitive task by providing objective measurements; we can reasonably assume that it will encourage some cooperative atmosphere during the appraisal process, and that it enables radiographers to commit to work. Besides, we think that a developmental approach will empower not only managers, but also radiographers by providing them with a tool to uncover objectively their own performance shortcomings, which may enable them to strive for their own development.

We have developed models for a developmental performance appraisal's decision support system, and for the changes required in the PACS-RIS information environment. We have also argued that the decision support system model can be extended and used in other areas, such as patient safety; undeniably, a reduced dose to patients is a major concern in patient safety.

Figure 4. An information flow model for the developmental performance appraisal of radiographers

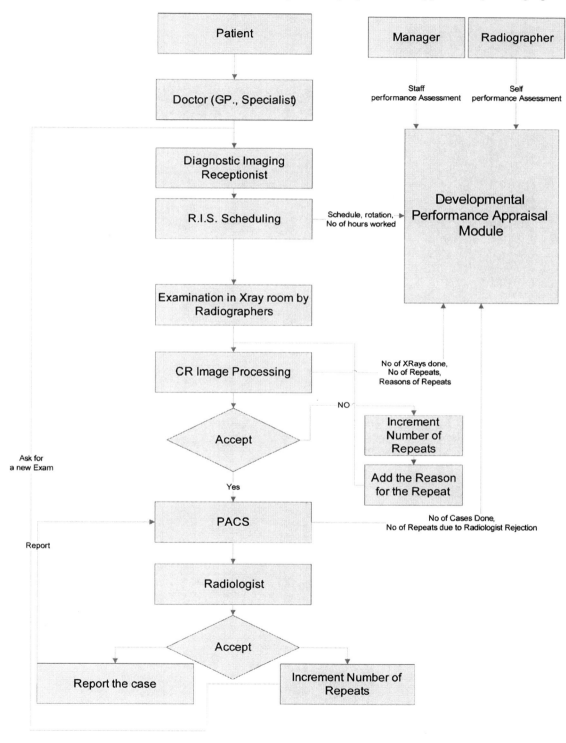

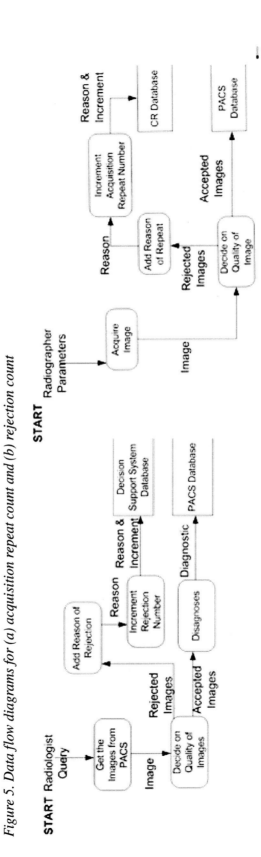

Figure 5. Data flow diagrams for (a) acquisition repeat count and (b) rejection count

We conclude that PACS and RIS can be used as basis to develop a DSS that supplies a developmental performance appraisal approach in the radiology department. The capabilities of the PACS/RIS and medical imaging modalities integration has not been fully explored; further research is required to explore other managerial aspects of this digital environment.

REFERENCES

Abujudeh, H. H., Kaewlai, R., Asfaw, B. A., & Thrall, J. H. (2010). Quality initiatives: Key performance indicators for measuring and improving radiology department performance. *Radiographics*, *30*(3), 571–580. doi:10.1148/rg.303095761 PMID:20219841.

Boswell, R., & Boudreau, W. (2000). Employee satisfaction with performance appraisals and appraisers: The role of perceived appraisal use. *Human Resource Development Quarterly*, *11*(3), 283–299. doi:10.1002/1532-1096(200023)11:3<283::AID-HRDQ6>3.0.CO;2-3.

Coates, G. (1996). Image and identity: Performance appraisal in a trust hospital. *Health Manpower Management*, *22*(3), 16–22. doi:10.1108/09552069610125883 PMID:10161774.

Crowe, B., & Sim, L. (2005). An assessment of the effect of the introduction of a PACS and RIS on clinical decision making and patient management at Princess Alexandra Hospital Brisbane, Australia. *International Congress Series*, *1281*, 964–967. doi:10.1016/j.ics.2005.03.347.

Daft, R., & Marcic, D. (2001). *Understanding management* (3rd ed.). Hercourt.

Donnelly, L. F., Gessner, K. E., Dickerson, J. M., Koch, B. L., Towbin, A. J., & Lehkamp, T. W. et al. (2010). Quality initiatives: Department scorecard: A tool to help drive imaging care delivery performance. *Radiographics*, *30*(7), 2029–2038. doi:10.1148/rg.307105017 PMID:20801869.

Dowd, S. B., & Tilson, E. (1996). The benefits of using CQI/TQM data (continuous quality improvement/total quality management). *Radiologic Technology*, *67*(6), 533–535. PMID:8827822.

Edmonstone, J. (1996). Appraising the state of performance appraisal. *Health Manpower Management*, *22*(6), 9. doi:10.1108/09552069610153071 PMID:10164227.

Edwards, D. (1986). *Out of the crisis*. Cambridge, MA: MIT Center for Advanced Engineering Studies.

Fletcher, C. (1993). Appraisal: An idea whose time has gone? *Personnel Management*, *25*(9), 34.

Gellerman, S. W., & Hodgson, W. G. (1988). Cyanamid's new take on performance appraisal. *Harvard Business Review*, *66*(3), 36.

Grote, D. (2000). Performance appraisal reappraised. *Harvard Business Review*, *78*(1), 21.

Hackman, J. R., & Wageman, R. (1995). Total quality management: Empirical, conceptual, and practical issues. *Administrative Science Quarterly*, *40*(2), 309. doi:10.2307/2393640.

Handy, C. (1993). *Understanding organisation* (4th ed.). London: Penguin.

Health Level 7. (2006). *Health level 7*. Retrieved June 28th 2007, from http://www.HL7.org

Hu, M., Pavlicek, W., Liu, P. T., Zhang, M., Langer, S. G., Wang, S., & Wu, T. T. (2011). Informatics in radiology: Efficiency metrics for imaging device productivity. *Radiographics, 31*(2), 603–616. doi:10.1148/rg.312105714 PMID:21257928.

Huczynski, A., & Buchanan, D. (2001). *Organizational behaviour: An introductory text* (4th ed.). Englewood Cliffs, NJ: Prentice Hall.

Johnson, J. R. (1991). No excuses performance appraisals. *Harvard Business Review, 69*(1), 188.

Kimura, M. (1991). *PACS, RIS, HIS - Each as a part of allied healthcare information system.*

Kruskal, J. B., Anderson, S., Yam, C. S., & Sosna, J. (2009). Strategies for establishing a comprehensive quality and performance improvement program in a radiology department. *Radiographics, 29*(2), 315–329. doi:10.1148/rg.292085090 PMID:19168762.

Lawrence, P. (2005). Preparing a cultural strategy for PACS. *Radiology Management, 27*(1), 21–29. PMID:15794374.

Man, E. (2005). A functional approach to appraisal and retention scheduling. *Records Management Journal, 15*(1), 21–33. doi:10.1108/09565690510585402.

McGregor, D. (1972). An uneasy look at performance appraisal. *Harvard Business Review, 50*(5), 133.

Meyer, H. H., Kay, E., & French, J. R. P. (1989). Split roles in performance appraisal. *Harvard Business Review, 67*(1), 26.

Mulvaney, J. (2002). The case for RIS/PACS integration. *Radiology Management, 24*(3), 24–29. PMID:12080929.

Nagy, P. G., Warnock, M. J., Daly, M., Toland, C., Meenan, C. D., & Mezrich, R. S. (2009). Informatics in radiology: Automated web-based graphical dashboard for radiology operational business intelligence. *Radiographics, 29*(7), 1897–1906. doi:10.1148/rg.297095701 PMID:19734469.

Palmer, K. T., McElearney, N., & Harrington, M. (2004). Appraisal standards in occupational medicine. *Occupational Medicine, 54*(4), 218–226. doi:10.1093/occmed/kqh068 PMID:15190157.

Papp, J. (2006). *Quality management in the imaging sciences* (3rd ed.). MOSBY.

Rogoski, R. R. (2003). PACS as an enterprise resource: Digital imaging comes of age, as improved web, storage, network and EMR technologies support its extended reach throughout the healthcare enterprise. *Health Management Technology, 24*(11), 14–16, 20. PMID:14608707.

Rubin, D. L. (2011). Informatics in radiology: Measuring and improving quality in radiology: Meeting the challenge with informatics. *Radiographics, 31*(6), 1511–1527. doi:10.1148/rg.316105207 PMID:21997979.

Ryan, C. (2003). Understanding performance appraisal. *Journal of Community Nursing, 17*(8), 9–14.

Torres, L. S., Dutton, A. G., & Norcutt, T. A. L. (2003). *Basic medical techniques and patient care in imaging technology* (6th ed.). Philadelphia: Lippincott, Williams and Wilkins.

Wilson, J., & Cole, G. (1990). A healthy approach to performance appraisal. *Personnel Management, 22*(6), 46.

Winstanley, N. B. (1980). Legal and ethical issues in performance appraisals. *Harvard Business Review, 58*(6), 186–192.

Worthy, S., Rounds, K. C., & Soloway, C. B. (2003). Strengthening your ties to referring physicians through RIS/PACS integration. *Radiology Management*, *25*(2), 18–22. PMID:12800559.

KEY TERMS AND DEFINITIONS

Decision Support Systems: A Decision Support System (DSS) is an information system that uses computing powers to analyze a set of data and provide information to users in order for them to make decisions. A DSS supplies decision makers with insight in order to make decision but never makes the decision itself.

Employee Performance Appraisal: A procedure that allows managers and employees to discuss employee's performance, and set performance objectives for a period of time.

Informatics: An area of research and development that investigates the use of information and communication technologies in the healthcare system.

Information Management: A field that investigates how information can be collected, stored and used to meet organizational targets.

PACS: Picture archiving and communication systems that allows medical imaging data to be collected, stored, communicated throughout the radiology department. Radiologists use the PACS to report the images.

RIS: Radiology Information Systems are computer systems that will allow patient tracking and scheduling, and reporting in the radiology department.

Quality Control: Quality Control is a process to ensure that proper standards are maintained in an organization.

Chapter 5
Using Case Costing Data and Case Mix for Funding and Benchmarking in Rehabilitation Hospitals

Grace Liu
York University, Canada

ABSTRACT

The concern for Ontario hospitals in Canada is that the funding model has recently changed from global- to activity-based funding, which will affect hospitals' operational budget and cost management. Hospitals will be reimbursed based on a pre-set payment price for each patient type or case mix treated. Specifically, the purpose of this chapter is to describe how case costing data and case mix information are collected and used for funding. A framework is proposed for health administrators, policy makers, and researchers to understand the input variables for determining resource utilization and long stay trim point. A clinical decision-making tool is demonstrated to assist hospital administrators to define admission criteria and predict length of stay and volumes with clinical teams. The chapter highlights the importance of data quality and use of comparative data and concludes with 10 key success factors for better funding and benchmarking for rehabilitation hospitals.

INTRODUCTION

Case costing and case mix are widely used in health care systems internationally. In Ontario, Canada, case costing and case mix will be used as the funding model has recently changed from global funding to service based funding. Given this funding approach, it is crucial that hospitals manage their case costs and understand their vari-

ous patient populations (or case mix). As case mix of patients will determine the funding allocated, hospital administrators need to admit appropriate case mix of patients, manage their costs and monitor the volume of services provided. The chapter will describe and analyze case costing data and case mix and to optimize funding and benchmarking in rehabilitation hospitals. A "Shrub" framework will be provided to understand the input variables for determining resource utilization and long stay trim point. A clinical decision-making tool

DOI: 10.4018/978-1-4666-4321-5.ch005

is demonstrated for defining admission criteria and predict length of stay and volumes. It is important health administrators, policy makers and researchers considers data quality when analyzing case costing data and case mix for funding and benchmarking.

The objectives of the chapter are:

1. To describe data collection systems:
   a. Ontario Healthcare Reporting Standard Data.
   b. Adult Inpatient Rehabilitation Minimum Data.
2. To provide a "Shrub" framework to understand the factors that impact funding:
   a. Describe "Input Variables for Determining Resource Utilization" and "Long Stay Trim Point Illustration for a particular Rehab Patient Group (RPG)".
   b. Clinical implications for rehabilitation hospitals.
3. To demonstrate a clinical decision-making tool:
   a. Defining admission criteria for rehabilitation hospitals.
   b. Predicting length of stay and volumes with clinical teams.
4. How to optimize funding and benchmarking:
   a. Ensuring data accuracy and quality.
   b. Using comparative data with peer groups.
   c. Collecting data across the continuum of care.

BACKGROUND

Ontario Case Costing Initiative

"In the early 1990s, the Ministry of Health and Long Term Care (MOHLTC) began considering moving to a rates and volume reimbursement system for hospitals" (Murray et al, 2005, p 6). The Ontario Case Costing Project (OCCP) was initi-ated in 1992 to develop case weights for Ontario hospitals. The OCCP was renamed the Ontario Case Costing Initiative (OCCI) in April 2000 to collect case costing data and develop hospital funding methodologies. Ontario has adopted an approach known as "micro costing or bottom-up" (Murray et al., 2005, p 6). "In this method individual patient activities and resources associated with each activity are added together to arrive at the total" (Murray et al., 2005, p 6).

The Ontario Case Distribution Methodology (OCDM) is primarily based on the Ontario Healthcare Reporting Standards (OHRS), which is the mandatory reporting framework for the financial and statistical information. The Ontario Case Costing Methodology is based on activity-based accounting, and provides instruction on how to take hospital costs by department and assign them to individual patients to obtain a case-specific total cost" (Murray et al, 2005, p 7). According to Sutherland (2011), "activity-based funding (ABF) is associated with higher volumes of hospital care, shorter lengths of stay and has not been linked to poorer quality of care" (p. 2). As per Canadian Institute for Health Information, Institute of Health Economics and Canadian Health Services Research Foundation (2011), "ABF model encourages providers to treat more people, they may also result in a reduction in the number of services a person receives if the model used isn't sufficiently sensitive to issues of severity" (p. 5).

Case Mix System in Inpatient Rehabilitation

In fall of 2002, Ontario MOHLTC mandated the collection of National Rehabilitation Reporting System (NRS) in all designated adult inpatient rehabilitation beds. The minimum dataset and reporting system was developed and is maintained by the Canadian Institute for Health Information (CIHI). Contained within the minimum dataset is the Functional Independence Measure (FIM™)[1], which is the property of the Uniform Data System for Medical Rehabilitation, a division of UB Foundation Activities, Inc. (1997). FIM™ is a standardized 18 item tool to assess patients' motor and cognitive function. The higher the scores, the more independent the patients are, and the lower the scores, the more dependent the patients are. In 2004, the Ontario Joint Policy and Planning Committee (JPPC) was struck with the mandate to evaluate FIM™-based groupers and to develop cost weights reflective of Ontario inpatient rehabilitation costs (Sutherland & Walker, 2006, p 3).

When calculating cost for services and resource utilization, case mix classification systems, such as Diagnosis Related Groups (DRG), has been widely used in acute care settings. However, classification systems based on diagnosis does not describe the severity of the patients or resource utilization. In fact, the literature does not support classification systems based solely on diagnosis for inpatient rehabilitation (Sutherland & Walker, 2006, p 4). At the highest level, patients are assigned to a unique Rehabilitation Group (RC), which are collections of clinically similar patients (JPPC, 2006, p iv). Assignment to an RG was based on Rehabilitation Client Group code in the NRS data set. The Rehabilitation Patient Group (RPG) is a new case mix classification system, which groups patients that are clinically similar based on admission FIM™ motor and cognitive scores, and/or age (Sutherland & Walker, 2006, p 13). Generally, the higher RPGs reflect higher motor and/or cognitive function. Each RPG is associated with a specific diagnosis and severity, thereby it is assumed patients within a RPG usually receive similar treatments and have similar resource utilization and costs. CIHI (2012) created 21 RGs with 83 RPGs which patients could be assigned for assessing resource utilization and costs (p. 1).

DATA COLLECTION SYSTEMS

Ontario Healthcare Reporting Standard (OHRS) Data

The Ontario Healthcare Reporting Standard (OHRS) provides the framework to standardize the reporting of information to hospital administrators, policy-makers and researchers. Hospitals must follow the OHRS User Guide for coding to ensure consistency in accounting procedures. With OCCI, some rehabilitation hospitals volunteered to participate and submitted data to the MOHLTC. Hospitals have to capture the appropriate resources utilization, service intensity and all expenses related to patients' activities. For example, activities by nursing and allied health are captured from workload data, diagnostic imaging, and lab services are captured, as well as medical drugs expenditures. In rehabilitation, the data usually flows from the front line data entry to a data analysis decision support tool, with feeder data flow from finance to generate reports.

Adult Inpatient Rehabilitation Minimum Data

The Adult Inpatient Rehabilitation Minimum Data Set provides valuable health indicators to hospital administrators, policy-makers, and researchers. Hospitals must follow the NRS Rehabilitation Minimum Date Set Manual when coding socio-demographics, health characteristics, FIM™, and self-reported pain and health status. Important indicators can be generated from NRS data. Some examples of indicators include admission wait time, RPG case mix, Length Of Stay (LOS), active rehab LOS, number of clients discharged home compared to clients discharged, FIM™ score change, post-discharge living arrangement, and reasons waiting for discharge. These indicators were only made available by individual hospitals. In July 2009, CIHI introduced NRS eReports system, in which individual hospitals can search for the indicators most relevant and make comparisons with other hospitals across Canada.

"SHRUB" FRAMEWORK

Rehabilitation Cost Weight Based on Length of Stay Trim Point for Each RPG

The Ontario Joint Policy and Planning Committee (2006) as reported by Sutherland & Walker developed the RPG Case Mix Classification Methodology and Weighting System for Adult Inpatient Rehabilitation and recommended that LOS trim points be established (p. 13). Rehabilitation Cost Weight and LOS trim points are established to produce RPG resource utilization reports to determine hospitals' funding allocation. These reports summarize clinical and resource characteristics of patients' episodes based on facilities, which are useful for hospital administrators and management teams (CIHI, 2011, p 2).

There are three types of rehabilitation episodes which are: 1) Short-Stay, 2) Typical-Stay and 2) Long-Stay, quoted by CIHI (2011) "Case Mix RPG Grouping Methodology and Rehabilitation Cost Weight Information Sheet" (p.2). Depending on the type of episode, a different weighting method is applied. For a Typical-Stay, the Rehabilitation Cost Weight is used and for a Short-Stay, the Short-Stay Per Diem Rehabilitation Cost Weight is used. For a Long-Stay, the Rehabilitation Cost Weight and Long-Stay Per Diem Rehabilitation Cost Weight are applied.

Clinical Implications for Rehabilitation Hospitals

The "Shrub" Framework shows the "Input Variables for Determining Resource Utilization": The inputs are "Soil," "Water," and "Sun." The "Soil" is the foundation essential for case costing data collected from the Ontario Healthcare Reporting Standards. The input of the "Water" are variable as CIHI sets the LOS trim points for each RPG. The input of the "Sun" is also variable as the MOHLTC sets the Rehabilitation Cost Weight (RCW) for each RPG and may adjust the Base rate for each hospital annually (see Figure 1).

The "Roots" determine the RPG from NRS data. There are three types of rehabilitation episodes determined by RPG LOS trim points, which are described with clinical implications for hospitals: 1) Short-Stay Episode, 2) Typical-Stay Episode, and 3) Long-Stay Episode. Based on the LOS of a particular episode, the cost weight is then multiplied by a Base rate, which is a dollar amount per unit of cost weight, resulting in a dollar value for the price to be paid for the episode.

Short Stay Episode patients will receive the same RCW regardless of RPG. This will reduce the RCW and subsequently reduce funding, as these patients potentially are not ready for rehabilitation or signs-out against medical advice. Clinically, patients should be assessed for appropriateness to participate in rehabilitation phase in the acute care. Patients who are not medically stable to participate in rehabilitation or experience post-operative complications are readmitted to acute care are considered Short-Stay. For example, patients experiencing post-operative complications such as anesthetic effects (nausea or delirium) or are medically unstable (low hemoglobin or cardiac concerns) could be admitted to rehabilitation too early even though they follow the recommended

Figure 1. "Shrub" framework: input variables for determining resource utilization. Developed by G. Liu (2012).

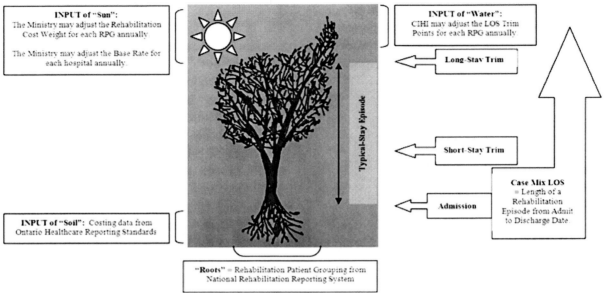

clinical pathway. Furthermore, patients who signs-out against medical advice may not have required rehabilitation or did not understood the purpose of rehabilitation. These scenarios will cause the hospital to receive less funding and essentially taking up beds for other more appropriate rehabilitation patients. It is recommended that the hospital administrators review the admission criteria and accept patients who are ready for rehabilitation.

Typical Stay Episode patients staying less than the established long stay trim point LOS will receive funding based on RPG. Clinically, most patients requiring rehabilitation will stay until the discharge date is set as per recommended by the rehabilitation team. In some cases, such as in Total Joint Replacement, there is a standardized clinical pathways for admission and discharge to community, which is highly cost-effective approach to contain costs without adverse consequence for patients (Brunenberg, van Styn, Sluimer, Bekebrede, Bulstra, & Joore, 2005, p 1). It is suggested that patients should be assessed for estimated LOS in rehabilitation phase while still in the acute care. Patients with pre-existing chronic health conditions (i.e. co-morbidities) could potentially be readmitted to acute care (i.e. service interruption) causing delay in their rehabilitation and affecting their LOS. In addition, patients with lack of social support (i.e. live alone) have difficulties returning to the community should have access to a Social Worker to assist in discharge planning. Furthermore, some of the RPGs do consider age, it is hypothesized patients who are older will tend to have a greater LOS, due to potentially lower pre-existing functioning. Therefore, hospital administrators should monitor and establish guidelines for typical stay patients based on the RPG LOS and make comparison with peer hospitals.

Long Stay Episode patients on the other hand will continue to receive funding; however, these patients should be evaluated to determine the cause of long stay episodes. Patients who will likely stay longer should be assessed early in the rehabilitation in order to facilitate their discharge to home or make arrangements for home care. If patients staying beyond the trim point cannot be discharged to home, the rehabilitation team should consider these patients as alternate level of care and/or make arrangements for admittance to other care facilities as deemed appropriate. Currently, the RPG does not include discharge FIM™, however, tracking the discharge FIM™ would be valuable, particularly if there is no functional gains extending the LOS beyond the trim point. The value of discharging these patients to alternate level of care setting is to free up inpatient rehabilitation beds for patients who require high-intensity rehabilitation. This ensures that the right rehabilitation patient is in the right bed at the right time.

The "Shrub" framework presented explains how the RPG case mix methodology is formulated, based on the "Roots" (for a specific RPG), "Soil" (case costing data from the Ontario Healthcare Reporting Standards), "Water" (LOS trim points for each RPG), and "Sun" (RCW set by the MOHLTC). As inputs of the soil, water and sun may be variable, the resulting "shrub" can grow larger or become stagnant depending on the right circumstances. The size of the "shrub" is important for calculating cost weight for a particular RPG, depending on the number of episodes that are short stay, typical stay and long stay.

As demonstrated in the "Long Stay Trim Point Illustration," the shrubs illustrates one particular RPG for comparison. The first scenario shows a shrub with extra long strands depicting variable length of stay greater than Long Stay Trim Point resulting in many Long Stay Episodes. The second scenario depicts length of stay less than Long Stay Trim Point resulting in Typical Stay Episodes. These 2 scenarios would produce different cost weight and impact on the number of weighted cases. The weighted cases will increase for long stay episode patients compared to typical stay episode patients according to the RPG. Short stay episode patients will significantly reduce the overall weighted cases (see Figure 2).

The challenge for hospitals is to ensure costs and resource utilization are in alignment with the care received for different episodes within the

same RPG or "shrub." Furthermore, hospitals need to evaluate length of stay and benchmark against peers for similar case mix of patients. Using eReports data for RPG case mix groups and LOS, hospitals can compare each RPG to LOS and benchmark against peer groups. As hospitals will be funded based on RPG and LOS; therefore, hospitals should establish target LOS for each RPG with the clinical teams who make decisions on admissions to rehab and discharge.

CLINICAL DECISION-MAKING TOOL

Defining Admission Criteria for Rehabilitation Hospitals

Due to an increased number of patients requiring rehabilitation and given that the number of rehabilitation beds have not increased, there are greater demands on inpatient rehabilitation beds. Hospitals must ensure the most appropriate rehabilitation patients are admitted to inpatient rehabilitation. Patients who do not require inpatient rehabilitation can be discharged home directly from acute care, with appropriate outpatient and/or home care services. The more complex patients may not be appropriate for inpatient rehabilitation should be referred to complex continuing care, long-term care, and/or alternate level of care temporarily (until they can participate in inpatient rehabilitation) (see Figure 3).

This clinical decision-making tool assessment can be done in acute care to direct patients to the most appropriate setting. In order to ensure consistency in clinical decision-making, the criteria is that clinicians should be certified to be a "NRS Assessor" by CIHI by a "NRS Trainer" in order to determine the cognitive and motor scores based on the FIM™. The FIM™ has 18 items, including Motor and Cognitive Function Scores, which the Assessor would score the patient depending on the level of independence. Functional status can be ranked using motor score and cognitive score. Utilizing this standardized system ranking patients

Figure 2. Long stay trim point illustration for a particular rehabilitation patient grouping. Developed by G. Liu (2012).

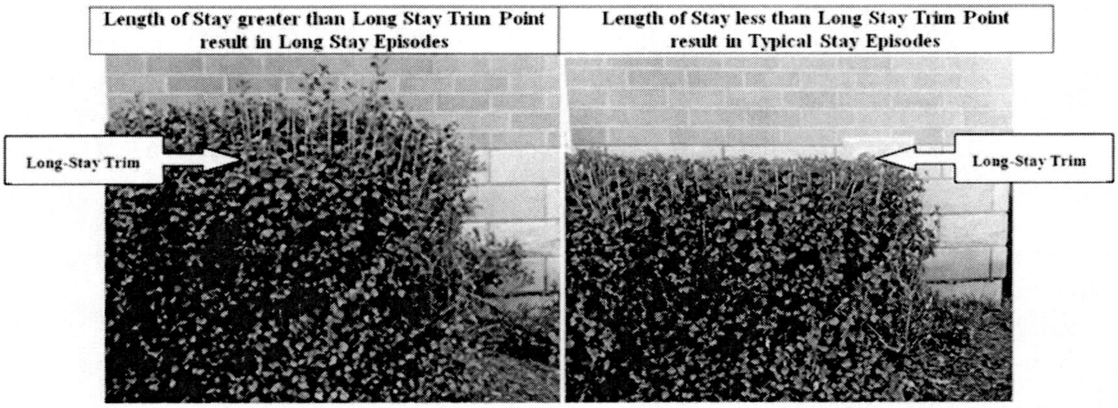

into high, moderate and low functional status, the NRS Assessor follows the algorithm and determines the patients' discharge designation (including home with outpatient services, home with home care, inpatient rehabilitation, or long term care facility temporary and then permanent). Patients who are high functioning, yet lack support (i.e. lives alone or unable to attend outpatients) will require home care.

With this clinical decision-making tool, only the most appropriate patients are admitted to inpatient rehabilitation. During the inpatient rehabilitation stay, if patients improve, they could be discharged home with home care to continue their rehabilitation. However, if patients are not improving in the inpatient rehabilitation within 2-4 weeks, they should be referred to long-term care or alternate level of care temporary. At the long-term care or alternative level of care, if there are no improvements within 3 months, patients should be referred to long-term care facility or complex continuing care permanently.

This algorithm is largely simplified for illustrative purposes and would require clinical decision-making input depending on the population and patients' specific condition (i.e. acuity), social living situation, health characteristics and goals for

rehabilitation. Furthermore, there are opportunities to standardize the care for commonly treated conditions (i.e. define the admission criteria, set targets for LOS, and set discharge criteria) to optimize resource utilization and funding. It would be in the hospitals' best interest to collaborate with acute care, and ambulatory care/home care to ensure smooth transition, create clinical decision-making tools for various case mix, and evaluate clinical outcomes across the continuum of care.

Predicting Length of Stay and Volumes with Clinical Teams

With the new case costing and case mix-funding model, the hospital administrators must involve the clinical teams, as they are the ones who predict LOS of patients. To optimize the funding, clinical staff and physicians will need to understand the new RPG case mix-funding model. Since the RPG case mix grouping is dependent upon LOS, clinical teams should review each RPG case mix and set target LOS based on previous data. The clinical team should be aware of case costing, and may have suggestions to cut costs down where possible along the continuum of activities. If the goal is to optimize the usage of rehabilitation beds, volumes

Figure 3. Clinical decision-making tool: admission criteria algorithm for rehabilitation. Developed by G. Liu (2012).

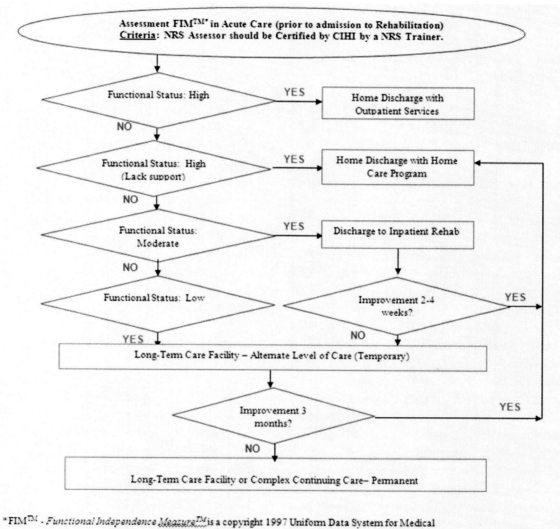

*FIM™ - Functional Independence Measure™ is a copyright 1997 Uniform Data System for Medical Rehabilitation, a division of UB Foundation Activities, Inc.

may increase along with workload, impacting on the clinical teams. Case mix can be beneficial as it creates transparency and clinical teams can share best practices on quality, innovation and cost management (CIHI, IHE & CHSRF, 2011, p. 12).

Involvement of clinicians is critical in affect the case mix LOS. For example, Johnson, Richards, Pink and Campbell (1998, p 129) commented that one hospital was able to make dramatic re-

ductions in its average LOS for one stroke case mix grouping. It will be important to evaluate the appropriate case mix of patient conditions who benefit most from rehabilitation. For example, the GTA Rehab Network used data from CIHI's Discharge Abstract Database and NRS Database to assess the flow of severe stroke patients and compare it with stroke best practices guidelines. It was discovered the earlier admission to rehabilitation improves clinical outcomes, reduces LOS and Alternate Level of Care days (CIHI, 2012, p 6). Further research into best practices around benchmarking, evaluation, administrative practices and measurement will support quality and productivity improvements (CIHI, IHE, & CHSRF, 2011, p. 12).

OPTIMIZE FUNDING AND BENCHMARKING

Ensuring Data Accuracy and Quality

Case costing and case mix data must be submitted accurately, particularly if funding aligned with current expenditures and resource utilization. Furthermore, given this funding approach, "it is crucial that the MOHLTC has valid and reliable data on which to formulate costs for services" (Murray et al, 2005, p 1). Similarly, hospitals themselves will need to better understand and manage their case costs and ensure that patient care provided is evidence-based. Therefore, hospitals have to involve several departments, including finance, decision-support, and clinical teams to determine treatment intensity and resource utilization to achieve the best outcomes for each RPG case mix grouping.

Data quality in coding is particularly important, when classifying patient into Rehabilitation Client Groups, and determining RPGs. CIHI provides many educational workshops to define and promote guidelines and standards for data elements submitted to the NRS. Hospitals can also ensure data quality by doing internal audits or validation. For example, the days waiting for admission is an important wait times indicator for admission into rehabilitation. If this is data element is missing, the number of days waiting for admission cannot be calculated, limiting the ability to use NRS data for meaningful analysis of rehabilitation admission wait times indicator (CIHI, 2012, p 3). More accurate reporting by hospitals will in turn improve the case mix methodology.

Efforts aimed at assisting clinicians to increase their understanding of the case mix methodology may lead to improvements in data quality. It is suggested by Johnson, Richards, Pink and Campbell (1998, p 127) that users can influence the enhancement of existing tools. In specific clinical areas, there are improvements that could be made in coding to improve data quality. For example, trauma patients could not be assigned to the appropriate clinical category and users were concerned that the methodologies were weak (Johnson, Richards, Pink & Campbell, 1998, p 128). In specialty programs, such as burns, there are variation in patients' LOS because patients require greater expertise and care by specialized clinical professionals. Clinical teams must be involved in the implications of case mix tools applications and relate them to their roles and responsibilities (Johnson, Richards, Pink & Campbell, 1998, p 128).

Using Comparative Data with Peer Groups

With this newly established system using RPG Case Mix Classification methodology and weighting system, hospital administrators, policy-makers, and researchers will have to be vigilant and even reassess the funding formula annually. As of September 1, 2011, record-level files containing data from NRS that has been grouped to RPGs are available via eNRS. These files contain facilities own data only and include a subset of NRS data elements related to the RPG case-mix and cost weight methodologies (CIHI, 2011, p 1). CIHI is supporting the Ministry's new Health Based Allocation Model funding methodology under the Health Systems Funding Strategy (CIHI, 2011, p 1). In addition, since RCWs and LOS trim points are being adjusted annually, the funding calculations will need to be adjusted.

It is in the best interest to predict several scenarios to ensure funding is appropriately adjusted considering the case mix of patients admitted and volumes. Furthermore, benchmarking with peer groups will be needed continuously to evaluate the LOS trim point and hospitals should then set their own targets for LOS trim point for various RPGs. Due to the new RPG case mix methodology, there will be constant monitoring, adjustments and updating. Hospital administrators should look at peer group data from E-Reports, who treat similar RPGs and compare their LOS. Using the "Clinical Decision-Making Tool", clinical pathways can be established based on RPGs case mix throughout the continuum of care.

Collecting Data across the Continuum of Care

From an inpatient rehabilitation perspective, there are challenges and limitations in collecting and calculating all direct and indirect cost related to patients' full episode of care. For example, it is challenging to gather data from the acute care hospital on preoperative (i.e. orthopedic consultation fee) and admission care in acute care hospital (i.e. surgical fees). In rehabilitation, it is possible to collect data from feeder departments (Nursing, Allied Health, Diagnostic Imaging, Laboratory, Pharmacy, etc.) with use of data flow mapping and integration to merge the data sources, using appropriate hardware and software system, to retrieve the case costing data and generate reports.

With the current method of data collection, there are different systems utilized as patients flow from inpatient acute care, to inpatient rehabilitation and to outpatient services or home care. Even in some instances, the outpatient data is not captured, as it is not mandatory to collect data in outpatient settings. There needs to be a consistent way of collecting the same set of data through the continuum of care, from inpatient acute care, to inpatient rehabilitation and to outpatient or home care. With several acute care and rehabilitation hospitals being merged as one entity, there will be opportunities to collaborate and improve data collection to capture the full episode of care from acute care to rehabilitation.

SOLUTIONS AND RECOMMENDATIONS

Better Data Equals Better Funding and Benchmarking in Hospitals

With case costing and case mix data, there is potential to improve hospital performance and efficiency with collaboration of clinicians, administrators and decision-support (Johnson, Richards, Pink & Campbell, 1998, p 128). To ensure robust data collection process from all feeder areas requires commitment from all areas of the organization. Regular data quality review includes representatives from key areas, namely Nursing, Laboratory, Pharmacy, Diagnostic Imaging, Allied Health, Health Records and Information Technology. A number of factors affect the use of case costing data for internal decision including CEO and senior management commitment, investment in decision support, continuing education for staff on case costs and establishment of the value of costing data with front line, middle managers and clinicians (Murray, Hannam, & Wong, 2004, p 22). Furthermore, the collection of robust case costing data from all areas promotes a culture of shared evidence-based decision-making.

There is a lack of research on case costing using RPG Case Mix Classification methodology and weighting system. The Ontario JPPC developed the RPG Case Mix Classification methodology and Weighting System for Adult Inpatient Rehabilitation. However, there are areas for improvement such as identifying co-morbid conditions and service interruptions, which have significant impact on variation in LOS (Sutherland & Walker, 2006, p 3). There will be ongoing changes with this new methodology.

CIHI has demonstrated that it is committed to continually improve its methodologies to better meet the needs of the users of case mix tools and to better understand reflecting current patterns of practice in health care (Johnson, Richards, Pink & Campbell, 1998, p 128).

The appropriate cost data and case mix data are essential for analysis used in program planning, resource allocation and utilization management. It is possible to collect data in one organization to compare costs and case mix. However, the challenge is that there is variation and lack of consistently in data collection amongst all the external stakeholders in acute care, rehabilitation, outpatients and/or home care. Several rehabilitation hospitals are starting to track outpatient data. Therefore, it is difficult to track patient costs from acute care, to rehabilitation, to outpatients and/or home care. Ideally, patients who are discharged directly home from acute care should be analyzed for resource utilization and outcomes, compared to similar patients who were admitted to inpatient rehabilitation services. Without consistent data across the continuum of care, it is difficult to determine the best resource utilization in producing the best outcomes.

Key Success Factors for Better Funding and Benchmarking in Hospitals

1. **Educate Stakeholders on the New Funding Model:** CIHI (2010) suggested "user education is required regarding the new system" (p 3). Use "Shrub" Framework describing the input variables for determining resource utilization to educate hospital administrators and clinicians on the new RPG case mix methodology and to increase awareness of the clinical implications of the new funding model for inpatient rehabilitation, specifically Short-Stay, Typical-Stay, and Long-Stay Episodes.

2. **Collaborate with Acute Care Partners:** Hospitals in acute care, rehabilitation, and ambulatory care/home care should collaborate to ensure smooth referral process and access to services. Use "Clinical Decision-Making Tool" to enhance the utilization of

inpatient rehabilitation beds for the most appropriate patients. This tool should be completed by the referring facility by a NRS Assessor to ensure the right patient is referred to the right bed and/or home care.

3. **Develop Clinical Pathways Based on RPGs Case Mix:** CIHI (2010) suggested that "case mix groups must be clinically meaningful to review the pathways of care and staffing to ensure cost efficiency" (p 5). Hospitals could establish target LOS for each RPG with the clinical teams who make decisions on discharge (i.e. define the admission criteria and set targets for LOS).

4. **Involvement of Clinical Teams:** With case costing, there are opportunities to improve resource utilization for specific patient groups or compare variations in resource use to increase overall quality (MOHLTC, 2006, p 3). The clinical team should be aware of case costing, and may have suggestions to cut costs down where possible along the continuum of activities. Clinical teams can also provide input on resource utilization and treatment intensity to achieve the best outcomes for each RPG case mix.

5. **Involvement of Finance and Decision Support:** Case costing provides answers to important management and planning questions that cannot traditionally be answered with departmental management and financial information alone (MOHLTC, 2006, p 3). In answering the question, "What are the cost impacts of admitting patients with a particular case mix?", involvement of finance and decision-support, along with clinical teams is critical to determine funding and resource utilization for each RPG case mix.

6. **Benchmarking with Peers:** CIHI (2010) has made the case mix group transparent to hospital administrators (p 5). The common questions raised by administrators are "How do we compare to our peers for case costs

similar patients?" and "Why are there differences in costs (due to different treatments or therapy intensity)?" Hospitals should use eReports data for making comparisons for each RPG to LOS and volumes of patients to admit and benchmark against peer groups.

7. **Improve Data Accuracy and Quality in Coding:** Data quality in coding is important, when classifying patient into Rehabilitation Client Groups, and determining RPGs. More accurate reporting by hospitals following CIHI guidelines and standards for data elements will in turn improve the case mix methodology. With the implementation of activity-based funding, CIHI (2010) indicated "it is imperative that coding practice be monitored to guard against attempts by hospitals to increase their payment revenue through coding practices that aggrandize their patient episode" (p 4).

8. **Develop Consistency in Data Collection Across the Continuum of Care:** Develop consistency in data collection and/or similar systems to track the flow of patients throughout the continuum of care. By improving data collection capturing the full episode of care, it is possible to manage costs and evaluate clinical outcomes across the continuum of care. Due to changes in the funding to activity-based, there could be potential changes in the flow of patients in the entire system. CIHI (2010) suggested that "it is critical to assess changes across hospitals and among the different health sectors to determine if the observed changes are desirable in terms of quality of care or allocation of health care resources" (p 6).

9. **Reassess the Funding Formula Annually:** The jurisdiction will make refinements to ensure alignment with its reimbursement system or its health policy goals (CIHI, 2010, p 5). The weighted cases will increase

for long stay episode patients compared to typical stay episode patients according to the RPG. In calculating cost weights, it requires accuracy and fine-tuning (CIHI, 2010, p 5). Since RCWs and LOS trim points are adjusted annually, hospital administrators will have to evaluate the LOS and volumes for each case mix each year.

10. **Further Research for Developing the RPG Case Mix Methodology:** There are advantages and disadvantages and favourable and unfavourable changes for activity-based funding in hospitals. Research on case costs and use of the RPG case mix is needed to support the new funding model. CIHI suggested that "for jurisdictions undertaking implementation of activity-based funding, there may be benefits to collaborate with one another and with CIHI in attaining a national case mix system" (CIHI, 2010, p 6).

FUTURE RESEARCH DIRECTIONS

In terms of implications for practice and policy, it is necessary to focus not only on clinical outcomes, but consider case costing throughout the entire system. It was suggested by DeJong, Tian, Smout, Horn, Putman, Hsieh, Gassawy, and Smith (2009, p 1) in the US, that clinicians and policy makers need to consider the entire post acute pathway and assess costs associated with each. In a study by Stineman, Escarce, Tassoni, Goin, Granger, and Williams (1998, p 1) in the US, they concluded that medical costs, rather than LOS may be more appropriate measure the effect of coexisting medical illness on resource use. Therefore, it will be important to collect cost data, however, there are challenges to collect direct patient costs and workload from acute care hospitals, due to various cost systems used or it could be a different referral hospital site.

With linkages in computer systems, acute care and rehabilitation hospitals can collect data from all feeder areas, including frontline, finance, system support, and decision support. As data entry from all the feeder departments are seamlessly interface between each area and the main costing system, the data can be used on an ongoing basis by CEO and senior management for decision making. However, there must be regular data quality reviews to ensure validity of data at hand. For research, the data collected could be systematically transferred to other software for further statistical analysis. As well, clinical and administrative data could be incorporated with case costing data for making comparative analysis, such as benchmarking with peer facilities, or creating management reports for funding purposes.

CONCLUSION

The book addresses the potential of health informatics to provide a platform that support health management and policy decisions. Specifically, this chapter provides insight showing how existing cost data and case mix information collected can be used and translated into health decision-making, service delivery, and cost management for hospitals. Given the Ministry's new Health Based Allocation Model funding methodology, hospitals will be reimbursed for the care they give to their various patient populations based on expected case costs and volumes of services given, which will impact on hospitals' operational budget and cost management. It is crucial that hospitals understand their case mix of patients and manage their case costs. A "Shrub" framework and clinical decision-making tool is provided in this chapter to understand case cost and case mix to enable hospital administrators, policy makers, and researchers to analyze and optimize funding and benchmarking with peers in a rehabilitation setting.

The "Shrub" framework presented in this chapter explains how the RPG case mix methodology is formulated, based on the "Roots" (for a specific RPG), "Soil" (case costing data from the Ontario Healthcare Reporting Standards), "Water" (=LOS trim points for each RPG), and "Sun" (RCW set by the MOHLTC). The "Clinical Decision-Making Tool" presented facilitates the acceptance of most appropriate patients to inpatient rehabilitation, due to increasing demands on inpatient rehabilitation beds. Patients with who do not fit into the short duration rehabilitation should be considered for alternate level of care in a long-term care facility. Patients who are not ready for rehabilitation should not be admitted pre-maturely to rehabilitation. Furthermore, patients who do not wish to participate in inpatient rehabilitation should be referred to outpatient services and/or home care. This "Clinical Decision-Making Tool" should be done acute care to ensure the right patients are admitted to right bed at the right time.

Accuracy and quality of data is critical for evidence-based decision-making and for appropriate funding of hospital services. Furthermore, better data equals better funding and benchmarking in hospitals. Since there are only scant research on case costing data and application of the case mix methodology on funding, 10 key success factors for better funding and benchmarking in hospitals are presented.

REFERENCES

Brunenberg, D. E., van Styn, M. J., Sluimer, J. C., Bekebrede, L. L., Bulstra, S. K., & Joore, M. A. (2005). Joint recovery programme versus usual care: An economic evaluation of a clinical pathway for joint replacement surgery. *Medical Care, 43*(10), 1018–1026. doi:10.1097/01. mlr.0000178266.75744.35 PMID:16166871.

Canadian Institute for Health Information. (2010). *Choice of a case mix system for use in acute care activity-based funding options and considerations* (Discussion Paper: Activity-Based Funding Unit). Ottawa, Canada: Canadian Institute for Health Information.

Canadian Institute for Health Information. (2011a). *Funding models to support quality and sustainability: A pan Canadian dialogue summary report*. Ottawa, Canada: Canadian Institute for Health Information, Institute of Health Economics, & Canadian Health Services Research Foundation.

Canadian Institute for Health Information. (2011b). *Case mix RPG grouping methodology and rehabilitation cost weights information sheet*. Ottawa, Canada: Canadian Institute of Health Information.

Canadian Institute for Health Information Update. (2012). *National rehabilitation reporting system*. Ottawa, Canada: Canadian Institute for Health Information Update.

DeJong, G., Tian, W., Smout, R., Horn, S., Putman, K., & Hsieh, C. et al. (2009). Long-term outcomes of joint replacement rehabilitation patients discharged from skilled nursing and inpatient rehabilitation facilities. *Archives of Physical Medicine and Rehabilitation, 90*. PMID:19651264.

Johnson, L. M., Richards, J., Pink, G. H., & Campbell, L. (1998). *Case mix tools for decision making in healthcare*. Ottawa, Canada: Canadian Institute for Health Information.

MOHLTC. (2006). *Ontario guide to case costing*. MOHLTC.

Murray, G., Hannam, R., & Wong, J. (2004). *Case costing in Ontario hospitals: What makes for success*. Toronto, Canada: The Change Foundation.

Ontario Joint Policy and Planning Committee. (2006). *Evaluation and selection of a group and weighting methodology for adult inpatient rehabilitation care*. Reference Document RD10-10.

Stineman, M. G., Escarce, J. J., Tassoni, C. J., Goin, J. E., Granger, C. V., & Williams, S. V. (1998). Diagnostic coding and medical rehabilitation length of stay: Their relationship. *Archives of Physical Medicine and Rehabilitation, 79*. PMID:9523773.

Sutherland, J. (2011). *Hospital payment mechanisms: An overview and options for Canada*. Ottawa, Canada: Canadian Health Services Research Foundation Series of Reports on Cost Drivers and Health System Efficiency.

Sutherland, J., & Walker, J. (2006). *Technical report: Development of the rehabilitation patient group (RPG) case mix classification methodology and weighting system for adult inpatient rehabilitation*. Toronto, Canada: Ontario Joint Policy and Planning Committee.

ADDITIONAL READING

Baker, H. (2002). *RD9-6 evaluation and selection of a classification/assessment took for rehabilitation care in Ontario*. JPPC Reference Article.

Benoit, D., Shea, W., & Mitchell, S. (2000). Developing cost weights with limited costs data – Experiences using canadian cost data. *Casemix Quarterly, 2*(3), 88–96.

Boltz, C. K., Sutherland, J., & Lawrenson, J. (2006). Cost weight compression: Impact of cost data precision and completeness. *Health Care Financing Review*, 27(3), 111–122. PMID:17290652.

Carter, G.M., & Totten, M. (2005). *Preliminary analysis for refinement of the tier comorbidities in the inpatient rehabilitation facility prospective payment system*. RAND Technical Report.

Dukett, S. J. (2008). Design of price incentives for adjunct policy goals in formula funding for hospitals and health services. *BMC Health Services Research*, 8(72).

Ellis, R. P., & Vidal-Fernandez, M. (2007). Activity-based payments and reforms of the English hospital payment system. *Health Economics, Policy, and Law*, 2(4), 435–444. doi:10.1017/S1744133107004276 PMID:18634644.

Farrar, S., Yi, D., & Sutton, M. et al. (2009). Has payment by results affected the way that English hospitals provide care? Difference-in-differences analysis. *British Medical Journal*, 339(7790), 554–556. PMID:19713233.

Forgione, D. A., Vermeer, T. E., & Surysekar, K. et al. (2004). The impact of DRGs in health care payment systems on quality of health care in OECD countries. *Journal of Health Care Finance*, 31(1), 41–54. PMID:15816228.

Goldfield, N. (2010). The evolution of diagnosis-related groups (DRGs), from its beginnings in case-mix and resource use theory, to its implementation for payment and now for its resource allocation in the acute hospital sector current utilization for quality within and outside the hospital. *Quality Management in Health Care*, 19(1), 3–16. PMID:20042929.

Jackson, T. (2001). Using computerized patient-level costing data for setting DRG weights: The Victorian (Australia) cost weight studies. *Health Policy (Amsterdam)*, 56(2), 149–163. doi:10.1016/S0168-8510(00)00148-2.

Kastberg, G., & Silverbo, S. (2007). Activity-based financing of health care – Experience from Sweden. *The International Journal of Health Planning and Management*, 22(1), 25–44. doi:10.1002/hpm.868 PMID:17385331.

Leister, J. E., & Stausberg, J. (2005). Comparison of cost accounting methods from different DRG systems and their effect on health care quality. *Health Policy (Amsterdam)*, 74(1), 46–55. doi:10.1016/j.healthpol.2004.12.001 PMID:16098411.

Ljunggren, B., & Sjoden, P. O. (2003). Patient-reported quality of life before, compared with after a DRG intervention. *International Journal for Quality in Health Care*, 15(5), 433–440. doi:10.1093/intqhc/mzg066 PMID:14527987.

Lowthian, P., Disler, P., Ma, S., Eagar, K., & Green, J., & de Graaff. (2000). The Australian national subacute and non-acute patient casemix classification (AN-SNAP), its application and value in a stroke rehabilitation programme. *Clinical Rehabilitation*, 14, 532–537. doi:10.1191/0269215500cr357oa PMID:11043880.

Marchildon, G.P. (2005). *Health systems in transition: Canada*. Copenhagen, Denmark: World Health Organization on behalf of the European Observatory on Health Systems and Policies.

McAllister, J. (2010, January/February). A better way of funding hospitals. *Canadian Healthcare Manager*, 17-21.

McNutt, R., Johnson, T. J., & Odwazny, R. et al. (2010). Changes in MSDRG assignment and hospital reimbursement as a result of centres for medicare & medicaid changes in payment for hospital-acquired conditions: Is it coding or quality? *Quality Management in Health Care, 19*(1), 17–24. PMID:20042930.

Mikkola, H., & Hakkinen, U. (2002). The effects of case-based pricing on length of stay for common surgical procedures. *Journal of Health Services Research & Policy, 7*(2), 90–97. doi:10.1258/1355819021927737 PMID:11934373.

Miller, H. (2009). From volume to value: Better was to pay for health care. *Health Affairs, 28*(5), 1418–1428. doi:10.1377/hlthaff.28.5.1418 PMID:19738259.

Or, Z. (2009). Activity based payment in France. *Euro Observer, 11*(4), 5–6.

Polverejan, E., Gardiner, J. C., Bradley, C. J., Holmes-Rovner, M., & Rovner, D. (2003). Estimating mean hospital cost as a function of length of stay and patient characteristics. *Health Economics, 12*, 935–947. doi:10.1002/hec.774 PMID:14601156.

Preya, C. (2004). Coding response to a case mix measurement system based on multiple diagnosis. *Health Services Research, 39*(4), 1027–1045. doi:10.1111/j.1475-6773.2004.00270.x PMID:15230940.

Relles, D.A., Ridgeway, G., Carter, G.M., & Beeuwkes Buntin, M. (2005). *Possible refinements to the construction of function-related groups for the inpatient rehabilitation facility prospective payment system.* RAND Technical Report.

Rosenberg, M. A., & Browne, M. J. (2001). The impact of the inpatient prospective payment system and diagnostic-related groups: A survey of the literature. *North American Actuarial Journal, 5*(4), 84–94. doi:10.1080/10920277.2001.10596020.

Scheller-Kreinsen, Geissler, A., & Busse, R. (2009). The ABC of DRGs. *Euro Observer, 11*(4), 1–5.

Siciliani, L. (2006). Selection of treatment under prospective payment system in the hospital sector. *Journal of Health Economics, 25*(3), 479–499. doi:10.1016/j.jhealeco.2005.09.007 PMID:16542741.

Silverman, E., & Skinner, J. (2004). Medicare upcoding and hospital ownership. *Journal of Health Economics, 23*(2), 369–389. doi:10.1016/j.jhealeco.2003.09.007 PMID:15019762.

Steinbusch, P. J., Oostenbrink, J. B., & Zuurbier, J. J. et al. (2007). The risk of upcoding in case-mix systems: A comparative study. *Health Policy (Amsterdam), 81*(23), 289–299. doi:10.1016/j.healthpol.2006.06.002.

Stineman, M. (2002). Prospective payment, prospective challenge. *Archives of Physical Medicine and Rehabilitation, 83*, 1802–1805. doi:10.1053/apmr.2002.36067 PMID:12474191.

Street, A., & Maynard, A. (2007). Activity based financing in England: The need for continual refinement of payment by results. *Health Economics, Policy, and Law, 2*(4), 419–427. doi:10.1017/S174413310700429X PMID:18634642.

Sutherland, J., & Preyra, C. (2006). A mixture model approach to updating payment weights with an application to ICD-10 implementation. *Health Care Management Science, 9,* 349–357. doi:10.1007/s10729-006-9999-7 PMID:17186770.

Sutherland, J. M., Benoit, D., & Gallant, V. et al. (2001). Analysis of the impact of using Canadian cost data as the sole source to develop Canadian cost weights. *Casemix Quarterly, 3*(3), 88–96.

KEY TERMS AND DEFINITIONS

Activity-Based Funding: Bottom-up approach to funding by defining the cost of activities required to provide a particular service.

ALC Days: Number of days assigned to alternate level of care (ALC) patient service during the patient's hospitalization.

Case Mix Funding: Patients' disease and complexity are taken to account based on resource intensity of the services provided.

Evidence-Based Practice: Practice based on the best available evidence from research.

FIM™: Functional Independence Measure™ is a copyright 1997 Uniform Data System for Medical Rehabilitation, a division of UB Foundation Activities, Inc.

Global Funding: A set amount given to a hospital for providing services, which is non specific to the patient population.

Long-Stay Episode: Case Mix LOS greater than the Long-Stay Trim (Trim$_{LS}$) for a given RPG.

Long-Stay Per Diem Rehabilitation Cost Weight (PDRCW$_{LS}$): Weight each patient day for NRS Long-Stay episodes. Note: Long-Stay PDRCW is different for each RPG.

NRS Assessor: Certified by CIHI to complete National Rehabilitation Reporting System FIM™.

NRS Trainer: Certified by CIHI to train NRS Assessors to complete FIM™.

Outliers: Cases with length of stay beyond the Trim LOS.

Rehabilitation Cost Weight (RCW): Average relative resource utilization for inpatients in a given RPG.

Rehabilitation Patient Groups (RPGs): RPGs are categorized by the Canadian Institute for Health Information which classifies patients into statistically and clinically homogeneous groups.

Short-Stay Episode: Case Mix LOS less than or equal to Short-Stay Trim (Trim$_{SS}$) for a given RPG.

Short-Stay Per Diem Rehabilitation Cost Weight (PDRCW$_{SS}$): Weight each patient day for NRS Short-Stay episodes. Note: Short-Stay PDRCW is the same for each RPG.

ENDNOTES

[1]   FIM™: *Functional Independence Measure™* is a copyright 1997 Uniform Data System for Medical Rehabilitation, a division of UB Foundation Activities, Inc.

Chapter 6
Implementation of Case Costing with Ontario Case Costing Initiative (OCCI)

Thuy Thi Thanh Hoang
York University, Canada

ABSTRACT

Over the past decade there has been a tremendous spread of computerized systems in hospitals. The advancement provided an opportunity for hospitals to gain access to computerized clinical, financial, and statistical data. Case costing information is the integration of clinical, financial, and statistical data to provide costing information at the patient level. Ontario Case Costing Initiative (OCCI) is an undertaking of the Ontario Ministry of Health and Long-Term Care (MOHLTC). This chapter focuses on the implementation of case costing using OCCI as a guideline for a hospital. It addresses the process of implementation by discussing proposals for planning, implementing, transitioning, and evaluation of case costing. The adoption of the OCCI allows health care professionals to analyze integrated health information and further enables evidence-based decision making.

INTRODUCTION

Over the past decade, there has been a tremendous spread of computerized systems in hospitals. The advancement provided an opportunity for hospitals to gain access to computerized clinical, financial, and statistical data.

Clinical data sources include all the medical data such as patient records, laboratory results and others which are needed for health service delivery to the patients (Mettler & Vimarlund,

2009). Administrative data sources contain all the business data, which includes statistical data, and financial data, which are required for running the organization (Mettler et al, 2009). The integration of clinical, financial and statistical data provides the opportunity for hospitals to present case costing information at the patient level. Ontario Case Costing Initiative (OCCI) is an undertaking of the Ontario Ministry of Health and Long-Term Care (MOHLTC). The primary goals of the OCCI are the collection of case costing data in support of improved management decision making and the development of hospital funding methodologies (OCCI, 2012).

DOI: 10.4018/978-1-4666-4321-5.ch006

As the health care system evolves, health care providers are finding themselves under increasing levels of financial risk for effective patient management, while at the same time being held more accountable for demonstrating their ability to provide and document appropriate cost-effective high quality care (Rosenstein, 1999). In order to accomplish this objective, providers have taken dramatic steps in collaborating informatic information applications to allocate patient specific case costing data to identify opportunities to improve patient outcomes. The successful implementation of the OCCI necessitates appropriate people with committed resources, information access, and technical support.

This chapter will focus on the implementation of case costing using OCCI as a guideline for a hospital. The objective of this chapter is to address the process of implementation by discussing proposals for planning, implementing, transitioning, and evaluation of case costing. The adoption of the OCCI will allow health care professionals to analyze integrated health information and will further enable evidence-based decision-making.

BACKGROUND

Case Costing and the Ontario Case Costing Initiative (OCCI)

According to Andru and Botchkarev (2008) a Case is an "instant of a disease that led to the individual's inpatient stay, which has been registered by the health service organization, reported to the Canadian Institute for Health Information (CIHI) Discharge Abstract Database (DAD), database and eventually has a corresponding record with all appropriate attributes in the Provincial Health Planning Database (PHPDB)." Case Cost is "expenditures (direct and indirect) incurred by the health service facility relating to the treatment of a specific patient-level case...the Case Cost

dollar value of a specific case is always an approximation of the 'real-life' hospital expenses" (Andru et al, 2008).

Overall, Case Costing is a "process of allocating expenditures of various hospital departments to each individual Case with an objective to determine the Case Cost. The process is performed according to the OCCI methodology" (Andru et al, 2008). Case costing data can play an important role in making cooperation a success. Gaining access to all available data and using sophisticated analytics to move towards case costing provides the means to achieve new levels of efficiency that can help them control costs and enhance revenue while improving the quality of care being delivered.

The OCCI was created for the collection of case costing data in support of improved management decision-making and the development of weights used in hospital funding methodologies as well as hospital funding methodologies (MOHLTC, 2012). The OCCI is collecting case cost data from hospitals for acute inpatient, day surgery ambulatory care cases and complex continuing care (MOHLTC, 2012). Participating hospitals have implemented a standardized case costing methodology developed by the OCCI and have participated in a series of Milestone Reviews conducted by the OCCI and MOHLTC to ensure the quality of the data.

The standardized case costing methodology contains two sources of data that make up the case cost record. The first is the cost data from the hospitals that has been produced, based on the OCCI costing methodology, and the second is the patient discharge abstract collected by CIHI (MOHLTC, 2012). The discharge abstract contains patient descriptive, demographic and clinical data having components such as patient classification systems (MOHLTC, 2012).

The goal of case costing is to allocate hospital costs to patient visits. The different category type of hospital costs are distributed into patient visits. Collaboratively, the cost, patient descriptive data and discharge abstract data files are merged based on the institution number, the patient's chart number, registration number, and the admission date. This information is then distributed by functional centre to patients (MOHLTC, 2012). Having cost information specific to patient level is the end product of case costing.

The integrated data abiding to the OCCI guidelines is sent by the hospital to the OCCI database. In the OCCI database, the cost data provides a resourceful analytical tool to examine costs from different perspectives. The hospital can access peer hospital data through the Costing Analysis Tool (CAT) on the Ontario Case Costing Initiative Website (www.occp.com). The integration of the various patient information databases provides an integrated view of both internal and external data. The process of implementing case costing is to help the hospital, the government, and the public understand the various costs of care for different types of patients, as well as the impact of new technology in health care.

Current Situation

The Ontario Case Costing Initiative is a way to collect case costing information from the hospitals. However, only 34% of the Ontario hospitals have been involved in the OCCI (OCCI, 2012). The low level of OCCI adoption alerts us that the majority of Ontario hospitals are in the process of planning the application case costing methodologies in their organization. With increasing pressure, the hospital leaders are looking for ways to perform cost-efficiency analyses to measure, report and sustain improvements in patient care as they respond to increased regulations, public scrutiny and demand for quality outcomes and data transparency (Fitzpatrick, 2006).

For example, requests for cost-efficiency analyses probes into areas such as hospital external and internal performance assessment, funding and budget planning and expense reimbursement

(Hawkins & Li, 2001). The issue is that hospital leaders have made substantial investments in departmental and transactional information systems that accomplish specific tasks, but they are not integrated (Fitzpatrick, 2006). It is necessary for hospitals to have access to case costing data reflecting patient specific level of information. The lack of integration of the data creates obstacles for hospital organizations when it comes to incorporating benchmarks to show internal and external comparisons of performance on a given set of indicators. It was recently announced that the Ontario MOHLTC is changing the way it funds hospitals. The Health Based Allocation Model (HBAM) is a new, methodology designed to promote the objectives of the Ontario health care system through funding policy. Once implemented, HBAM will support evidence-based distribution of funding that will move towards a "patient-based funding model" over time. As such, the application of health informatics applications such as the implementation of case costing will be important for the improvement of patient care in hospitals. The possibility to evaluate cost-efficiency is a powerful way to drive continued improvement and optimization in hospitals.

Advantages of Case Costing

Advantages are evident with the implementation of case costing. The benefits associated with case costing includes more consistent master data, significantly more efficient business through a complete view; improved efficiency in change management processes, and improved return on information technology investment (Kerr, 2008). The power of case costing data for improving the quality of care is boundless. It generates accurate analysis in which effective interventions can be deployed, outcomes of care enhanced and overall costs reduced (Fickenscher, 2005). Case costing data facilitates better informed decision making at all levels in the hospital.

Challenges of Case Costing

Like other initiatives, case costing also has a many implementation challenges. The technical and organizational challenges include: new technology, new way of doing business, focus on "learning", buy-in by front-line users regarding technical and procedural changes needed in feeder systems to meet the needs of the corporate system, developing hospital confidence in cost data, systems training, coordinating the collection, and entry of data where interfaces do not exist so that information is entered on a timely and accurate basis such as nursing workload and various episodic area data (MOHLTC, 2012).

IMPLEMENTATION OF CASE COSTING WITH THE ONTARIO CASE COSTING INITIATIVE

Purpose

The purpose of the implementation of OCCI at a hospital is to gather patient-specific cost and workload data that generates case costs by integrating financial, clinical, and statistical data. This data produce new views that will help answer operational management and planning questions, while still providing the necessary departmental management information that the hospital is accustomed to using.

Stakeholders

Case costing stakeholders include employees and unions, patients, board, management, medical staff, Ministry of Health and Long-Term Care and others. To ensure the success of the case cost project, it is critical to promote case costing to all stakeholders so that they will invest the extra effort both in the short and long term to produce the additional data needed (MOHLTC, 2012).

Stakeholders are the key to success of the OCCI implementation. The collaboration of the stakeholders is the driver for case costing.

Applications: External Assessment – STEEP

Social

In the absence of clear contextualized research on case costing, the culture of case costing is underdeveloped. Efforts need to be made to ensure that case costing is not perceived simply as an information technology project, rather it should be perceived as an enabler to many clinical and health benefits (OHA, 2009). The understanding of core benefits of case costing is important for it to become a priority on stakeholder's agenda. In addition, the possibility of unanticipated "shocks to the system" may influence the case costing process. These may include sudden down or up swings in the economy, epidemic disease, and political or social upheaval (O'Brien-Pallas, 2002).

Technological

The health care sector is aligning its information technology approach with organizational goals in response to environmental pressures. From this perspective, information technology is used for the integration of information to maximize the value of organization's information. The integration of information technology systems shows some promise of being able to improve the health care delivery system while containing costs (Wang, Wan, Burke, Bazzoli, & Lin, 2005).

Environmental

Environmental factors include managed care pressure, competition, and community demand (Wang et al, 2005). Environmental uncertainty, complexity, and diversity increases demand on the organizational information system to take appropriate actions (Wang et al, 2005). Subsequently, hospital organizations have to strategically align themselves to the meet the demands of the environment and competitors.

Economic

With economic instability, there is an increasing pressure on health care providers to control health care costs, the overriding emphasis of health care restructuring has been to reduce health care expenses (Rosenstein, 1999). The lack of funding in hospital is a barrier for case costing implementation projects. Economic environmental pressure is one of the main sources of influence on priorities for the hospital.

Political

Case cost data is important for hospital decision-making. Case costing can be used to perpetuate health care system reform efforts by providing support to hospital funding, research and policy development initiatives (MOHLTC, 2012). Case cost information may be used by the government to facilitate and allocate funding models within the province and between the Local Health Integration Networks (LHINs).

Roles and Responsibilities

For a successful implementation project, a strong team is required. Case costing implementation project include roles such as project manager, financial data analyst, financial case cost analyst, decision support analyst, data extract programmer and a super user.

A project manager is required to oversee the day-to-day activity of the project. The project manager is responsible for communication of project mandates, project organization, project planning process, ensure appropriate participation by all required users, perform audit and change control, communicate project progress, and ensure that project charges are appropriate (MOHLTC, 2012).

The financial data analyst and decision support analyst are responsible for data loading and reconciliation. The financial case costing analyst is responsible for cost model support, calculation and reconciliation. The data extract programmer will be responsible for the development and maintenance of data extracts. Lastly, the super user will aid in building and maintaining cost models, report generation, and others.

The case costing implementation project will affect most hospital departments. Ongoing data collection is required for a robust case costing data set. The Chief Executive Officer (CEO) of the hospital must be committed to the project through involvement in the implementation effort, assignment of resources, and commitment of necessary investments in information systems, and active participation in identifying executive information needs (MOHLTC, 2012). A strong supportive team will help to facilitate acceptance of the case costing project and maintains its sustainability.

Planning

The OCCI has summarized the case costing methodology into four steps:

1. Gather the data.
2. Allocate indirect costs.
3. Calculate functional centre unit.
4. Distribute costs to patients.

The standardized OCCI methodology of case costing simplifies and summarizes the task of patient-specific costing for planning and implementation purposes. The successful accomplishment of each step is critical, since the results of each step feeds into the next step.

Timeline and Project Tasks

A timeline is allocated for the case costing project implementation. The project schedule outlines the project tasks and duration that the hospital can expect for their implementation.

Data Resources

In preparation for the case costing project, the hospital should save data from their source data systems. The hospital must have 12 months of cost data in order meet the project deliverables.

Implementing

Step 1: Gathering Data

Ontario Case Costing Initiative outlined a series of six steps associated with Step 1: Gathering Data of the implementation. The first step is reviewing of current work methods. Different hospital costs areas (e.g. health records, pharmacy, lab, etc.) are collected and will be distributed. The second step is identifying workload elements. The third step is assigning time unit values. The fourth step is ongoing data collection. The fifth step is establishing productivity target. The last and sixth step is monitoring key relationships (MOHLTC, 2012).

The two forms of data are financial data and cost distribution data. Firstly, hospital financial data is defined according to the MIS (Management Information System) Standards. Hospitals must adhere to the account structure presented in the MIS Standards and the account codes presented in the Ontario Hospital Reporting System (OHRS) Chart of Accounts (MOHLTC, 2012). This provides a framework for the compilation and comparison of financial and statistical data.

Secondly, cost distribution data is based on workload. Workload is used to distribute nursing costs of the hospital. Workload data recording should adhere to the National Workload Measurement System (NWMS) and it serves as the

cost distribution base for order entry and results reporting for cost accounting in departmental and intermediate products which are translated into workload units by functional centre for each patient (MOHLTC, 2012). Gathering data is the first step in the case costing process. The OCCI standards for the collection of financial, statistical and patient descriptive data ensure the comparability of data.

Step 2: Allocate Indirect Costs

The second step of the case costing process is allocating indirect costs. The Simultaneous Equation Allocation Methodology (SEAM) is the OCCI standard method for indirect cost allocation. A formula is used to allocate costs of the Administrative and Support functional centres to the patient care functional centres (MOHLTC, 2012).

Step 3: Calculate Functional Centre Unit Costs

The third step of the case costing process involves calculating unit costs for services provided by each nursing functional centre. This approach is referred to as the Functional Centre Unit Cost method. The Functional Centre Unit Cost method tracks patient-specific unit costs to calculate separate unit costs for direct and indirect costs using Nursing Workload data (MOHLTC, 2012). Calculation of functional centre unit costs should be based on annual statistics and expenditures.

Step 4: Distribute Costs to Patients

The fourth and last step in the case costing process entails the distribution of costs to patients. The calculation of the functional centre costs for a case requires the following information:

1. Service recipient workload units received by the patient from the functional centre during the period.

2. Functional centre unit direct cost and unit indirect cost for the period.

3. Total cost of patient-specific supplies provided to the patient from the functional centre during the period.

4. Total cost of other non-workload distributed products and services delivered to patients (MOHLTC, 2012). Functional centre costs are distributed to patients based primarily on the proportion of service recipient workload.

Transitioning

The completion of the implementation stages at the hospital results in case costing data that follows the OCCI methodology. The case costing data is now available for analysis. The transitioning process addresses the stakeholders. Education, promotion, and orientation are provided to stakeholders to address the benefits of case costing from different levels from the hospital, health care system, and individual. This transition will control expectations, address contentious issues, and focus on improving existing services (MOHLTC, 2012). The transition will be communicated through workshops, newsletters, education sessions, and orientation sessions.

Evaluation

The evaluation process is a review and assessment of the current environment to the target environment. The evaluation seeks to find whether or not the implemented case costing is consistent with all applicable standards and guidelines. The primary objective of this is to evaluate case costing system in terms of identifying the validity and reliability of the data and identifying any constraints that may hinder the sustainability of case costing. The evaluation analysis is conducted with the collaboration of the case costing project manager, case costing team, department managers, information systems staff and others. The case

costing evaluation process allows the assessment of performance levels creating opportunities for improvement.

Case Costing at The Scarborough Hospital (TSH)

The Scarborough Hospital (TSH) is one of the hospitals that implemented case costing under the OCCI. TSH is a recognized large community hospital in Ontario. It operates more than 550 beds with about 110,624 emergency visits and 30,052 inpatient admissions a year (The Scarborough Hospital [TSH], 2012). The Scarborough Hospital implemented case costing in 1998 (TSH, personal communication, August 22, 2012). The undertaking of OCCI by TSH was strategic from a planning perspective. In an interview with Kully Singh, a senior case costing business analyst from TSH, she explained that TSH uses case costing information for workforce planning, the annual budgeting processes, monthly budget monitoring, ensuring matched budget and actual costs to the clinical needs of patients, assist in relating care delivered to clinical outcomes, and identify opportunities for work-flow improvement and skill mix decisions (TSH, personal communication, August 22, 2012). There are four OCCI Milestones which are audited by MOHLTC and OCCI. All four OCCI Milestones were passed in 2010 (TSH, personal communication, August 22, 2012).

To develop workload data for patient unit, TSH implemented the GRASP workload system. It is now in use across all inpatient and outpatient areas for both nursing and allied health professionals (TSH, personal communication, August 22, 2012). In the past few years, TSH successfully expanded the workload instrument into rehabilitation, emergency department areas, and chronic care (TSH, personal communication, August 22, 2012).

In moving forward with the next steps for OCCI, TSH will focus on enhancing data quality (TSH, personal communication, August 22, 2012). Case costing application and the integration of workload data are critical for ongoing sustainability of workload measurements at the service, program and corporate levels. The data will also allow TSH to compare its performance with other hospitals.

The Scarborough Hospital has recognized that case costing information can serve as the backbone for evidence-based internal resource allocation related to the annual budgeting process, identification of potential efficiencies and internal allocation of new, volume related funding. Case cost information is used by the hospital to facilitate informed decision-making.

Case Costing and Research

Successful implementation of OCCI has created a new tool for information called the OCCI Costing Analysis Tool available on the OCCI Website. The general public and health professionals have full access to the OCCI Costing Analysis Tool. This tool enables case costing data analysis from different perspectives. Data can be viewed by patient type, fiscal year, hospital, Case Mix Grouper (CMG), principle procedure, most responsible diagnosis, age group and case type. Certainly, the OCCI Costing Analysis Tool has been increasingly used by researchers to facilitate the case costing information piece of their research.

A research study by Menzies, Lewis, and Oxlade (2008) focused on the cost of tuberculosis (TB) care in Canada. This research compared spending costs of different activities by various jurisdictions and in different regions. This study collected patient data from CIHI and cost data from OCCI. OCCI was used to retrieve case costing data based on average per diem cost for the 14 most common medical causes of acute care hospitalization in Ontario (Menzies et al, 2008). Using OCCI's data, Ontario costs data were adjusted to average Canadian costs using relative costs published in the Hospital Financial Performance Indicators report from the Canadian Institute for Health Information (CIHI) (Menzies et al, 2008). The results of the study indicated that total TB-related expenditures in Canada were $74 million, equivalent to $47,290 for every active TB case diagnosed (Menzies et al, 2008). In addition, using the case costing information helped them identify regional differences in TB-related expenditures.

Results of the study showed that the highest expenditures were in the Northern Territories with $72,441, followed by the four Western provinces with $35,914, and lowest in the Atlantic Provinces with $28,259 per active TB case (Menzies et al, 2008). As evident, case costing data retrieved from the OCCI is useful for identifying cases at micro level. This level of data will help the government in making decisions on how to allocate TB-related care services within the different jurisdictions and regions. For instance, the high costs associated with care of active TB could be addressed by the government implementing initiatives such as prevention measures. In essence, preventative measures will reduce the overall rate of tuberculosis care in the community. This is an example of case costing data being used in research and policy developments. Case costing data is very valuable in driving evidence-based changes in the community.

FUTURE RESEARCH DIRECTIONS

There are many opportunities for the expansion and research of case costing. In 2010, Ontario Institute for Cancer Research (OICR) and Cancer Care Ontario (CCO) announced $6 million in funding for the Health Services Research Program (HSRP) to improve the delivery of cancer care in Ontario. The funding went to several projects, one of which involved the case costing of cancer in Ontario. For the next few years, one of the focus areas for HSRP will be case costing and economic evaluation (OICR, 2012). This project will develop methods to use Ontario's hospital administrative data for economic evaluation. It will also study the determinants of cost for cancer care in Ontario. The future and emerging trend is moving towards using data to inform cancer service innovations, evaluate technologies, and optimize patient care.

CONCLUSION

The practical implication of adopting case costing with OCCI is very germane to hospitals' strategy and performance. Future health care informatics research should be conducted to investigate how case costing data affect efficiency and quality of hospital care. The demand for case costing information will continue to increase. There is always the demand to advance analytical capabilities to create applications to assist with decision making to meet the needs of our Canadian health care.

REFERENCES

Andru, P., & Botchkarev, A. (2008). *Using financial modelling for integrated health care databases.* Retrieved December 18, 2012 from http://www.gsrc.ca/1569094939.pdf

Fickenscher, K. (2005). The new frontier of data mining. *Health Management Technology, 26*(10), 26–30. PMID:16259138.

Fitzpatrick, M. (2006). Using data to drive performance improvement in hospitals. *Health Management Technology, 27*(12), 10–16. PMID:17256646.

Hawkins, J., & Li, J. (2001). *A system for evaluating inpatient care cost-efficiency in hospital.* Retrieved December 18, 2012, 2012 from http://www.ncbi.nlm.nih.gov/pmc/articles/PMC2243448/pdf/procamiasymp00002-0408.pdf

Kerr, K. (2008). Metadata repositories in health care. *Health Care and Informatics Review Online, 12*(3), 37–44.

Menzies, D., Lewis, M., & Oxlade, O. (2008). Cost for tuberculosis care in Canada. *Canadian Journal of Public Health, 5*(99), 391–396.

Mettler, T., & Vimarlund, V. (2009). Understanding business intelligence in the context of health care. *Health Informatics Journal, 15,* 254–264. doi:10.1177/1460458209337446 PMID:19713399.

Ministry of Health and Long-Term Care (MOHLTC). (2012a). *Health analyst's toolkit.* December 18, 2012 from http://www.health.gov.on.ca/english/providers/pub/healthanalytics/health_toolkit/health_toolkit.pdf

Ministry of Health and Long-Term Care (MOHLTC). (2012b). *Ontario case costing guide. Data Standards Unit, Health Data Branch.* MOHLTC.

O'Brien-Pallas, L. (2002). Where to from here? *Canadian Journal of Nursing Research, 33*(4), 3–14. PMID:11998195.

Ontario Case Costing Initiative (OCCI). (2012a). *About the OCCI.* Retrieved on December 18, 2012 from http://www.occp.com

Ontario Case Costing Initiative (OCCI). (2012b). *OCCI costing analysis tool (CAT).* Retrieved December 18, 2012 from http://www.occp.com

Ontario Case Costing Initiative (OCCI). (2012c). *Ontario case costing facilities.* Retrieved December 18, 2012 from http://www.occp.com

Ontario Health Association (OHA). (2009). *Supporting transformation: A vision for e-health human resources for Ontario.* Retrieved December 18, 2012 from http://www.oha.com/KnowledgeCentre/Library/Documents/Supporting_Transformation_FINAL.pdf

Ontario Institute for Cancer Research (OICR). (2012). *Ontario institute for cancer research.* Retrieved December 18, 2012, 2012 from http://oicr.on.ca/files/public/OICR%20Slidedeck%2010Feb12%20revised%207%20August%202012.pdf

Rosenstein, A. (1999). Measuring the benefits of clinical decision support: Return on investment. *Health Care Management Review, 24*(2), 32–43. PMID:10358805.

The Scarborough Hospital (TSH). (2012). *Key facts and figures.* Retrieved December 18, 2012 from http://www.tsh.to/pages/Key-Facts--Figures

Wang, B., Wan, T., Burke, D., Bazzoli, G., & Lin, B. (2005). Factors influencing health information system adoption in American hospitals. *Health Care Management Review, 30*(1), 44–51. doi:10.1097/00004010-200501000-00007 PMID:15773253.

KEY TERMS AND DEFINITIONS

Case Costing: Is a process of allocating expenditures of various hospital departments to each individual *Case* with an objective to determine the *Case Cost.*

CAT: Costing Analysis Tool is an analytical tool to examine costs.

CIHI: Canadian Institute for Health Information.

HBAM: Health Based Allocation Model is a new, methodology designed to promote the objectives of the Ontario health care system through funding policy.

MOHLTC: Ministry of Health and Long-Term Care.

OCCI: Ontario Case Costing Initiative.

TSH: The Scarborough Hospital.

Chapter 7
Informatics and Health Services:
The Potential Benefits and Challenges of Electronic Health Records and Personal Electronic Health Records in Patient Care, Cost Control, and Health Research – An Overview

Nelson Ravka
York University, Canada

ABSTRACT

Personal electronic health records are seen as a key component to improved health care for patients, empowering motivated patients by giving them access to their own records resulting in increased self-care, shared decision making, and better clinical outcomes. Benefits through electronic record keeping would also accrue to health care providers through the availability and retrievability of data, reduced duplication of medical tests, more effective physician diagnosis and treatment, reduced incidence of prescription errors, and flagging inappropriate drug combinations. Utilizing information technology could also moderate the cost of health care services. Electronic health records would also improve clinical research through access to a large database of patient electronic records for research and determining best practices. Although potential benefits are considerable, many challenges to implementation must be addressed and resolved before this potential of improved health care provision and cost efficiency can be realized.

INTRODUCTION

Personal Health Records (PHRs) and Electronic Health Records (EHRs) are seen as key components to improving health care to patients as well as promoting wellness to the public at large

DOI: 10.4018/978-1-4666-4321-5.ch007

(Tang, Ash, Bates, Overhage, & Sands, 2006). Electronic health records are digital depositories for clinician records and managed by clinicians or health institutions. Hayrinen et al. describe EHRs as repositories of patient data in digital form, stored and exchanged securely, and accessible by multiple authorized users that contain retrospective, concurrent, and prospective information. Their primary purpose is to support continuing, efficient, and quality orientated health care (Hayrinen, Saranto, & Nykanen, 2008). An advisory panel to the U.S. government's Health Information Technology Adoption Initiative has listed the functions of EHRs as 1) having the ability to electronically collect and store data about patients, 2) having the ability to supply that information to health providers on demand, 3) having the ability to allow physicians to enter patient care orders on the computer, and 4) having the ability to provide health professionals with health care decision making support (Blumenthal & Glasor, 2007). Garde et al. describe EHRs as having the following necessary characteristics:

- **Patient-Centred:** The EHR relates to the patient, not an encounter with an institution.
- **Longitudinal:** A long-term record of patient care.
- **Comprehensive:** Record of care from all health care providers and institutions.
- **Prospective:** Plans, goals, orders, and evaluations are recorded (Garde, Knaup, Hovenga, & Heard, 2007).

Conceptually, PHRs are digital health information vehicles that can be managed by individuals (patients or surrogates) compared to EHRs that are managed by health providers or clinical institutions. Although there is no absolute consensus on what defines PHRs, a description suggested by the Markle Foundation's working group on policies for information sharing between doctors and patients is useful. It describes PHRs as: "an electronic application through which individuals can access, manage and share their health information...in a private, secure and confidential environment" (Markle Connecting for Health, 2004). The National Alliance for Health Information Technology further clarifies an idealized model of PHRs as "an electronic record of health-related information that conforms to a common interoperability standard allowing information to be drawn from multiple sources while being managed, shared and controlled by the individual" (Kahn, Aulakh, & Bosworth, 2009, p. 369).

There is a range of formats that PHRs can be classified. The simplest is a stand-alone patient-initiated application that is not linked with any other system. The patient enters their own health data using commercial applications. Google Health and Microsoft Health Vault are examples of companies that have introduced such systems. However there is a concern that patients would not keep records up to date in a stand-alone PHR (Tang et al., 2006). Consequently these PHRs could be unreliable instruments for conveying information to clinicians or health institutions. Tang, et al. suggest that although some information can be supplied by patients, clinicians must have access to their own past inputs to assist in decision making. They stated; "[T]he reliability of patient-entered data depends on the nature of the information per se, the patient's general and health literacy, and the specific motivations for recording the data." (Tang et al., 2006, p. 122) In a study conducted by Ira C. Denton, 1000 patients were offered their medical information in a stand-alone PHR system. Only 330 accepted. After 10 months, of those who responded to a survey, 37% continued to use the electronic record (Denton, 2001). According to Linda Reed, chief information officer, Atlantic Health; "[M]any people are more willing to keep their Facebook page updated than their medical records" (Page, 2010).

Acknowledging the limitations of stand-alone PHRs that depend on patient-only inputs, a more information reliable model would involve health records that are stored in the patient's EHR. Such a 'tethered' system of provider owned and maintained PHR would consist of a summary of clinically relevant health information that is made available to patients. These systems can include functionalities such as appointment requests and prescription renewals. There can also be an opportunity for patient input that can be uploaded and saved to the provider's EHR (Tang et al., 2006). A still more complex system involves the linking of different health care data sources in a seamless interoperative functionality to allow for the transfer of patient data from all sources to the provider's EHR and patient PHR (Tang et al., 2006). This most complex system consists of a portable, interoperable digital file in which selected, clinically relevant health data can be managed, secured and transferred. With this level of functionality, Steinbrook wrote in the New England Journal of Medicine:

Online repositories will allow patients to store, retrieve, manage, and share their health data— such as lists of medical problems, medical history, medications, allergies, immunizations, test results, insurance information, and doctors' visits over the internet (Steinbrook, 2008, p. 1653).

In a February 2005 symposium sponsored by the American College of Medical Informatics, participants concluded that PHRs that were linked to EHRs either through tethering or interconnectivity would provide much greater benefits than stand-alone PHRs (Tang et al., 2006). Tethered PHR adoption would be tied to the growth in EHR adoption (especially by primary care physicians who are the main source of patient data) and would have the additional role of advising and supporting patients in their health care and self-management (Archer, Fevrier, Lokker, McKibbon, & Straus, 2011).

BENEFITS OF PHRS AND EHRS

There is growing public interest for access to health records and a general belief that this access would be useful in allowing patients to assume more responsibility and decision-making for their own health-care (Tang & Lansky, 2005). This electronic modality would empower motivated patients by giving them access to their own records

and allow them to manage and share their health information in a private, secure and confidential environment. Pagliari et al. list the functions of these PHRs that include:

- Access to providers' electronic clinical record which includes history, drugs and test results.
- Access to a personal health organizer (can include information on clinics, doctors, tests, dates, non-prescribed treatments and scanned documents).
- Access to self-management support such as care plans, graphing of symptoms, passive biofeedback, instructive or motivational feedback, decision aids and reminders.
- Enablement of secure patient-provider communication for booking appointments, reordering prescriptions, and seeking advice through patient-doctor e-mail.
- Easily accessed links to information concerning illness, treatments or self-care.
- Links to sources of support such as patient organizations or virtual peer networks.
- Improve or facilitate the capture of symptoms or health behaviour data by self-reporting or link to electronic monitoring devices. (Pagliari, Detmer, & Singleton, 2007)

Detmer et al. also include in PHR potential functionality the ability to review insurance eligibility and benefits, the processing of claims and payments and automated checking for drug interactions (Detmer, Raymond, Tang, & Bloomrosen, 2008).

The potential of PHRs accrues to both patients and providers. Pagliari et al. suggest that the potential functionalities of PHRs can provide patient empowerment through access to their personal data, health information and communication opportunities. They note that the potential exists for increased self-care, shared decision making and better clinical outcomes and that patient involvement can improve safety through flagging diagnostic and drug errors, recording non-prescribed medications or improving accessibility to test results or drug alerts (Pagliari, Detmer, & Singleton, 2007). Hayrinen et al. state that PHRs can:

...reduce geographic barriers to patient care and act as a point of record integration, particularly in fragmented health systems, thus improving continuity of care and efficiency. Although the number and quality of studies remains limited, existing research suggest improvements in communication and trust between patients and professionals, confidence in self-care, compliance in chronic disease, and accuracy of records. Patients particularly value online reordering of prescriptions, laboratory results, disease management plans, trend charts, drug lists and secure messaging (Hayrinen et al., 2008, p. 293).

Pagliari et al. summarize the benefits derived from the use of PHRs. Patient empowerment creates distinct benefits through better health and quality of life. Increased personal responsibility can drive health maintenance and self-care. Motivation to comply with treatment through increased participation in decision-making and acquisition of health knowledge can result from the use of PHRs. Quality of care improves with improved relationships with health care providers through better communication. Patients have more flexible access to services such as appointments, tests and electronic consulting. Patient safety is enhanced through reduced errors, quicker access to results and drug alerts. Patient care can be improved with knowledge of otherwise unreported health behaviours and drug use and potentially better collaboration between caregivers and health care providers (Pagliari et al., 2007).

Examples of the advantages of PHRs can be informative. Tang and Lee describe a common scenario:

Mary is 68 years old, has four chronic conditions, takes seven medications, and averages 12 visits per year to her six physicians. In between visits, she spends a lot of time on the telephone with them or their staff—making appointments, requesting prescription renewals and referrals, seeking test results, and asking questions that she forgot to bring up in person....What if Mary could view her test results within hours after her blood was drawn? What if she could upload her home glucometer and blood-pressure readings so she could graph them and see how changes in her behaviour affect them? What if her health care team received copies of her readings and could recommend dose adjustments for her medications? And what if it all happened without an office visit (Tang & Lee, 2009, p. 1276)?

Wolter et al. illustrates another scenario of how a PHR can improve information sharing between health care providers:

A patient is visiting a cardiologist for the first time. The physician asks the patient what medications he is taking. This is not a simple question, and the patient has trouble recalling all the necessary information: which medications he takes, the dosage for each, how often he takes them, how long he has been taking them, and the prescribing physician for each. He is not entirely sure why he has been prescribed one of them (Wolter & Friedman, 2005, p. 28).

Demand is growing among the public for access to their health records (Detmer et al., 2008). A 2003 survey by the Markle Foundation found that 65% of respondents were interested in electronically accessing their own personal health records. 90% believed it was important to be able to track their symptoms or changes in health care on-line. 71% stated that PHRs would be helpful in clarifying doctors' instructions. 65% believed that it would help in preventing medical mistakes. 54% believed it would change the way they managed their own health. 60% thought it would improve care. When asked about specific features, 75% of respondents indicated PHRs would be useful to e-mail their doctor, 69% believed it would be useful to store immunization records, 65% would use it to transfer information to specialists, 63% would look up test results and 62% would track medication use. The survey found that those with chronic illnesses, frequent health care users and caregivers had the greatest interest in PHRs (Markle Connecting for Health, 2003). A second survey by the Markle Foundation in 2006 reconfirmed public interest (Markle Connecting for Health, 2006).

A case study by Chen et al. illustrates the benefits of PHRs to health care providers. Following the installation of an EHR system with PHR functionalities that included secure patient-provider messaging, the total office visit rate among Kaiser Permanente patients decreased by 26.2%. (Kaiser health care providers are salaried employees. Their salaries are not dependent on the number of patient visits.) Comparing before and after implementation of the EHR and PHR system, office visits decreased from 99.6% of all ambulatory care contacts to 66%. Scheduled telephone visits accounted for 30% of contacts post-installation and secure messaging accounted for 4%. Although marginal or unnecessary office visits were reduced, the new modalities of care allowed an increase in patient contacts of 8%. Additionally, benefits involved reduced direct costs to patients through reduced cost of travel and parking and reduced school or work time loss. Surveys showed that patients' overall satisfaction with the new system were at least as high as previously. They perceived that the interest taken in their care by their health care providers was as good after implementation of EHRs and PHRs (Chen, Garrido, Chock, Okawa, & Liang, 2009).

Pagliari et al. suggest that the potential benefit to health care providers goes beyond unnecessary consultations and corresponding reduced waiting lists. They see the possibility of lower costs through better health and reduced use of services and treatments. Finally, health care providers could benefit from reduced provider liability through increased safety and patient self-management of their own health issues (Pagliari et al., 2007).

However Dunn and Wynia question whether care providers are better off with the addition of patient information input through their PHRs. The line between empowering and overwhelming patients and doctors with data may create its own problems. They suggest:

[W]ith too much information, decisions may be inappropriately delayed. Information overload can occur and some information may be pushed out; usually, more recently acquired information is retained and used, even if it is not the most relevant. Information will also tend to be retained if it supports a preconceived notion. Mental fatigue or decision fatigue can occur from the labour of sifting through information, and fatigued decision makers might make fast, careless decisions or suffer from decision paralysis (Dunn & Wynia, 2010, p. 67).

Innovative design and functioning of PHRs could rescue the users from these issues. It is possible that large amount of information can be converted into a summary format that would also generate recommendations (Dunn et al., 2010). Development of such decision support functions would enhance the value of PHRs to health care providers, avoiding the potential of overwhelming information interfering with appropriate or timely decision making (Dunn et al., 2010).

Electronic health records provide the digital link to PHRs and the benefits to patients that can come of it. Benefits of electronic records would also accrue to health care providers. Menachem and Collum suggest potential advantages over paper-based record systems that include:

- Improved legibility, availability and retrievablity of records and data.
- Reduced likelihood of duplication or unnecessary medical tests.
- Shorter patient waiting lists.
- More effective physician diagnosis and treatment through real time access to current best practices.
- Reduced incidence of prescription errors.
- Improved management and monitoring of multiple prescriptions.
- Improved flagging of inappropriate drug combinations that can cause adverse drug reactions.
- Increased efficiency in the delivery of health services (Menachemi & Collum, 2011).

EHRs can also be beneficial in clinical research (Diamond, Mostashari, & Shirky, 2009). Compiling information from a large data base of patients' electronic records would allow for assessments of treatment choices and determining best practices, enhance clinical research processes, and determine the incremental benefits of new medicines as well as documenting the frequency and severity of adverse events (Lumpkin, 2007). EHRs can improve efficiency and contain costs through innovative designing and conducting of global clinical trials (EHR4CR, 2011).

The goals of the Electronic Health Records for Clinical Research project (EHR4CR) are examples of the potential of EHRs for clinical research. This EU research project jointly run be academics and industrial partners is intended to; "build, validate and deploy a Europe-wide innovative technological platform to re-use EHRs data for clinical research purposes" (EHR4CR, 2011). Its goals are to attract research and development investments in Europe, to increase access to innovative medicines and to improve health outcomes while accomplishing these objectives within applicable legal, ethical and privacy protections of patients. The initiative would seek to moderate the cost of clinical trials by more efficiently evaluating patient populations, improving protocol design and identifying suitable patients for clinical trials thus eliminating unnecessary repetitive re-entry of data, confirming reliability of data sources and rendering easier the detection and reporting of rare adverse events. The realization of these objectives would create significant efficiency gains, faster access to new drugs and improve health outcomes (EHR4CR, 2011).

There are difficult obstacles that interfere with these goals. They include patient privacy, autonomy and consent, and interoperability across institutions, countries and continents (Jensen, Jensen, & Brunak, 2012). West et al. note three requirements that would allow EHRs to be useful for clinical research:

1. The ability to assemble patient clinical information from all providers to assess care quality.
2. The standardizing of entry procedures for recording patient care to optimize text mining of information and facilitate the use of data for research and assessing care quality.
3. The means to avoid using patient identifiers in sections of EHRs related to clinical data to conform to privacy requirements (West et al., 2009).

The potential advantages conferred to clinical research from EHRs are exciting in its scope. However it will take time and research to develop the protocols and technical standards to realize this potential.

CHALLENGES TO THE USE OF PHRS AND EHRS

Interoperability

The promise of better health care through shared health care and clinical research that are the potential benefits of EHRs can only be realized if information can be distributed efficiently to authorized stakeholders (Taylor, Bower, Frederico, & Bigelow, 2005). Taylor et al. state that; "[E]ffective connectivity is required to avoid redundant tests; improve safety and coordination among providers; increase administrative efficiency; and improve consumers' compliance with prevention, disease management, and care guidelines" (Taylor, Bower, Frederico, & Bigelow, 2005). The Institute of Electrical and Electronics Engineers defines interoperability as the "ability of two or more components to exchange information and to use the information that has been exchanged" (Institute of Electrical & Electronics Engineers, 1990). If information technology does not allow for a systematic processing of information, clinicians will bear unnecessary costs and workload as well as compounding the chance of introducing data errors. Garde et al. state:

Captured data must be of high quality (i.e. correct and complete), high reliability and high flexibility. This requires a mixture of free text entries and highly structured and standardized data items and the use of integrity constraints and plausibility checks. Different information systems used by the various health care providers of shared care must be able to interoperate, so that one system can understand the context and meaning of information provided by another system" (Garde et al., 2007, p. 333).

Unfortunately, as Thomas Beale argues, many systems have proprietary software that makes them expensive to modify and extend (Garde et al., 2007). The key to the widespread use of EHRs is standardization (Garde et al., 2007). This is not an easy goal. With technological and scientific advancements, changes are constantly needed to increase the scope and application of EHRs as medical knowledge expands. Standardization must include the means to incorporate change (Garde et al., 2007). To be fully beneficial EHRs that currently differs not only from each proprietary system within jurisdictions but also from country to country must be harmonized (Begoyan, 2007).

Harmonization must address two areas of interoperability—functional and semantic (Garde et al.,2007. Functional interoperability involves the exchange of information between different EHR systems that is readable by humans (Begoyan, 2007). Semantic interoperability refers to the exchange of information between systems that is computer processable by the receiving system (Begoyan, 2007). Begoyan lists the requirements to achieve semantic interoperability as follows;

- The utilization of a standardized EHR Reference Model to define and coordinate the semantics of EHR information structures.
- Use of a standardized service interface to define and coordinate the semantics of interfaces between EHR and other services.
- Utilization of a standardized set of domain-specific concept models to address needs dealing with archetypes and templates for different domain concepts.
- Use of standardized terminologies to define the language that is used in archetypes (The first two prerequisites also apply to functional interoperability) (Begoyan, 2007, p. 3).

Begoyan identifies a number of national and international organizations responsible for developing standards for EHRs. They include ISO (International Organization for Standardization) whose activities are limited to the structure and function of the EHR and the systems that processes EHR; CEN (European Committee for Standardisation) that oversees the development of multi-disciplinary standards including the interoperability of EHRs; HL7 (Health Level Seven) that is involved in providing standards between different types of healthcare computer applications including incorporating clinical and administrative data; and DICOM (Digital Imaging and Communications in Medicine) that has developed the standard for medical image communication allowing an independent exchange between medical images and related information (Begoyan, 2007). At the time of his review, Begoyan suggested that HL7 version3; "can be the foundation of future health care environments" (Begoyan, 2007, p. 7). However until semantic interoperability is achieved, full EHR utilization will be hampered by incompatible EHR systems purchased by different users (Begoyan, 2007).

Taylor et al. contend that the low rate of EHR adoption and the lack of interoperability in systems not designed for sharing of health information is a major barrier to connectivity. They identify four market failures that perpetuate these barriers:

1. The disconnect between those that pay for the technology and those who benefit from it.
2. The lack of pressure to adopt a standards-based EHR system.
3. The lack of incentives to develop a standards-based system or share detailed electronic patient data with competitors.
4. The lack of widespread access to standardized patient care data that could improve general health care performance (Taylor et al., 2005).

Interoperability is the backbone to efficient use of health information technology (Taylor et al., 2005; Garde et al., 2007). It is also a formidable technical challenge to overcome (Hersh, 2004). Its importance for fulfilling the potential of EHRs is

driving research in standardization that adequately addresses the harmonization issues of semantics and functionality (Begoyan, 2007).

Access and Literacy Challenges

The potential for PHR use can only be realized if the modality is accessible (Pirtle & Chandra, 2011). This requires a public that is computer competent, has access to the internet and has a degree of health literacy. It is estimated that 50% of U.S. adults would not comprehend the information that could be made available to them for the purpose of allowing them to make better health choices (Pirtle & Chandra, 2011). In the U.S. only 44% of low- income households have computers and only 34% have an internet connection (Beacom, 2010). Computer literacy and internet access are necessary conditions for on-line communications and accessing information. These criteria are least available to low income individuals. In addition, identified groups with low health literacy are populations over age sixty five, members of minorities or immigrant groups and those with chronic physical conditions (Kahn et al., 2009). Groups that are among the largest users of health care are the elderly and those with chronic conditions (Bodenheimer & Fernandez, 2005). As well, since poverty is a known determinate of ill health (McCally, et al., 1998) the poor can be included as disproportionate users of health-care (Wolter & Friedman, 2005; Wagstaff, 2002). If costs are not a barrier to accessing health care (as is the case in OECD countries with universal health care), then people of lower socio-economic status use more health care services than wealthier people (Asada & Kephart, 2007). It is likely that the largest users of health care resources are also the most health illiterate and the least likely to have computer or internet access. They would be excluded from the potential benefits of PHRs (Eyserbach, 2008).

This lack of access prevents disadvantaged groups from participating in social networking, denying them the ability to confer with peers and informing themselves of relevant information and what others are doing (Eyserbach, 2008). Thus the utilization of the power of the internet as a source of motivation and self-help is unavailable to the computer illiterate or those without access. These factors present a cautionary warning. Health maintenance and health recovery are multi-dimensional concepts that are related to many disciplines. Without addressing tangentially related issues, PHRs will be beneficial to a privileged part of the population and thus realize only a fraction of their potential.

Thus far those without computer or internet access have been excluded as candidates for PHR benefits (Pirtle & Chandra, 2011). However smart phones are becoming ubiquitous. This may be the future entry point to PHRs for disadvantaged groups who would otherwise not have access. Paglieri suggests; "[T]he emergence of mobile and wireless applications that allow remote submission of data to a shared record offer new possibilities and real time decision support" (Pagliari et al., 2007, p. 331). Much development work must be done to realize the potential of this way forward.

Denton has shown that many patients may not want to take the personal responsibility that PHRs allow (Denton, 2001). Therefore it may be a modality that is most suitable for certain motivated patients and caregivers (Tang et al., 2006). Paglieri et al. suggest that although surveys indicate that most people would like access to their health records, the most likely users and therefore the ones who would gain the most from PHRs would be those with long term conditions who have ongoing incentives to track their illness and treatments and patients experiencing periodic need for care that triggers an interest in information and communication (Pagliari et al., 2007). Caregivers and relatives of elderly parents or children in hospitals can benefit from PHRs by developing a partnership with health care providers through information sharing that could impact the patient's care (Pagliari et al., 2007).

Privacy and Security Challenges

Privacy and security are serious concerns for most people. The Personal Health Working Group of the Markle Foundation stated in 2003 that 91% of people reported that they were very concerned about the privacy and security of their personal health information (Kaelber, Jha, Johnston, Middleton, & Bates, 2008). Halanka et al. studied three functioning PHR systems that were clinic or institutional owned and maintained. A number of privacy and security challenges were common to all three systems. These include:

- Should the entire problem list be shared?
- Should the entire medication list and allergy list be shared?
- Should all laboratory and diagnostic test results be shared with the patient?
- Should clinical notes be shared with the patient?
- How should patients be authenticated to access the PHR?
- Should minors be able to have their own private PHR and should patients be able to share access to their PHRs via proxies?
- Should the PHR include secure clinician-patient messaging (Halamka, Mandl, & Tang, 2008)?

The authors noted that all three systems chose to share the entire problem list with patients and facilitated patient understanding by using full text descriptions of problems. One provided hyperlinks to provide explanatory information of diagnoses. All shared the entire medication list. All shared laboratory and diagnostic tests (where not restricted by jurisdictional laws) and established protocols so that disturbing information could first be conveyed by personal communication with a health care provider. All decided not to share clinical text notes. All implemented username and password protocols to ensure privacy. As to policy regarding PHRs and minors, each system determined their own unique policy. Although concerns existed about a lack of reimbursement involving secure messaging, all three provided the service. The authors noted that with careful attention to policy concerning privacy, security, data stewardship and personal control, PHRs can be successfully deployed (Halamka et al., 2008).

Further research is needed to develop a standard protocol for ensuring appropriate PHR privacy and security (Kaelber et al., 2008). Answers to questions such as who controls sharing of and access to a PHR of minors and non-competent patients and what would be an acceptable trade-off between verification of authenticity of a user and the interests of legitimate patient proxies must be debated and a policy consensus developed. A balance must be agreed on how much security is needed to allow easy patient access but difficult enough to prevent security breaches. Consideration must be given to the possibility of unintentially limiting PHR use if access is too difficult. Answers to what common procedures can be developed to allow access if passwords are forgotten or if the patient is incapacitated must be found. Kaelbe et al., referring to issues of privacy and security, ask what authentication methods would "ensure both privacy and security yet in doing so do not present a major barrier to access." (Kaelber et al., 2008, p. 731) How would the use of patient records for research be allowed while still protecting patient privacy? PHRs will only become commonplace when these privacy and security issues are resolved (Kaelber et al., 2008).

Adoption and Attitude Challenges for PHR Utilization

Use of PHRs will hinge on overcoming attitudinal and physical adoption barriers among patients and care providers (Kaelber et al., 2008). As previously noted, some limited research has shown interest among patients. However adoption has been low when access is available even when it was provided free of charge (Kaelber et al., 2008; Denton, 2001). The attitudes of physicians are even less well documented. Some studies show that providers are hesitant about adopting PHRs (Witry, Doucette, Daly, Levy, & Chrischilles, 2010). Physicians are concerned about any additional work that would be required that would not be compensated (Kaelber, Jha, Johnston, Middleton, & Bates, 2008). Witry et al. observed; "While providers believe PHRs have the potential to decrease errors and increase efficiency, they are concerned about how to integrate PHRs into patient appointments that are already too short" (Witry et al., 2010, p. 8). Archer et al., suggest a number of adoption issues among healthcare providers. These include; " new workflow demands and resistance to change, inadequate technology literacy, responsibility for ensuring the accuracy and integrity of health information across multiple interconnected data systems, and confidentiality and privacy risks" (Archer et al., 2011, p. 518). Physicians' limited view of PHR functions and benefits and their perception of barriers to its use may inhibit support for PHR use (Witry et al., 2010).

Cost many also be a barrier to PHR adoption (Tang et al., 2006). There is some data to indicate that motivated patients may be willing to pay $2-$5 per month (Archer et. Al., 2011). How would PHRs be subsidized? Archer and Fevrier-Thomas state:

[T]he diffusion of ePHRs to those who are genuinely motivated to adopt them will be a significant cost if done effectively. Until solid information can be collected and the future of such systems is decided, support for ePHRs will be a major public policy issue for healthcare systems administrators and funding agencies (Archer & Fevrier-Thomas, 2010).

The financial aspects of PHR and EHR integration in health care must be addressed and sufficient value to all participants must be apparent to justify their use (Tang et al., 2006).

THE BUSINESS CASE FOR PHRS AND EHRS

Adoption of PHRs will be affected by how much the various stakeholders would be willing to support it (Tang et al., 2006). There must be advantages in the PHR model that would make business sense to health care providers and patients. Walker and Carayon state that; "substantial evidence suggests that achieving the goal of higher-quality patient outcomes at decreased cost per outcome requires improved, patient-centered care processes" (Walker & Carayon, 2009, p. 475). The various providers and health care support services that must cooperate to supply the data and contribute to the functionality of the PHR must see where they will profit either through efficiency gains or remuneration for their involvement from their investment in time and software and hardware expenses (Tang et al., 2006). The introduction of provincial subsidies in Canada and allocation of funds towards healthcare information technology in the USA in the American Recovery and Reinvestment Act of 2009 (ARRA) are incentives to accelerate the use of EHRs that may hasten adoption in both countries (Blumenthal, 2009) (Webster, 2010).

The ARRA provided $17 billion as financial incentives to physicians and hospitals to adopt and use EHRs (Blumenthal, 2009). Blumenthal notes that; "[S]tarting in 2011, physicians can receive extra Medicare payments for the 'meaningful use' of a 'certified' EHR that can exchange data with other parts of the health care system" (Blumenthal, 2009, p. 1478). Meaningful use refers to the use of EHRs in a way that will improve quality and efficiency in the health care delivery system. Blumenthal states:

...if EHRs are to catalyze quality improvement and cost control, physicians and hospitals will have to use them effectively. This means taking advantage of embedded clinical decision supports that help physicians take better care of their patients (Blumenthal, 2009, p. 1479).

If PHRs are also to become widespread, patients will have to see significant value if they are to demand and support implementation. To some, empowerment in sharing in their health care with providers may prove to be sufficient incentive. Others may appreciate the communication functionalities of PHRs. Still others will value the savings in time and expenses by eliminating some physical visits to their health care providers (Kaelber & Pan, 2008). All these various advantages are intuitively self-serving and may only require education of the public that this new modality of care is available.

Enlisting the less motivated is more problematic. A study by Fosyth et al. showed that some patients did not want to understand their own medical information let alone contribute to its contents. They did not feel comfortable with even possessing their own medical records (Forsyth, Maddock, Iedema, & Lassere, 2010). A strategy for engaging these patients may revolve around convincing them of the merit of having these records available at medical appointments and emergency care visits. Those with limited English skills could appreciate the advantage of PHRs in reducing communication issues (Forsyth et al., 2010). (As previously noted, the problems of a lack of access to computers and computer illiteracy of disadvantaged groups are symptoms of larger social issues. The potential benefits of PHRs for these groups must be addressed through effective social policies that strive for equitable opportunity.)

A critical economic criterion for successful implementation involves the compensation to providers to enlist their cooperation in the communication functionality of PHRs (Blumenthal,

2009). Tethered PHR systems can allow for secure e-mail access between patient and physician as well as the facilitation of telephone appointments in lieu of office visits (Chen et al., 2009). Many current reimbursement models do not compensate physicians for these methods of communication (Blumenthal, 2009). In advance of determining changes in the payment to providers, research will be required to determine if these modalities of patient care are advantageous in:

1. Utilization of time.
2. Satisfaction by patients in their perception of care received.
3. Effectiveness of care and health outcomes compared to standard models of care (Yau, Williams, & Brown, 2011).

Answers to these questions through appropriate research would provide insight in the economic (as well as health) benefits that could drive the implementation of PHRs. Kaelber and Pan note that any cost savings and value to stakeholders including patients has yet to be demonstrated (Kaelber & Pan, 2008). Kaelber et al. state; "[I]n considering reimbursement reform, policymakers need additional information about the benefits of non-visit care to determine how best to compensate providers for it" (Kaelber et al., 2008, p. 733). These policy changes could affect one or more of the existing funding models of fee-for-service, salaried employment or capitation. As well, if PHR use can demonstrate improved health and health outcomes, a financial benefit can be accrued to the payer, which could provide an additional incentive to spread the system universally. Offering financial incentives to providers for utilizing EHR and PHR functionalities can be financed from the expected savings to the health care global budget.

PHR utilization in the fee-for-service funding model must address the new communication modalities. Currently, the fee-for-service funding model does not compensate providers for time spent in phone or e-mail communications with patients. If research confirms that the overall time needed to treat patients is reduced, the availability of extra time in the working day through substituting non-visit care for some office visits can allow an added flow of income from additional patients. This may balance a significant amount of the loss of income from reduced office visits. However, this theoretical scenario might not reflect any compelling reasons for providers to embrace the new modality. The time spent in voice or e-mail communications is still without compensation in the fee-for-service payment model. Working time is still expended without monetary reward. A new fee for voice or e-mail communications can reimburse providers for their time. If research also shows improved health and health outcomes using PHRs, a financial incentive involving increased fees to providers participating in the use of EHRs/PHRs may become a reasonable policy change. Any such policy changes must be based on health outcomes. Appropriate research and proof of concept demonstration initiatives must confirm whether the theoretical potential of PHRs is in fact translatable to actual improved health care, reduced appointments and reduced costs. A balance must be struck between additional fee payments and reduced global health care costs.

In payment models that involve salaried providers, there is less of a financial issue surrounding the utilization of PHRs. Providers will not be directly impacted monetarily if research shows improved health care outcomes with PHRs. Their working time and effort would not change if PHRs allow each provider to treat more patients. However salary levels may be altered to recognize the health care providers' role in improving health care efficiency. This salary adjustment may be a necessary incentive to reward providers for participating in the use of a more efficient and effective health care system.

Capitation models of provider compensation may be the most receptive of PHRs without requiring changes in the existing model. Capitation refers to a system of compensation to the provider that pays a fixed amount per patient per month without considering the amount of care or time each patient may require. If it can be shown that the use of PHRs can improve the health of patients and reduces the time required for each, there is an incentive for the provider to incorporate such a system into her practice. The outcome will be the same compensation while expending less time. Income can be maintained with less work or increased if more patients are added to the patient roster to fill the additional clinic time created through the use of PHRs.

If the use of PHRs can provide better health maintenance, improved health outcomes when care is needed and reduced use of resources, policy initiatives could be used to pursue the potential benefits of PHRs. A shift in funding amounts or funding methods to encourage providers to adopt the use of PHRs would further the goals of administrators in health care funding. Each compensation model would require some use of financial incentives to encourage the adoption of PHRs. However, the capitation model may be the method that provides the greatest natural incentive for adoption. Striving for efficiency is a characteristic of the capitation model and those working in that system would be the least resistant to utilize a tool that could improve efficiency. Their own financial interest in PHRs would be an incentive to encourage patients to utilize them. Government policy that encourages doctors to adopt a capitation remuneration model and include PHRs in their patient care strategy could be part of the effort to control health care costs.

Taylor et al. have attempted to monetize the potential benefits of incorporating Health Information Technology (HIT). Although referring specifically to the American system of health care, they estimate that $81 billion can be saved annually by using EHR systems. They estimate the cost of implementation for inpatient and outpatient systems of $7.6 billion per year during the adoption period. To attain these savings they note three requirements;

1. There must be widespread provider adoption of a standard-based EMR system.
2. There must be effective connectivity between providers and between providers and patients.
3. There must be intense efforts to improve quality and efficiency performance (Taylor et al., 2005).

Obstacles to attaining these benefits would be the cost of acquiring and implementing these systems, the uncertainty of financial benefits to providers, and the high initial physician time requirements to implement the system (Taylor et al., 2005).

Shekelle et al., examining five cost-benefit analyses involving the use of EHRs, reported that all predicted significant savings (Shekelle, Morton, & Keeler, 2006). Not all potential benefits are theoretical. The case study by Chen et al. examining the effects of Kaiser Permanente's utilization of EHRs and PHRs showed improvement in patient care efficiency through reduced office visits (Chen et al., 2009). This suggests cost benefits although the study did not examine per patient time savings accrued to providers through the introduction of health information technology. Documentation of actual financial benefits is largely unavailable. Chaudhry et al. concluded:

[P]ublished evidence of the information needed to make informed decisions about acquiring and implementing health information technology in community settings is nearly nonexistent. For example, potentially important evidence related to initial capital costs, effect on provider productivity, resources required for staff training (such as time and skills), and workflow redesign is difficult to locate in the peer-reviewed literature. Also lacking are key data on financial context, such as degree of capitation, which has been suggested as a model to be an important factor in defining the business case for electronic health record use (Chaudhry, et al., 2006, p. 748).

Chaudhry et al. showed evidence does exist that health information technologies do improve quality and efficiency. Examining the effects on health care in four benchmark research institutions following the installation of multifunctional health information technology systems that included decision support, they documented five effects:

1. More care was provided that was in adherence to guidelines and protocols.
2. Surveillance and monitoring for disease conditions and care delivery was improved.
3. Medication errors decreased.
4. Less patient care was required.
5. Utilization of time was inconclusive (Chaudhry, et al., 2006).

Oliver has reported on the improvement in the health record performance of the Veteran Health Administration (VHA) in the United States following the installation of an EHR system. He observed, "[T]he system increased the availability of patient-charts at the point of clinical encounter from 60% to 100% between 1995 and 2004. At least one in five medical tests in the US is repeated because of lost patient records, but lost records are no longer a problem in the VHA" (Oliver, 2008, p. 1213). Hurricane Katrina demonstrated the benefit of EHRs. Many New Orleans evacuees found themselves without their medical records. Brown et al. noted that; [T]he outcome was different for enrolled veterans. Their complete electronic clinical records were available from the rehosted VistA [VHA electronic records] system to authorized users with access to VA's secure network" (Brown, et al., 2007, p. S138).

The UK's Department of Health launched a project, the Whole System Demonstrator program, to determine whether ehealth would live up to the expectations claimed for it as part of a transformational delivery of health care. In their findings released December, 2011 the Department of Health stated:

....if used correctly telehealth can deliver a 15 percent reduction in A&E [ambulatory and elective] visits, a 20 percent reduction in emergency admissions, a 14 percent reduction in elective admissions, a 14 percent reduction in bed days and an 8 percent reduction in tariff costs. More strikingly they also demonstrate a 45 percent reduction in mortality rates" (KPMG International Cooperative, 2012, p. 13).

Further research is needed to quantify the cost savings of these effects within the global health care budget. Cost-benefit analyses projections are encouraging (Chaudhry, et al., 2006). The potential for savings through either reduced need for health care or more efficient provision of care is so compelling that agencies responsible for funding have embraced the technology as a method of controlling health care spending in an environment of aging societies, accelerating drug costs and increasingly sophisticated and costly health care (Blumenthal, 2009).

THE STATE OF RESEARCH ON PHRS

Too little is known about the actual benefits of PHRs. So little research has been initiated that Kaelber et al. warn; "....we believe the lack of evaluation and the current rudimentary understanding of how PHRs can specifically contribute to health care quality, safety, efficiency and patient satisfaction threatens the viability and sustainability of these systems" (Kaelber et al., 2008, p. 730). The authors note four areas of research opportunities for PHRs: function evaluation, adoption and attitudes, privacy and security and architecture. They suggest that currently function evaluation may be the most important area of research. This includes information collecting (retrieving from external sources), sharing, exchanging (two-way sharing), and self-management. These areas of functionality should be explored to assess their importance with respect to health care quality, safety, efficiency, cost, and patient and provider satisfaction (Kaelber et al., 2008).

Several issues regarding PHR privacy and security require investigation. Who controls sharing and access to a PHR of minors and non-competent patients requires further inquiry. Consensus must be found on acceptable trade-offs between verification of authenticity of a user and the interests of legitimate patient proxies. Research that would aid in establishing acceptable protocols is necessary to encourage widespread use of PHRs (Mandl et. al., 2001).

Research is needed to determine the model of PHR design of data collection, infrastructure and applications that will best support patient-centred health care. The issue of interoperability is a critical element of PHR functionality and standards for architecture compatibility must be explored (Kaelber & Pan, 2008).

Research to assess the business case for PHRs is critical to determine the viability of PHRs and whether the investments made in this field is warranted. Many current reimbursement models do not compensate providers for the new modalities of communication that PHRs provide (Kaelber & Pan, 2008). In advance of determining changes in the payment to providers, research must determine if these modalities of patient care are advantageous in utilization of time, satisfaction by patients in their perception of care received and effectiveness of care and health outcomes compared to standard models of care (Witry et. al., 2010). The research that would provide the necessary insight in the economic (as well as health) benefits will drive the progress in PHR implementation (Kaelber & Pan, 2008).

EHR AND PHR UTILIZATION: A WORLD VIEW

In 2011, a consortium of five of the largest health care providers in the U.S.—Kaiser Permanente, the Mayo Clinic, Geisinger, Intermountain Health-

care and Group Health, each with established EHR systems, committed to share patient records through an open source and make available the infrastructure to all health care providers in the U.S. to ensure general interoperability and connectivity. To further systemic integration of health care delivery, national content and exchange standards as set out by government would be followed to allow for interoperability with government systems (KPMG International Cooperative, 2012).

Oliver notes that the U.S. Veterans Health Administration provides an open source, public domain adaptable platform to allow any health care institution to access at no cost the EHR system that was developed for their own use (the Veterans Health Information Systems and Technology Architecture). The system engages all U.S. veterans and was developed over two decades developing from a hospital-based to a broader health-care system over that period. It provides stored information on medical charting, provider orders and patient progress notes (Oliver, 2008).

Denmark has an advanced IT system through "a public web-based portal that collects and distributes key healthcare information to citizens and healthcare professionals, and empowers patients to access the healthcare system more effectively" (KPMG International Cooperative, 2012, p. 11). The interface is adaptable to the needs of specific users. Patients have their own unique webpage that allows access to diagnosis and treatment information, booking of appointments, secure emails to health providers, ordering medications, monitoring self-compliance with medication and access to disease management systems (KPMG International Cooperative, 2012).

The United Kingdom embarked on a nationwide EHR project in 2002. The program was intended to integrate patient records, prescription services, secure email communications and support archiving radiology images with the purpose of improving patient access to their health care providers and improve satisfaction with the service. However the project was delayed and scaled back in 2011, a result of insufficient clinical engagement, gaps in stakeholder expectations and problems with technology. The U.K. experience highlights the challenges in implementing EHRs. A critical component for successful implementation of the project involves the cooperation and collaboration between the various stakeholders. The differences in values, priorities and methodology between the political, clinical, academic, technical, and commercial players were a barrier to the ambitious initial expectations (KPMG International Cooperative, 2012).

The Australian state and territorial governments established a national authority to develop a system based on national standards for collecting, exchanging and securing health information. The intention from the outset was to attain full interoperability based on national standards. Engagement with all stakeholders was a strategic priority that fostered adoption and utilization (KPMG International Cooperative, 2012).

In 2011 Singapore began a coordination of information project of patient health care records that was available in providers' widely adopted individual EHR systems. The new National effort was to consolidate the information to form an integrated patient centred health care record that include diagnoses, allergies, immunizations, medications, treatment, referrals and care plans (KPMG International Cooperative, 2012).

The experience of the province of Ontario, Canada provides a cautionary tale. In 2002 the province of Ontario established the Smart Systems for Health Agency (SSHA) that was charged with overseeing the creation of a secure electronic network connecting the medical community. Between 2002 and 2008 approximately $1 billion was spent on this project (Office of the Auditor General of Ontario, 2009). In 2009 an audit by the Auditor General's office was released. It found that Ontario did not yet have an electronic record system that met the needs of health providers or the public. The report stated that the private IT network that was created remained underutilized because "there is insufficient health related information

on it" (Office of the Auditor General of Ontario, 2009, p. 8). No thought had been given to how this private network would provide secure access to the public. The Auditor General criticized the endeavor for its lack of upfront strategic planning and overall lack of effective oversight as well as unrealistic timelines, inadequate integration of various components of the system, the inability of the end product to meet user requirements and the lack of cost-effective management.

MACRO AND MICRO FACTORS IN THE SUCCESSFUL IMPLEMENTATION OF EHR TECHNOLOGY

EHR and PHR models are exceedingly complicated to create and implement. Venkatramen et al., observed:

[W]hile there are hundreds of vendors currently serving the EMR systems market, there is limited data standardization across these systems. Further, these systems are so fine-tuned and built for a specific function that integration with other systems (for example, computerized patient order entry systems [CPOE], automated drug dispensing systems [ADDS], and accounting/billing systems) becomes a nightmare (Venkatraman, Bala, Venkatesh, & Bates, 2008, p. 141).

Without proper protocols and planning the end result can be disappointing. Venkatraman et al. examined the VHA's IT systems and architecture and from this case study suggests six strategies to help in the development of EHR systems;

1. Develop a common operational database and application interface.
2. Use an interoperable system based on common standards and architecture to allow the seamless transfer of patient information.
3. Align clinical and administrative processes.

4. Develop a Web-based interface to allow access to patient data from any location.
5. Develop enterprise data warehouse and business intelligence systems as part of EHRs to allow for better clinical decisions and medical research.
6. Develop clinical decision support capabilities as part of EHR architecture (Venkatraman et al., 2008).

As important as the architecture and operational systems are to the successful use of EHRs, the actual process of implementation at the health provider's location is equally critical (Smith, 2003). Smith reported on the installation of an EHR system in a medical clinic. The ultimate success of the project was summarized by seven key factors;

- Clear definition of goals.
- Strong project leadership team to run the implementation.
- Project manager with sufficient, dedicated time.
- Strong physician leader to champion the project.
- Detailed analysis of work flow.
- High level of staff flexibility.
- Commitment to "plan for the worst; hope for the best" (Smith, 2003, p. 41).

Studer reviewed the literature examining the effect of organizational factors on successful EMR system implementation. A number of critical factors were identified:

1. Management support for the project and the communication of that support to the entire provider organization is essential.
2. A physician champion for the project must be identified.
3. Financial resources to purchase and implement the project and provide for ongoing maintenance must be budgeted. This must also include compensation for the reduction of productivity during and after implementation and financial incentives and rewards to members of the health provider team.
4. The organization must provide adequate initial and ongoing training for EHR system users and sufficient dedicated time must be scheduled for this training. This training must address any unrealistic expectations and emphasize the goals and benefits of the enterprise.
5. Ongoing and on-site technical support must be made available.
6. All members of the organization must have input in the design and implementation of the EHR system.
7. All physicians must be supportive of the goals, anticipated benefits and implementation process of the EHR system.
8. The system must be easy to learn and use and not interfere with the physician-patient interaction.
9. The system must have effective redundancy and backup safeguards (Studer, 2005).

It is only with sufficient planning and forethought that the implementation of a EHR system can be successfully achieved.

CONCLUSION

It is widely believed that the use of EHR's and PHR's will help provide better health care and do so more cost efficiently than present systems (Walker & Carayon, 2009). Witry et. al., state; "[D]evelopment of a national HIT [Health Information technology] infrastructure, including

Electronic Medical Records (EMRs), Personal Health Records (PHRs), and medical record interoperability, has the potential to increase efficiency, decrease medical errors, and improve healthcare quality" (Witry et. al., 2010). At this point in the development and implementation of IT systems these beliefs are largely unproven (Kaelber & Pan, 2008). Little in the way of case studies has shown that the potential is indeed realizable. It is imperative that further research be undertaken in the various components of EHR and PHR systems development. This would include efforts to perfect the architecture and interoperability of electronic health record technology. Case studies must be completed to demonstrate that cost efficiency and health improvement are real benefits of EHRs and PHRs. Many stakeholders are invested in the belief that these systems will be transformative in the provision of health care and controlling health costs. It is critical for the widespread adoption of EHRs and PHRs to show that these assumptions are valid.

REFERENCES

Archer, N., Fevrier, U., Lokker, C., McKibbon, K., & Straus, S. (2011). Personal health records: A scoping review. *Journal of the American Medical Informatics Association, 18,* 515–522. doi:10.1136/amiajnl-2011-000105 PMID:21672914.

Archer, N., & Fevrier-Thomas, U. (2010). An empirical study of Canadian consumer and physician perceptions of electronic personal health records. In *Proceedings of the Annual Conference, Administrative Sciences Association of Canada* (pp. 512-522). Regina, Canada: ASAC.

Asada, Y., & Kephart, G. (2007). Equity in health services use and intensity of use in Canada. *BMC Health Services Research.* doi:10.1186/1472-6963-7-41 PMID:17349059.

Beacom, A. M. (2010). Communicating health information to disadvantaged populations. *Family & Community Health, 33*(2), 152–162. doi:10.1097/FCH.0b013e3181d59344 PMID:20216358.

Begoyan, A. (2007). An Overview of interoperability standards for electronic health records. *Integrated Design and Process Technology,* 1-8.

Berk, M., & Monkeit, A. (2001). The concentration of health care expenditures, revisited. *Health Affairs, 20*(2), 9–18. doi:10.1377/hlthaff.20.2.9 PMID:11260963.

Blumenthal, D. (2009). Stimulationg the adoption of health information technology. *The New England Journal of Medicine, 260,* 1477–1479. doi:10.1056/NEJMp0901592.

Blumenthal, D., & Glasor, J. (2007). Information technology comes to medicine. *The New England Journal of Medicine, 356*(24), 2527–2534. doi:10.1056/NEJMhpr066212 PMID:17568035.

Bodenheimer, T., & Fernandez, A. (2005). High and rising health care costs: Part 4: Can costs be controlled while preserving quality? *Annals of Internal Medicine, 143*(1), 26–31. doi:10.7326/0003-4819-143-1-200507050-00007 PMID:15998752.

Bourgeois, F., Taylor, P., Emans, S., Nigrin, D., & Mandl, K. (2008). Whose personal control? Creating private, personally controlled health records for pediatric and adolescent patients. *Journal of the American Medical Informatics Association, 15*(6), 737–743. doi:10.1197/jamia.M2865 PMID:18755989.

Brown, S., Fischetti, L., Graham, G., Bates, J., Lancaster, A., McDaniel, D.,... Kolodner, R. (2007). Use of electronic health records in disaster response: The experience of department of veterans affairs after hurricaine Katrina. *American Journal of Public Health, 97*(S1), S136-S141. doi:102105/AJPH 2006.10494B

Buckley, B., Murphy, A., & MacFarlane, A. (2011). Public attitudes to the use in research of personal health information from general practitioners' records: a survey of the Irish general public. *Journal of Medical Ethics, 37*(1), 50–55. doi:10.1136/jme.2010.037903 PMID:21071570.

Chaudhry, B., Wang, J., We, S., Maglione, M., Mojica, W., Roth, E., & Morton, S. (2006). Systematic review: Impact of health information technology on quality, efficiency, and costs of medical care. *Annals of Internal Medicine, 144*, 742–752. doi:10.7326/0003-4819-144-10-200605160-00125 PMID:16702590.

Chen, C., Garrido, T., Chock, D., Okawa, G., & Liang, L. (2009). The kaiser permanente electronic health record: Transforming and streamlining modalities of care. *Health Affairs, 28*(2), 323–333. doi:10.1377/hlthaff.28.2.323 PMID:19275987.

Coffield, R., DeLoss, G., & Mooty, G. (2008). The rise of the personal health record: panacea or pitfall of health information. *Health Law News. University of Houston. Health Law and Policy Institute, 12*(10), 8–13.

Cushman, R., & Froomkin, A. (2010). Ethical, legal and social issues for personal health records and applications. *Journal of Biomedical Informatics, 43*(5), S51–S55. doi:10.1016/j.jbi.2010.05.003 PMID:20937485.

Denton, I. (2001). Will patients use electronic personal health records? Responses from a real-life experience. *Journal of Healthcare Information Management, 15*(3), 251–259. PMID:11642143.

Detmer, D., Raymond, B., Tang, P., & Bloomrosen, M. (2008). Integrated personal health records: transformative tools for consumer-centric care. *BMC Medical Informatics and Decision Making, 8*(45). doi: doi:10.1186/1472-6947-8-45 PMID:18837999.

Diamond, C., Mostashari, F., & Shirky, C. (2009). Collecting and sharing data for population health: A new paradigm. *Health Affairs, 28*(2), 454–466. doi:10.1377/hlthaff.28.2.454 PMID:19276005.

Dunn, K., & Wynia, M. (2010). Dreams and nightmares:practical and ethical issues for patients and physicians using personal health records. *The Journal of Law, Medicine & Ethics, 38*(1), 64–73. doi:10.1111/j.1748-720X.2010.00467.x PMID:20446985.

EHR4CR. (2011). *EHR4CR executive summary.* EHR4CR.

Eyserbach, G. (2008). Medicine 2.0: Social networking, collaboration, participation, apomediation, and openness. *Journal of Medical Internet Research, 10*(3), e22. doi:10.2196/jmir.1030 PMID:18725354.

Follen, M., Castaneda, R., Mikelson, M., Johnson, D., Wilson, A., & Higuchi, K. (2007). Implementing health information technology to improve the process of health care delivery: A case study. *Disease Management, 10*(4), 208–215. doi:10.1089/dis.2007.104706 PMID:17718659.

Forsyth, R., Maddock, C., Iedema, R., & Lassere, M. (2010). Patient perceptions of carrying their own health information: Approaches towards responsibility and playing an active role in their own health--Implications for a patient-held health file. *Health Expectations*, *13*(4), 416–426. doi:10.1111/j.1369-7625.2010.00593.x PMID:20629768.

Gans, D. (2005). Medical groups' adoption of electronic health records and information systems. *Health Affairs*, *24*(5), 1323–1333. doi:10.1377/hlthaff.24.5.1323 PMID:16162580.

Garde, S., Knaup, P., Hovenga, E., & Heard, S. (2007). Towards semantic interoperability for electronic health records: Domain knowledge governance for open EHR archetypes. *Methods of Information in Medicine*, *46*(3), 332–343. PMID:17492120.

Gaylin, D., Moiduddin, A., Mohamoud, S., Lundeen, K., & Kelly, J. (2011). Public attitudes about health information technology, and its relationship to health care quality, costs, and privacy. *Health Services Research*, *46*(3), 920–938. doi:10.1111/j.1475-6773.2010.01233.x PMID:21275986.

Halamka, J., Mandl, K., & Tang, P. (2008). Early experiences with personal health records. *Journal of the American Medical Informatics Association*, *15*(1), 1-7. doi:10.1197/jamia M2562

Hayrinen, K., Saranto, K., & Nykanen, P. (2008). Definition, structure, content, use and impacts of electronic records: A review of the research literature. *International Journal of Medical Informatics*, *77*(5), 291–304. doi:10.1016/j.ijmedinf.2007.09.001 PMID:17951106.

Hersh, W. (2004). Health care information technology: Progress and barriers. *Journal of the American Medical Association*, *292*(18), 2273–2274. doi:10.1001/jama.292.18.2273 PMID:15536117.

Heubusch, K. (2008). IT standards for PHRs: Are PHRs ready for standards? Are standards ready for PHRs? *Journal of American Health Information Management Association*, *79*(6), 31–36. PMID:18604973.

Hillestad, R., Bigelow, J., & Bower, A. (2005). Can electronic medical record systems transform health care? Potential health benefits, savings, and costs. *Health Affairs*, *24*, 1103–1117. doi:10.1377/hlthaff.24.5.1103 PMID:16162551.

Honeyman, A., Cox, B., & Fisher, B. (2005). Potential impacts of patients access to their electronic records. *Informatics in Primary Care*, *13*, 55–60. PMID:15949176.

Institute of Electrical & Electronics Engineers. (1990). *IEEE standard computer dictionary: A compilation of IEEE standard computer glossaries*. New York: IEEE.

Jensen, P., Jensen, L., & Brunak, S. (2012). Mining electronic health records: Towards better research applications and clinical care. *National Review*, *13*, 395–405. doi:10.1038/nrg3208 PMID:22549152.

Kaelber, D., Jha, A., Johnston, D., Middleton, B., & Bates, D. (2008). A research agenda for personal health records. *Journal of the American Informatics Association*, *15*(6), 729-736. doi:10.1197/jamia. M2547

Kaelber, D., & Pan, E. (2008). The value of personal health record (PHR) systems. In *Proceedings of AMIA Annual Symposium* (pp. 343-347). AMIA.

Kahn, J., Aulakh, V., & Bosworth, A. (2009). What it takes: Characteristics of the ideal personal health record. *Health Affairs, 28*(2), 369–376. doi:10.1377/hlthaff.28.2.369 PMID:19275992.

Kharrazi, H., Chisholm, R., VanNasdale, D., & Thompson, B. (2012). Mobile personal health records: An evaluation of features and functionality. *International Journal of Medical Informatics, 81*(9), 579–593. doi:10.1016/j.ijmedinf.2012.04.007 PMID:22809779.

Kim, M., & Johnson, K. (2002). Personal health records: evaluation of functionality and utility. *Journal of the American Medical Informatics Association, 9*(2), 171–180. doi:10.1197/jamia.M0978 PMID:11861632.

Koppel, R., Metlay, J., & Cohen, A. (2005). Role of computerized physician order entry systems in facilitating medical errors. *Journal of the American Medical Association, 293*, 1197–1203. doi:10.1001/jama.293.10.1197 PMID:15755942.

KPMG International Cooperative. (2012). *Accelerating innovation: The power of the crowd.* KPMG.

Lee, R., & Garvin, T. (2003). Moving from information transfer to information exchange in health and health care. *Social Science & Medicine, 56*, 449–464. doi:10.1016/S0277-9536(02)00045-X PMID:12570966.

Liederman, E., & Morefield, C. (2003). Web messaging: a new tool for patient-physician communication. *Journal of the American Medical Informatics Association, 10*, 260–270. doi:10.1197/jamia.M1259 PMID:12626378.

Lumpkin, J. (2007). Archimedes: A bold step into the future. *Health Affairs, 26*(2), w137–w139. doi:10.1377/hlthaff.26.2.w137 PMID:17259195.

Maloney, F., & Wright, A. (2010). USB-based personal health records: an analysis of features and functionality. *International Journal of Medical Informatics, 79*, 97–111. doi:10.1016/j.ijmedinf.2009.11.005 PMID:20053582.

Mandl, K., Kohame, I., & Brandt, A. (1998). Electronic patient-physician communication: problems and promise. *Annals of Internal Medicine, 129*, 495–500. doi:10.7326/0003-4819-129-6-199809150-00012 PMID:9735088.

Mandl, K., Szolovits, P., & Kohane, I. (2001). Public standards and patients' control: how to keep electronic medical records accessible but private. *British Medical Journal, 322*(7281), 283–287. doi:10.1136/bmj.322.7281.283 PMID:11157533.

Markle Connecting for Health. (2003). *Americans want benefits of personal health records.* New York: Markle Foundation.

Markle Connecting for Health. (2004). *Connecting Americans to their healthcaare: Final report of the working group on policies for electronic information sharing between doctors and patients.* New York: Markle Foundation.

Markle Connecting for Health. (2006). *Survey finds Americans want electronic personal health information to improve own health care.* New York: Markle Foundation.

McCally, M., Haines, A., Fein, O., Addington, W., Lawrence, R., & Cassel, C. (1998). Poverty and ill health: Physicians can and should make a difference. *Annals of Internal Medicine, 129*(9), 726–733. doi:10.7326/0003-4819-129-9-199811010-00009 PMID:9841606.

McCray, A. (2005). Promoting health literacy. *Journal of the American Medical Informatics Association, 12*, 153–163. PMID:15561782.

Menachemi, N., & Collum, T. (2011). Benefits and drawbacks of electronic health record systems. *Risk Management and Healthcare Policy, 4,* 47–55. doi:10.2147/RMHP.S12985 PMID:22312227.

Middleton, B., Hammond, W., Brennan, P., & Cooper, G. (2005). Accelerating U.S. EHR adoption: How to get there from here: Recommendations based on the 2004 ACMI retreat. *Journal of the American Medical Informatics Association, 12,* 13–19. doi:10.1197/jamia.M1669 PMID:15492028.

Miller, R., West, C., Brown, T., Sim, I., & Ganchoff, C. (2005). The value of electronic health records in solo or small group practices. *Health Affairs, 24,* 1127–1137. doi:10.1377/hlthaff.24.5.1127 PMID:16162555.

Office of the Auditor General of Ontario. (2009). *Ontario's electronic health records initiative, special report.* Toronto, Canada: Office of the Auditor General of Ontario.

Oliver, A. (2008). Public-sector health-care reforms that work? A case study of the US veterans health administration. *Lancet, 371*(9619), 1211–1213. doi:10.1016/S0140-6736(08)60528-0 PMID:18395583.

Page, D. (2010, September). The two paths to PHRs. *Hospital and Health Networks Magazine.*

Pagliari, C., Detmer, D., & Singleton, P. (2007). Potential of electronic personal health records. *British Medical Journal, 335*(7615), 330–333. doi:10.1136/bmj.39279.482963.AD PMID:17703042.

Pirtle, B., & Chandra, A. (2011). An overview of consumer perceptions and acceptance as well as barriers and potential of electronic personal health records. *American Journal of Health Sciences.*

Poon, E., Blumenthal, D., Jaggi, T. H. M., Bates, D., & Kaushal, R. (2004). Overcoming bariers to adopting and impementing computerized physician order entry systems in U.S. Hospitals. *Health Affairs, 23*(4), 184–190. doi:10.1377/hlthaff.23.4.184 PMID:15318579.

Poon, E., Jha, A., Christino, M., Honour, M., Fernandopulle, R., Middleton, B., & Kaushal, R. (2006). Assessing the level of healthcare information technology adoption in the United States: A snapshot. *BMC Medical Informatics and Decision Making, 6*(1). doi:10.1186/1472-6947-6-1 PMID:16396679.

Powell, J., Fitton, R., & Fitton, C. (2006). Sharing electronic health records: the patient view. *Informatics in Primary Care, 14,* 55–57. PMID:16848967.

Pyper, C., Amery, J., Watson, M., & Crook, C. (2004). Patients' experiences when accessing their on-line electronic patient records in primary care. *The British Journal of General Practice, 54,* 38–43. PMID:14965405.

Shekelle, P., Morton, S., & Keeler, E. (2006). *Costs and benefits of health information technology.* Rockville, MD: Agency for Healthcare Research and Quality.

Smith, P. (2003). Implementing an EMR system: One clinic's experience. *Family Practice Management, 10*(5), 37–42. PMID:12776405.

Steinbrook, R. (2008). Personally controlled online health data--The next big thing in medical care. *The New England Journal of Medicine, 358*(16), 1653–1656. doi:10.1056/NEJMp0801736 PMID:18420496.

Studer, M. (2005). The effect of organizational factors on the effectiveness of EMR system implementation--What have we learned? *Electronic Healthcare, 4*(2), 92–97.

Tang, P., Ash, J., Bates, D., Overhage, J., & Sands, D. (2006). Personal health records: Definitions, benefits, and strategies for overcomming barriers to adoption. *Journal of the American Medical Informatics Association, 13*(2), 121–126. doi:10.1197/jamia.M2025 PMID:16357345.

Tang, P., & Lansky, D. (2005). The missing link: Bridging the patient-provider health information gap. *Health Affairs, 24*, 1290–1295. doi:10.1377/hlthaff.24.5.1290 PMID:16162575.

Tang, P., & Lee, T. (2009). Your doctor's office or the internet? Two paths to personal health records. *The New England Journal of Medicine, 360*(13), 1276–1278. doi:10.1056/NEJMp0810264 PMID:19321866.

Taylor, R., Bower, A., Frederico, G., & Bigelow, J. (2005). Promoting health information technology: Is there a case for more-aggressive government action? *Health Affairs, 24*(5), 1234–1245. doi:10.1377/hlthaff.24.5.1234 PMID:16162568.

Venkatraman, S., Bala, H., Venkatesh, V., & Bates, J. (2008). Six strategies for electronic medical records systems. *Communications of the ACM, 51*(11), 140–144. doi:10.1145/1400214.1400243.

Waegemann, C. (2005). Closer to reality: Personal health records represent a step in the right direction for interoperability of healthcare IT systems and accessibility of patient data. *Health Management Technology, 26*, 16–18. PMID:15932068.

Wagstaff, A. (2002). Poverty and health sector inequalities. *Bulletin of the World Health Organization*, 97–105. PMID:11953787.

Walker, J., & Carayon, P. (2009). From tasks to processes: The case for changing health information technology to improve health care. *Health Affairs, 28*(2), 467–477. doi:10.1377/hlthaff.28.2.467 PMID:19276006.

Wang, S., Middleton, B., & Prosser, L. (2003). A cost-benefit analysis of electyronic medical records in primary care. *The American Journal of Medicine, 114*, 397–403. doi:10.1016/S0002-9343(03)00057-3 PMID:12714130.

Webster, P. (2010). United States to compel physicians to make meaningful use' of electronic health records. *Canadian Medical Association Journal, 182*(14), 1500–1502. doi:10.1503/cmaj.109-3361 PMID:20837690.

Weitzman, E., Kaci, L., & Mandl, K. (2010). Sharing medical data for health research: The early personal health record experience. *Journal of Medical Internet Research, 12*(2), e14. doi:10.2196/jmir.1356 PMID:20501431.

Weitzman, E., Kelemen, S., Kaci, L., & Mandl, K. (2012). Willigness to share personal health record data for care improvement and public health: A survey of experienced personal health record users. *BMC Medical Informatics and Decision Making, 12*(39). PMID:22616619.

West, S., Blake, C., Liu, Z., McKoy, J., Oertel, M., & Carey, T. (2009). Reflections on the use of electronic health record data for clinical research. *Health Informatics Journal*, *15*(2), 106–121. doi:10.1177/1460458209102972 PMID:19474224.

Witry, M., Doucette, W., Daly, J., Levy, B., & Chrischilles, E. (2010). Family physician perceptions of personal health records. *Perspectives in Health Information Management*, *7*(Winter), 1–12. PMID:20697465.

Wolter, J., & Friedman, B. (2005). Health records for the people: Touting the benefits of the consumer-based personal health record. *Journal of American Health Information Management Association*, *76*(10), 28–32. PMID:16333941.

Yamin, C., Emani, S., Williams, D., Lipsitz, S., Karson, A., Wald, J., & Bates, D. (2011). The digital divide in adoption and use of a personal health record. *Archives of Internal Medicine*, *171*(6), 568–574. doi:10.1001/archinternmed.2011.34 PMID:21444847.

Yau, G., Williams, A., & Brown, J. (2011). Family physicians' perspectives on personal health records. *Canadian Family Physician Medecin de Famille Canadien*, *57*(5), e178–e184. PMID:21642732.

ADDITIONAL READING

Bourgeois, F., Taylor, P., Emans, S., Nigrin, D., & Mandl, K. (2008). Whose personal control? Creating private, personally controlled health records for pediatric and adolescent patients. *Journal of the American Medical Informatics Association*, *15*(6), 737–743. doi:10.1197/jamia. M2865 PMID:18755989.

Buckley, B., Murphy, A., & MacFarlane, A. (2011). Public attitudes to the use in research of personal health information from general practitioners' records: a survey of the Irish general public. *Journal of Medical Ethics*, *37*(1), 50–55. doi:10.1136/jme.2010.037903 PMID:21071570.

Coffield, R., DeLoss, G., & Mooty, G. (2008). The rise of the personal health record: panacea or pitfall of health information. *Health Law News. University of Houston. Health Law and Policy Institute*, *12*(10), 8–13.

Cushman, R., & Froomkin, A. (2010). Ethical, legal and social issues for personal health records and applications. *Journal of Biomedical Informatics*, *43*(5), S51–S55. doi:10.1016/j.jbi.2010.05.003 PMID:20937485.

Follen, M., Castaneda, R., Mikelson, M., Johnson, D., Wilson, A., & Higuchi, K. (2007). Implementing health information technology to improve the process of health care delivery: A case study. *Disease Management*, *10*(4), 208–215. doi:10.1089/dis.2007.104706 PMID:17718659.

Gans, D. (2005). Medical groups' adoption of electronic health records and information systems. *Health Affairs*, *24*(5), 1323–1333. doi:10.1377/hlthaff.24.5.1323 PMID:16162580.

Gaylin, D., Moiduddin, A., Mohamoud, S., Lundeen, K., & Kelly, J. (2011). Public attitudes about health information technology, and its relationship to health care quality, costs, and privacy. *Health Services Research*, *46*(3), 920–938. doi:10.1111/j.1475-6773.2010.01233.x PMID:21275986.

Heubusch, K. (2008). IT standards for PHRs: are PHRs ready for standards? Are standards ready for PHRs? *Journal of American Health Information Management Association*, *79*(6), 31–36. PMID:18604973.

Hillestad, R., Bigelow, J., & Bower, A. (2005). Can electronic medical record systems transform health care? Potential health benefits, savings, and costs. *Health Affairs, 24*, 1103–1117. doi:10.1377/hlthaff.24.5.1103 PMID:16162551.

Honeyman, A., Cox, B., & Fisher, B. (2005). Potential impacts of patients access to their electronic records. *Informatics in Primary Care, 13*, 55–60. PMID:15949176.

Kharrazi, H., Chisholm, R., VanNasdale, D., & Thompson, B. (2012). Mobile personal health records: An evaluation of features and functionality. *International Journal of Medical Informatics, 81*(9), 579–593. doi:10.1016/j.ijmedinf.2012.04.007 PMID:22809779.

Kim, M., & Johnson, K. (2002). Personal health records: evaluation of functionality and utility. *Journal of the American Medical Informatics Association, 9*(2), 171–180. doi:10.1197/jamia.M0978 PMID:11861632.

Koppel, R., Metlay, J., & Cohen, A. (2005). Role of computerized physician order entry systems in facilitating medical errors. *Journal of the American Medical Association, 293*, 1197–1203. doi:10.1001/jama.293.10.1197 PMID:15755942.

Lee, R., & Garvin, T. (2003). Moving from information transfer to information exchange in health and health care. *Social Science & Medicine, 56*, 449–464. doi:10.1016/S0277-9536(02)00045-X PMID:12570966.

Liederman, E., & Morefield, C. (2003). Web messaging: A new tool for patient-physician communication. *Journal of the American Medical Informatics Association, 10*, 260–270. doi:10.1197/jamia.M1259 PMID:12626378.

Maloney, F., & Wright, A. (2010). USB-based personal health records: an analysis of features and functionality. *International Journal of Medical Informatics, 79*, 97–111. doi:10.1016/j.ijmedinf.2009.11.005 PMID:20053582.

Mandl, K., Kohame, I., & Brandt, A. (1998). Electronic patient-physician communication: Problems and promise. *Annals of Internal Medicine, 129*, 495–500. doi:10.7326/0003-4819-129-6-199809150-00012 PMID:9735088.

Mandl, K., Szolovits, P., & Kohane, I. (2001). Public standards and patients' control: How to keep electronic medical records accessible but private. *British Medical Journal, 322*(7281), 283–287. doi:10.1136/bmj.322.7281.283 PMID:11157533.

McCray, A. (2005). Promoting health literacy. *Journal of the American Medical Informatics Association, 12*, 153–163. PMID:15561782.

Middleton, B., Hammond, W., Brennan, P., & Cooper, G. (2005). Accelerating U.S. EHR adoption: How to get there from here: Recommendations based on the 2004 ACMI retreat. *Journal of the American Medical Informatics Association, 12*, 13–19. doi:10.1197/jamia.M1669 PMID:15492028.

Miller, R., West, C., Brown, T., Sim, I., & Ganchoff, C. (2005). The value of electronic health records in solo or small group practices. *Health Affairs, 24*, 1127–1137. doi:10.1377/hlthaff.24.5.1127 PMID:16162555.

Poon, E., Blumenthal, D., Jaggi, T. H. M., Bates, D., & Kaushal, R. (2004). Overcoming bariers to adopting and impementing computerized physician order entry systems in U.S. hospitals. *Health Affairs, 23*(4), 184–190. doi:10.1377/hlthaff.23.4.184 PMID:15318579.

Pyper, C., Amery, J., Watson, M., & Crook, C. (2004). Patients' experiences when accessing their on-line electronic patient records in primary care. *The British Journal of General Practice, 54,* 38–43. PMID:14965405.

KEY TERMS AND DEFINITIONS

Architecture Compatibility: Refers to the ability of the software components of EHR systems to work effectively together.

Business Intelligence System: A decision support system that transfers raw data into meaningful and useful information for the purpose of better decision-making and data analysis.

Capitation: System of payment for providing health care services that specifies a constant monthly amount for each patient regardless of how much care is provided.

Electronic Health Records (EHRs): Depositories of patient files in digital form created, stored and managed by health care providers or health institutions.

Enterprise Data Warehouse: A central repository of data created by integrating data from multiple sources that can be used for decision support in clinical decision-making and data mining for medical research.

Fee-For-Service: System of payment for providing health care services that specifies a fixed amount for each service provided.

Functional Harmonization: The exchange of data between different ERS systems that is readable by humans.

Interoperability: The ability to exchange information in digital form between various information sources.

Interoperative PHR: PHR that derives its content from all sources that is automatically transferred to a provider's EHR and patient PHR.

Personal Health Records (PHRs): Digital health records of an individual managed by that individual.

Semantic Harmonization: Exchange of data between EHR systems that is computer processable by the receiving system.

Tethered PHR: PHR that derives its content from information compiled and stored by the patient's health provider or health institution in their EHR system and is made available to the patient.

Section 2
Informatics and Health Policy Perspectives

Chapter 8
The Administrative Policy Quandary in Canada's Health Service Organizations

Grace I. Paterson
Dalhousie University, Canada

Jacqueline MacDonald
Annapolis Valley Health, South Shore Health and South West Health, Canada

Naomi Nonnekes Mensink
Dalhousie University, Canada

ABSTRACT

This chapter examines the process for administrative health service policy development with respect to information sharing and decision-making as well as the relationship of policy to decision making. The challenges experienced by health service managers are identified. The administrative health policy experience in Nova Scotia is described. There is a need for integrated policy at multiple levels (public, clinical, and administrative). The quandary is that while working to share health information systems, most Canadian health service organizations continue to individually develop administrative health policy, expending more resources on policy writing than on translation/education, monitoring, or evaluation. By exploring the importance and nature of administrative policy as a foundation for quality improvement in healthcare delivery, a case is made for greater use of health informatics tools and processes.

DOI: 10.4018/978-1-4666-4321-5.ch008

INTRODUCTION

In its simplest form, a policy tells people what to do and a procedure tells how to do it.(Cryderman, 1999, p. 17)

Policies provide structure to decisions. They allow consistent, informed decisions to be made about situations that have previously been encountered in health organizations, allowing clinicians, patients, users, and employees at any level to respond to a situation. Policies, based on the mission or purpose of the organization, provide the framework of objectives and measures that will allow decisions to be made and actions to be taken (Althaus, Bridgman, & Davis, 2007). Administrative policy is policy that: identifies the governing principle that enables or constrains decisions and action, is institution or group-wide, supports compliance with applicable law, and is mandated by the highest authority within the institution or group of institutions (University of Arizona, 2011).

According to the Canada Health Act, the primary objective of Canadian health care policy is "to protect, promote, and restore the physical and mental well-being of residents of Canada and to facilitate reasonable access to health services without financial or other barriers" (Nova Scotia Department of Health and Wellness, 2012, p. 9).

In this chapter, we explore the nature and purposes of administrative policy. We discuss the relationship of policy to decision making at both the administrative and clinical levels and the importance of well-developed policy for healthcare practice, as that relates to health information systems. We explore the importance and nature of administrative policy as a foundation for quality improvement in healthcare delivery through health informatics tools and processes such as electronic health records and health decision support systems; and for analysis for policy that focuses on the needs of policymakers.

We address the quandary that, while working to share health information systems, most Canadian health service organizations continue to individually develop administrative health policy, expending more resources on policy writing than on translation/education, monitoring or evaluation. Although policy can be most effective in bringing about improved health outcomes and organizational efficiencies, it is often difficult to see a relationship between health policy and health information systems. There is an absence of good policy-oriented data on which to base decisions. As an example, researchers found that Canada's wait-list information and management systems were inadequate and did not track outcomes to allow for continuous refinement of the criteria and weights used to prioritize patients in the wait-list policy (Lewis, Barer, Sanmartin, Sheps, Shortt, & McDonald, 2000). A systematic approach using health informatics skills and knowledge can empower policymakers to use data to develop policy, use information technologies to strategically communicate policy, and use outcomes data to monitor adherence to and effectiveness of policy.

Most research literature on health policy is concerned with public policy and clinical policy. There is a research-practice gap surrounding many aspects of administrative health policy (MacDonald, Bath, & Booth, 2008). The literature review for this chapter includes research on the relationship between policy and health informatics, and on health service managers' decision making at the administrative policy level. It focuses on what health service managers actually do rather than what they should do. We identify several challenges experienced by policymakers that provide opportunities for health informatics leadership and research. We also draw on experiences of OP3 (One Province, One Process, One Policy), a group working to share policies at the District Health Authority (DHA) level in Nova Scotia.

THE NATURE OF POLICY

With its many layers, health policy is more complex than "what to do" and "how to do it" (Cryderman, 1999, p. 17). The highest and most authoritative level is law or legislation. In Canada, the most general principles reside in the Canada Health Act where requirements for provincial and territorial government health service delivery are outlined. Each province or territory has legislation, such as the Nova Scotia Health Services and Insurance Act, that describes the "what". The regulations contained in the legislation describe the "how" with the attendant penalties listed. The process of passing Bills into laws is one of the main tasks of provincial legislative assemblies. A Bill becomes an Act, and thus provincial law, when it receives Royal Assent by the Lieutenant Governor. Acts are then translated into multi-organization policies for the levels of authority that apply the legislation to healthcare delivery in each geographic area or for specific patient groupings. The purpose of any policy is to guide corporate and individual decision-making at each level.

There is a complex set of historical, cultural, and socio-political forces that shape the policy environment (Bell, 2010). A fundamental policy assertion is that government should not solve a problem until it understands the problem. Being able to perceive the explicit, implicit and pragmatic dimensions of the policy problem is key to understanding the barriers and challenges associated with a particular policy goal and context.

Two frameworks for examining multi-layered health policy have been identified. Caldwell and Mays (2012) use macro-meso-micro frame analysis to study the transition of a policy from high-level idea to program in action where macro is national policy, meso is national programme and micro is local context. The Canadian Health Services Research Foundation (2000) identified three types of health policy decisions: public policy decisions that deal with determining what health services will be provided; administrative policy decisions that are concerned with operations including where specific health services will be located and how they will be offered; and clinical policy decisions that include determining criteria to identify who qualifies for specific services and how these services are to be managed. The informational uncertainty of clinicians is resolved more readily by research than is the informational uncertainty faced by government and managers (Canadian Health Services Research Foundation, 2000).

Provincial and federal governments, health researchers, and leaders of professional associations are more likely to be concerned with public policy and clinical policy than they are with administrative policy. Administrative and operating policies are more likely to be concerns at local levels, such as in hospitals and DHAs where, despite expected similarities, each health service organization has traditionally developed its own policy and procedure documents.

There has been little discussion in the literature of the differences between the above policy decision types and how they are integrated. There is a lack of understanding of their relationship with each other and with legislation and professional standards; and of whether the different types of health policy are best developed together or separately. It is not clear whether and how these policy decision types might relate to strategic, consequential, and far-reaching decisions; tactical, medium-range and moderate decisions that support strategic decisions; and operational decisions—the everyday decisions that support tactical decisions (Heller, Drenth, Koopman, & Rus, 1988).

RELATIONSHIP BETWEEN POLICY AND HEALTH INFORMATICS

As it pertains to curricula, the concept of "Health Informatics Policy" is usually considered to encompass topics such as leadership and ethics; information security; health communication; social implications of computing; and, negotiation and conflict resolution (Martz, Zhang, & Ozanich, 2007).

The form and characteristics of the system, the information exchange it enables, the permitted access and the permitted sharing are all based on policies within the organization or from multiple organizations that place enablers and constraints on the system since each participating organization has its own purposes. For example: who can enter prescriptions in a drug information system and whether the system is available near the bedside in a hospital (both policy based) often affects the quality of ordering and measurement of effectiveness. The policies, in turn, are based on the purpose and values of the organization. If improvement of patient health/condition is the over-riding purpose, health information systems have different characteristics and sharing procedures than if the over-riding purpose is risk management. Policies governing health information flow and use in one part of an organization may be different from those in another part of an organization based on unique purposes and constraints.

The concept of "Health Policy Informatics" as a subdiscipline of health informatics is emerging. It would tackle the challenges and problems arising from the multidimensional nature of information that is used for policy creation, dissemination, implementation, and evaluation; and would also address the challenges experienced by health service managers.

CHALLENGES EXPERIENCED BY HEALTH SERVICE MANAGERS

Knowledge Management

An organization's approach to knowledge management should be reflected in its culture, commitment to knowledge services, skills and use of information technology (Walton & Booth, 2004). The challenge is to ensure that information sys-tems are designed to enable clinical knowledge management—supporting clinicians (of any kind) with information about, critical analysis of, and learning-orientated dissemination of health related information about individuals and groups (Booth & Brice, 2004). A feedback loop that uses data from health records along with research evidence from clinical literature provides knowledge about what works in the local context (Zitner, Paterson, & Fay, 1998).

A study that examined health services managers' information behaviour found that managers rarely referenced external research-based information for their decision making. They were more often influenced by explicit organizational knowledge such as policies and guidelines (MacDonald, Bath, & Booth, 2008).

Multiple Communities of Practice

Policymakers need to address the multidimensional aspects of knowledge-making for policy (Bell, 2010). There are perspectival differences in how knowledge is acquired and understood by the multiple communities that are impacted by policy as described in the CHAMP (Clinicians, Health Informaticians, Administrators, Medical Educators, Patients) framework (Paterson, 2008). Communities of practice have vested interests in both the process and the outcomes. An assessment of needs should consider the advantage to be gained or lost in the planning process (Mensink, 2004). The authors' experience is that multiple communities of practice rarely work collaboratively to influence policy and legislation that affects all of them.

Researchers need to pay attention to the gaps in policy as these tell their own story. In Keshavjee et al.'s policy framework analysis for Electronic Medical Records (EMR), they acknowledge that policy at the macro (public policy) level lags client needs significantly (Keshavjee, Manji, Singh, & Pairaudeau, 2009). That framework focused on policies such as incentives for uptake of EMRs, engagement of key stakeholders from affected communities of practice, creation of suitable Information and Communication Technology (ICT) infrastructure, implementation of interoperability standards, and engagement of patients and their advocacy groups. To achieve interoperability with external systems in hospitals, laboratories and other health care provider communities, strong health information technology policies are required at the macro level.

Organizational Inertia

There are multiple and disparate processes for policy approval. A policy on the same topic, e.g., handheld devices, may come from multiple departments. In the experience of the authors, such policies may be identified as "universal" policy without reference to any approval process.

Embedding Policy in Information Systems

Whether or not to embed policy in information systems is a challenge, since an information system has a level of inertia inherent, such that it may continue to reflect outdated policy if no decision is made to systematically update it. This could lead to ignoring explicit policy because the current policy is not integrated with information systems and clinical workflow. This may result in workarounds by staff that are costly and a challenge to quality (Mensink & Paterson, 2010).

According to Grant et al., the health informatics research agenda should be dominated by the requirements for usable, useful and used systems (Grant, Moshyk, Kushniruk, & Moehr, 2003). If the effort needed to access policy resources at the clinician level is high, its usefulness will be diminished (Smith, 1996). A theoretical framework, the Normalisation Process Model, aims to identify factors that promote and inhibit the implementation of decision support technologies in routine practice (Elwyn, Légaré, van der Weijden, Edwards, & May, 2008).

There are programming challenges that may be difficult to overcome, including vendor agreements and information systems that do not fully fit with the purpose for which they were acquired. Collaboration is needed in the development and management of information resources to better ensure recognition of the differences in information structure and information needs based on varying philosophies of care and service as well as sites of care (Mohaghan & Cooke, 2004).

Protection of Health Information and Interprofessional Practice

A seamless integrated circle of care requires sharing of information across the settings of care, supported by legislation and policies at the local level. The regulatory and medico-legal barriers to interprofessional practice were identified (Lahey & Currie, 2005). Through collaboration between academics and policymakers the Regulated Health Professions Network Act was introduced (Lahey, 2012). Once passed, this legislation will enable interdisciplinary care and collaboration, and improve processes that may involve the different health professions involved in a patient's care (such as the investigation of a patient complaint for an adverse event, the sharing of competencies among the scopes of practice and the appeals process) (Wedlake, 2012). Policies that will be implemented need to be monitored to measure the impact of this Act.

At the macro level in Nova Scotia, the Personal Health Information Act, proclaimed on December 4, 2012 and effective June 1, 2013, "governs the collection, use, disclosure, retention, disposal and destruction of personal health information" (Nova Scotia Department of Health and Wellness, 2012). This act recognizes and supports the circle of care.

COACH, Canada's Health Informatics Association, publishes guidelines for the protection of health information. They state, "Health organizations must develop policies and procedures to protect the privacy, confidentiality, and security of personal health information under their control, to help mitigate the risk of unauthorized access, use or disclosure of such information, and to prevent against its loss or unnecessary destruction" (COACH, 2001). COACH publications are being continuously updated to align with changing legislation and new ways of delivering health information to patients and their caregivers.

Common Health Language

Policy committees need a standardized health glossary to achieve common policies and reduce the resource-intensive nature of administrative policy formulation. While there are medical dictionaries and online glossaries we are not aware of one that is specifically for health care professionals that melds written and spoken words and uses standardized health nomenclature that is grounded in a reference terminology. Access to a common language will support communication between professions, departments and health districts and help new health services staff. Use of a standardized health vocabulary is fundamental to both communications and information technology. It also enables semantic interoperability in ICT infrastructure (Paterson, 2008).

Generalization and Scaling Up of Policy

We need to pay systematic attention to how the benefits achieved in successful pilot or experimental projects can be expanded to serve more people more quickly and more equitably (Simmons & Shiffman, 2007). Policy is the articulation of

a government program. Program development requires an interactive, iterative, and process-oriented approach to be sustainable.

High-level policy may be overly detailed and rigid, creating challenges for those who are tasked with implementing those policies locally. Such policies may require elements or processes that may not be available locally. However, these high level policies do have the advantage of authority and support. "In contrast, decentralized approaches allow local initiative, autonomy, spontaneity, mutual learning and problem-solving. Their obvious disadvantage is that they do not have the reach of central authorities, and often do not command sufficient influence or resources to ensure appropriate policy reform" (Simmons & Shiffman, 2007, p. 15).

Since electronic information sharing has such a broad reach, central principles concerning this have to be clear and universally applied. This is especially true of information that is used for overall program quality management where policies and practices have to be consistent across different settings.

Creating/Developing a Learning Organization

A learning organization is one that creates and uses administrative policy to best manage changing conditions, and is not rigidly bound by rules that emphasize standardization (Simmons & Shiffman, 2007). Administrators of health information systems are responsible for enabling clinical care. They need to ensure that clinical knowledge management systems are available for clinicians and their patients where and when needed.

Despite lots of education and public discussion about the concept of a multi-disciplinary team involvement in care, formal hospital-based medical records that are used as a basis for sharing information with other clinicians may contain only information that has been approved by a central administrative committee that is primarily responsible for the legal status of the health record (Capital Health, 2011). Because of this approval process, there may be little information retained on the shared record from members of the team who are not hospital-based health practitioners. Examples include external (to the hospital) physiotherapists, family counselors, family caregivers and service staff who may have made important observations about the patient or been the most frequent confidant of the patient's wishes when in hospital. This affects not only the total care provided but also the richness of information available to researchers and others for quality improvement.

Shared Administrative Health Policy Development, Implementation, and Evaluation

There is an opportunity for efficiency if multiple organizations share policies. There must be a policy development framework with capacity, authority, and resourcing to achieve province-wide policy development, approval and distribution. In addition, policy readers need to be queried about their policy documentation needs and uses, and the barriers and challenges they encounter in finding and using institutional level policies.

Results arising from an evaluation of the effectiveness of program may identify policy issues. An independent evaluation of the Summary Care Records and HealthSpace programs in the UK (Greenhalgh, Hinder, Stramer, Bratan, & Russell, 2010) led to the closing of HealthSpace—a free, secure online health organizer—on December 14, 2012 and the destruction of all data in compliance with the Data Protection Act (NHS Connecting for Health, 2012). The findings raised questions about how this eHealth program in England was

developed and approved at the policy level. The evaluation revealed that the benefits anticipated by policy makers were not achieved.

HEALTH SERVICE MANAGERS, ADMINISTRATIVE POLICY, AND DECISION MAKING

Health services have been described as the most complex of organizations to manage (Glouberman & Mintzberg, 2001). Elsewhere they are referred to as "high velocity" environments "in which there is rapid and discontinuous change ... such that information is often inaccurate, unavailable, or obsolete" (Stephanovich & Uhrig, 1999, p. 198). Within this environment, health service managers are accountable for health service quality, resource use, employee effectiveness and wellbeing, and workplace safety and productivity.

Little research directly related to administrative health policy development has been identified. A mixed-methods study of 116 Australian health administrators' policy-related decision making practices used interviews and surveys to explore resource allocation decision situations (Baghbanian, Hughes, Kebriaei, & Khavarpour, 2012). Conclusions included that policy makers were "enlightened by" research that reached them indirectly. Managers made policy decisions by involving others with knowledge of the situation rather than by following formal procedures and reading primary research or systematic reviews. Decisions were characterized by ambiguity and complexity, short deadlines, incomplete information and significant unknowns. A UK study that used 21 interviews, document analysis and embedded research to assess understanding about national (macro level) policy translated to programs (meso level) and implemented locally (micro level) attributed differences to local contexts and different approaches to knowledge translation and concluded that a common understanding of purpose and objectives contributed to success (Caldwell & Mays, 2012).

Research on what health service managers actually do includes ten workplace studies of their information and decision making behavior. Five studies of health service managers and their workplace information access and use, each conducted in a different country and with a slightly different focus, found similar challenges related to information access and use (Head, 1996; Kovner & Rundall, 2006; Mbananga & Sekokotla, 2002; Moahi, 2000; Niedźwiedzka, 2003) despite difference in the wealth of the country (G8 or not), degree of computerization (desktop access to databases and the Internet, or not), single hospital or multi-site health service, and health service funding (whether public or private). These studies observed the importance of internal or local information to healthcare services. An additional five other studies of health service managers in their workplaces shared the finding that much of their work time was spent in meetings (Arman, Dellve, Wikström, & Törnström, 2009; Baghbanian, Hughes, Kebriaei, & Khavarpour, 2012; MacDonald, 2011; Moss, 2000; Tengelin, Arman, Wikström, & Delive, 2011).

The remaining literature on health service managers has tended to focus either on what they should do (Gray, 2009; Innvaer, Vist, Trommald, & Oxman, 2002; Innvær, 2009) or why they do not do what they should do (Kadane, 2005; Willis, Mitton, Gordon, & Best, 2012).

We do not know the cost to a health service organization of developing a single administrative policy or the potential return on investment of shared administrative policy development. OP3 members individually estimated the number of employees involved and the time needed to complete each task in the policy process model used by OP3. When tasks were totaled, the cost of developing a policy ranged from $10,000 to $200,000 with legal advice a factor contributing to higher policy development costs.

No research has been identified that explores how administrative policy decisions are made, how administrative policies are used or who uses them, whether policy development practices might be improved, or what the costs and benefits of shared policies are. Further research is needed to know whether problems solved and decisions made at health service managers meetings are shared within the organization and how they are shared, whether informally (either orally or through email) or formally (as administrative policy to support structured decision making).

ADMINISTRATIVE HEALTH POLICY IN CANADA

Through the 1980s and 1990s, Canadian hospitals were guided through policy and procedure manual development by Paula Cryderman (Cryderman, 1987). By the end of the 1990s, Cryderman recommended an overhaul to hospital policy manuals, citing forces of change that rendered manuals obsolete (Cryderman, 1999).

The Canadian Policy and Procedure Network (CPPN) has served since 2004 as "an informal forum for health care professionals to share and discuss policy and procedure topics for the improvement of health care" (Canadian Policy and Procedure Network, 2010). The CPPN is a moderated Yahoo Group with over 200 members. Members post an average 2,500 policy questions and requests for examples of policy and procedure documents per year.

The Canadian Association for Health Services and Policy Research (CAHSPR) is Canada's largest health services and policy research association. CAHSPR holds an annual conference and uses social media tools, such as Twitter, to build a community working towards evidence-based health care and health policy. "CAHSPR's mission is to improve health and health care by advancing the quality, relevance and application of research on health services and health policy" (Canadian

Association for Health Services and Policy Research, 2012). Annual conferences feature policy forums and panel discussions which encourage true dialogue and debate. Citizen participation is important to a democracy and to the development of health policies that reflect the type of society that citizens want.

Accreditations Canada has performance indicators to measure the degree to which a health care facility delivers health care services according to criteria. Personnel in charge of administrative health policy are often the ones who participate in the assessment, which makes visible to the reviewers how well a facility abides by its health policies. As part of the dissemination of knowledge, Accreditations Canada developed a searchable Leading Practices Database to recognize innovative solutions to improving the quality of healthcare services delivery (Accreditations Canada, 2012).

ADMINISTRATIVE HEALTH POLICY EXPERIENCE IN NOVA SCOTIA, 2007-2012

In 2005, recognizing the resource-intensive complexity of policy development within their DHAs, Chief Executive Officers (CEOs) of Nova Scotia's nine DHAs and the Izaak Walton Killam Health Centre (IWK, pediatric and obstetric health centre for the Maritime Provinces) commissioned a feasibility study of shared policy development. The study identified fifteen opportunities for efficiencies with shared policies (Table 1).

In response to the study, the DHA/IWK CEOs established a working group in 2007, initially with one representative from each organization. The group expanded to include representatives from the Nova Scotia Department of Health and Wellness Policy and Planning Branch, and from the Health Association of Nova Scotia Policy, Planning and Decision Support Unit. All members of this group, known as OP3, have full time responsibilities in their own organization. Two guides, Policy Development, Implementation and Evaluation (Capital Health, 2012) and Style Guide, provide standard approaches to writing and formatting policy documents (OP3: One Province, One Process, One Policy, 2011).

By the fall of 2012, the group accomplished five of the fifteen opportunities for efficiency (numbers 5, 8. 12, 13, and 14 in Table 1) including coordinated archiving and storage in the form of a Web-based platform for shared policy management (http://policy.nshealth.ca/). In 2012, although policy manuals for most DHAs remain

Table 1. Opportunities for efficiency for NS DHAs/IWK in shared policy development

Coordinated Policy Processes	Coordinated Policy Structures	Coordinated Policy Skills and Competencies	Coordinated Policy Technology/ Enablers
1. Coordinated issue identification. 2. Centralized research support. 3. Centralized policy development. 4. Centralized communication and education content development. 5. Coordinated archiving and storage. 6. Coordinated compliance monitoring. 7. Provincial coordination of practice guidelines and procedures.	8. Formalize the policy 'community of interest' or network. 9. Leverage existing provincial committees. 10. Create new policy development committees.	11. Provincial Policy researcher/ coordinator.	12. Common policy templates and formats. 13. Collaboration tools. 14. Document management tools. 15. Access to Common templates.

incomplete, an average of 500 policies per DHA is available on the site. Some DHAs have over 1,000 policies on the OP3 site.

In 2011, to inform strategic planning, OP3 members began considering evaluation of both group and policy process. A review of meeting minutes identified 45 tasks in the policy process that might be evaluated (Appendix A). To help explain the administrative policy development process to a DHA Policy Committee willing to develop a pilot evaluation survey, these 45 tasks

were grouped under 15 main headings, and arranged graphically as cogs in a policy process cycle (Figure 1).

In an effort to build a business case for a single office in Nova Scotia, OP3 members are considering how to best estimate or track the cost of developing a single policy in one DHA. Research is required to accurately calculate this cost. A suggested approach is to ask OP3 members to consider an estimated cost for a sample of policies in each DHA. By considering each of the 45 tasks

Figure 1. Administrative policy process: graphic representation of steps in the OP3 shared policy development process (©South Shore Health Authority and used with permission)

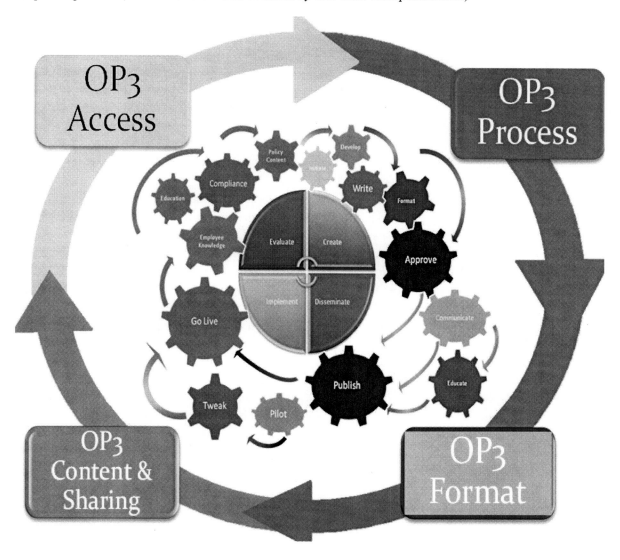

listed in Appendix A, OP3 members could estimate or track: 1) whether the task is routine in a DHA, 1a) if it is not routine, whether the member believes the task should be routine or 1b) if the task is routine, the number of employees typically engaged in the task, and 2) the average length of time required of a single employee engaged in the task.

DISCUSSION

Using the experience of one author with the OP3 working group process described above, we identified four particularly challenging areas that could benefit from an increased role of health informatics in health policy and management. We also discuss two additional areas where there is a relationship between health informatics research and administrative policy development at the health services level.

The Research Practice Gap

Managers need research to provide solutions to their problems rather than explanations of why things happen or instruction telling them what not to do. This "relevance gap" where either the research subjects or focus are not relevant to managers' needs has been suggested as the reason why managers make little use of research (Davies, 2006). Labadie uses the metaphor of a burning house to show how different the cultures are: "Decision makers put out fires, and researchers want to let the fire burn to understand how it spreads" (Labadie, 2005).

The research practice gap with respect to health policy generally, and in health informatics research specifically, can be expressed by the lack of administrative health policy research in several areas that impede OP3 working group progress.

A Variety of Sources for Rules

The relationship between provincial and federal legislation related to health, public health policy, clinical health policy, administrative health policy, professional standards, clinical competencies and practice guidelines is not clear. Typically various document types exist to address a subject, each created independently without reference to the others, each with their own sets of definitions and references. Administrative policy, intended to give clear policy guidance to practicing health professionals within a particular setting, must address local context while taking into consideration the full array of other influencing policies, practice guidelines and practice standards. This can leave health professionals and administrators confused so that they must rely on their own best judgment and hope that it is consistent with the purposes of the organization, congruent with current research and compliant with legislation and other rules.

Policy Contributor and Policy Approver

In the experience of the authors, the difference between the roles of these two stakeholder groups is not always clear and there is no system to support effective management of contributions and approvals. Historically, in single site health service organizations, tracking contributions during policy development has been accomplished through a printed one page tracking sheet. This documentation is handled separately from the approval process, with approvals managed through signatures on the original copies of printed policies. Multi-site, multi-organizational shared policy development requires an automated system or mechanism to track contributions from various sites and groups. There is a need to clarify for each policy the level of approval necessary for implementation in each organization and track whether that approval has been granted.

Shared Health Policy Language

A review of the 400 publicly available policies available on the OP3 policy site in April 2011 identified >1,000 terms defined within the policies. Some of these terms had as many as 18 different definitions created independently by the policy writer with inconsistencies between and within departments and DHAs. A study by a graduate student completed in 2012 identified terms defined as clinical, technical, administrative and general (Phinney, MacDonald, & Spiteri, 2012). The study concluded that of 26 potential policy languages examined, the best source of definitions for the variety of administrative health policy terms in Nova Scotia administrative health policies on the OP3 site was the Unified Medical Language System (U.S. National Library of Medicine, 2012). The best way to introduce and implement a standard language has not been identified.

A Critical Conflict Inherent in Health Informatics Policy: Privacy of Health Information

Health informatics policy implicitly affects two core values within healthcare delivery. One is the practice of patient-centered, collaborative healthcare through all parts and among all providers within the healthcare system. The other is protecting the privacy of patient information. Health informatics provides the tools, mechanisms and processes to share critical patient and patient-care information among the full range of healthcare providers and others critical to care and well-being of the patient. It also provides ready access to clinical research for evidence-based practice. Ideally, this information is also shared with the patient (or patient proxy) so that the patient is the

driver of his/her own health care. Appropriately applied, health informatics methods reduce the risk of "private" information becoming known to others outside of the care network.

Risk management is an important consideration. The risk of unwanted publicity or legal action against care providers and health organizations on the basis of information available must be managed through health informatics processes based on health informatics policy.

The Role of Administrative Health Policy in Education and Innovation

Another core value inherent in health care is that of innovation: continuous exploration into the best ways to deliver healthcare through complex systems of organizations and professionals. A sound health informatics policy encourages exploration and innovation by providing a statement of principles/values that encourages both exploration and its careful management. Such a policy also includes guidance and processes on introduction and integration of innovations, in care and professional practice, into the work of the organization and its associated care providers. Current areas of administrative innovation in this area are the use and dissemination of electronic health records, both within the organization and among related community healthcare providers.

Along with innovation (the introduction of new concepts and practices) comes the need for continuous learning among those who must change their practice and processes. Sound administrative policy related to health informatics and health information systems provides the framework and guidelines for what needs to be learned. Part of the administrative practice would then be to collaboratively learn new or varying practice principles and patterns. By learning together, administrative and clinical professionals discover the areas of potential challenge. By working through those challenges together in a continuous learning environment, the result is improved practice and health outcomes. Health services will be enabled by health information systems based on policy at all three levels: public, clinical and administrative.

CONCLUSION

The introduction and use of health information systems throughout health organizations and among members of multi-site organizations is still considered innovative. Health service organizations experience continuing change in practice and administration. Organization-wide innovations often require lengthy periods of time and iterative processes to accomplish (Rogers, 1983). Cost-effective shared administrative policy development to provide clear overall guidance for health services and for health informatics solutions designed to support health services is essential.

ACKNOWLEDGMENT

We acknowledge the assistance of Angela Clifton, South Shore Health Authority, for work on the administrative policy development cycle and task list. The work of the 2012 OP3 Working Group members is also acknowledged.

REFERENCES

Accreditations Canada. (2012). *Leading practice: Recognizing innovation and creativity in Canadian health care delivery*. Retrieved 12 16, 2012, from http://www.accreditation.ca/news-and-publications/publications/leading-practices/

Althaus, C., Bridgman, P., & Davis, G. (2007). *The Australian policy handbook* (4th ed.). Sydney, Australia: Allen & Unwin.

Arman, R., Dellve, L., Wikström, E., & Törnström, L. (2009). What health care managers do: Applying Mintzberg's structured observation method. *Journal of Nursing Management, 17*(6), 718–729. doi:10.1111/j.1365-2834.2009.01016.x PMID:19694915.

Baghbanian, A., Hughes, I., Kebriaei, A., & Khavarpour, F. A. (2012). Adaptive decision-making: How Australian healthcare managers decide. *Australian Health Review, 36*(1), 49–56. doi:10.1071/AH10971 PMID:22513020.

Bell, E. (2010). *Research for health policy*. Oxford, UK: Oxford University Press.

Booth, A., & Brice, A. (2004). Knowledge management. In Walton, G., & Andrew, B. (Eds.), *Exploiting knowledge in health services*. London, UK: Facet Publishing.

Caldwell, S. E., & Mays, N. (2012). Studying policy implementation using a macro, meso and micro frame analysis: The case of the collaboration for leadership in applied health research & care (CLAHRC) programme nationally and in North West London. *Health Research Policy and Systems, 10*(1), 32. doi:10.1186/1478-4505-10-32 PMID:23067208.

Canadian Association for Health Services and Policy Research. (2012). *About CAHSPR*. Retrieved 12, 16, 2012, from https://cahspr.ca/en/about

Canadian Health Services Research Foundation. (2000). *Health services research and evidence-based decision-making*. Ottawa, Canada: Canadian Health Services Research Foundation.

Canadian Policy and Procedure Network. (2010). *Canadian policy & procedure network*. Retrieved 12, 16, 2012, from http://ca.groups.yahoo.com/group/cppn/

Capital Health. (2011). *Health record forms management*. Retrieved from http://policy.nshealth.ca/Site_Published/DHA9/document_render.aspx?documentRender.IdType=6&documentRender.GenericField=&documentRender.Id=34962

Capital Health. (2012). *Policy development, implementation and evaluation*. Retrieved 12 16, 2012, from http://policy.nshealth.ca/Site_Published/DHA9/document_render.aspx?documentRender.IdType=6&documentRender.GenericField=&documentRender.Id=17121

COACH. (2001). *Guidelines for the protection of health information*. Edmonton, Canada: COACH - Canada's Health Informatics Association.

Cryderman, P. (1987). *Developing policy and procedure manuals*. Ottawa, Canada: Canadian Hospital Association.

Cryderman, P. (1999). *Customized manuals for changing times*. Ottawa, Canada: CHA Press.

Davies, H. (2006). Improving the relevance of management research: Evidence-based management: Design, science or both? *Business Leadership Review, 3*(3), 1–6.

Elwyn, G., Légaré, F., van der Weijden, T., Edwards, A., & May, C. (2008). Arduous implementation: Does the normalisation process model explain why it's so difficult to embed decision support technologies for patients in routine clinical practice. *Implementation Science; IS, 3*(1), 57. doi:10.1186/1748-5908-3-57 PMID:19117509.

Glouberman, S., & Mintzberg, H. (2001). Managing the care of health and the cure of disease-Part II: Integration. *Health Care Management Review, 26*(1), 70–84. doi:10.1097/00004010-200101000-00007 PMID:11233356.

Grant, A. M., Moshyk, A. M., Kushniruk, A., & Moehr, J. R. (2003). Reflections on an arranged marriage between bioinformatics and health informatics. *Methods of Information in Medicine, 42*(2), 116–120. PMID:12743646.

Gray, J. A. (2009). *Evidence-based healthcare and public health: How to make decisions about health services and public health*. London: Elsevier Health Sciences.

Greenhalgh, T., Hinder, S., Stramer, K., Bratan, T., & Russell, J. (2010). Adoption, non-adoption, and abandonment of a personal electronic health record: Case study of HealthSpace. *British Medical Journal, 341*, c5814. doi:10.1136/bmj.c5814 PMID:21081595.

Head, A. L. (1996). *An examination of the implications for NHS information providers of staff transferring from functional to managerial roles*. Aberystwyth, UK: University College of Wales.

Heller, F. P., Drenth, P., Koopman, P., & Rus, V. (1988). *Decisions in organizations: A three county comparative study*. London: Sage.

Innvær, S. (2009). The use of evidence in public governmental reports on health policy: An analysis of 17 Norwegian official reports (NOU). *BMC Health Services Research, 9*(1), 177. doi:10.1186/1472-6963-9-177 PMID:19785760.

Innvaer, S., Vist, G., Trommald, M., & Oxman, A. (2002). Health policy-makers' perceptions of their use of evidence: A systematic review. *Journal of Health Services Research & Policy, 7*(4), 239–244. doi:10.1258/135581902320432778 PMID:12425783.

Kadane, J. B. (2005). Bayesian methods for health-related decision making. *Statistics in Medicine, 24*(4), 563–567. doi:10.1002/sim.2036 PMID:15678444.

Keshavjee, K., Manji, A., Singh, B., & Pairaudeau, N. (2009). Failure of electronic medical records in Canada: A failure of policy or a failure of technology? In McDaniel, J. G. (Ed.), *Advances in Information Technology and Communication in Health* (pp. 107–114). Amsterdam: IOS Press BV.

Kovner, A. R., & Rundall, T. G. (2006). Evidence-based management reconsidered. *Frontiers of Health Services Management, 22*(3), 3–22. PMID:16604900.

Labadie, J.-F. (2005). Inter-regional front-line services knowledge brokering alliance. In *Proceedings of the Fourth Annual National Knowledge Brokering Workhop* (p. 8). Retrieved from http://www.cfhi-fcass.ca/migrated/pdf/event_reports/National_Workshop_Report_2005_e.pdf

Lahey, W. (2012, November 29). Collaboration vital to better health care, improved regulation. *The Chronicle Herald.*

Lahey, W., & Currie, R. (2005). Regulatory and medico-legal barriers to interprofessional practice. *Journal of Interprofessional Care, 19*(S1), 197–223. doi:10.1080/13561820500083188 PMID:16096156.

Lewis, S., Barer, M. L., Sanmartin, C., Sheps, S., Shortt, S. E., & McDonald, P. W. (2000). Ending waiting-list mismanagement: Principles and practice. *Canadian Medical Association Journal, 162*, 1297–1300. PMID:10813011.

MacDonald, J., Bath, P., & Booth, A. (2008). Healthcare services managers: What information do they need and use? *Evidence Based Library and Information Practice, 3*(3), 18–38.

MacDonald, J. M. (2011). *The information sharing behaviour of health service managers: A three-part study.* (Unpublished PhD Dissertation). Sheffield, UK: University of Sheffield Information School.

Martz, B., Zhang, X., & Ozanich, G. (2007). Information systems and healthcare XIV: Developing an integrative health informatics. *Communications of AIS, 19.*

Mbananga, N., & Sekokotla, D. (2002). *The utilisation of health management information in Mpumalanga Province.* Retrieved from http://www. hst. org. za/research

Mensink, N., & Paterson, G. (2010). The evolution and uptake of a drug information system: The case of a small Canadian province. *Studies in Health Technology and Informatics, 160*(Pt 1), 141–145. PMID:20841666.

Mensink, N. M. (2004). *Facilitating the development of a graduate-level university program using processes and principles of adult education.* (Unpublished MAdEd thesis). St. Francis Xavier University, Antigonish, Canada.

Moahi, K. H. (2000). *A study of the information behavior of health care planners, managers and administrators in Botswana and implications for the design of a national health information system (NHIS).* (Unpublished PhD dissertation). University of Pittsburgh, Pittsburgh, PA.

Mohaghan, V., & Cooke, J. (2004). The health and social care context. In Walton, G., & Andrew, B. (Eds.), *Exploiting knowledge in health services* (p. 16). London: Facet Publishing.

Moss, L. J. (2000). *Perceptions of meeting effectiveness in the capital health region.* (Unpublished MA thesis). Royal Roads University, Victoria, Canada.

NHS Connecting for Health. (2012). *HealthSpace.* Retrieved 12, 16, 2012, from http://www.connectingforhealth.nhs.uk/systemsandservices/healthspace

Niedźwiedzka, B. (2003). A proposed general model of information behaviour. *Information Research, 9*(1), Paper 164.

Nova Scotia Department of Health and Wellness. (2012,). *Overview and discussion paper, health services and insurance act.* Retrieved 12, 16, 2012, from http://www.gov.ns.ca/health/hsil/doc/ OverviewDiscussionDocument.pdf

Nova Scotia Department of Health and Wellness. (2012). *Personal health information act.* Retrieved 12, 16, 2012, from https://www.gov. ns.ca/dhw/phia/

OP3: One Province, One Process, One Policy. (2011). *Style guide for writers and developers of NS DHA and IWK policy documents.* Retrieved 12 16, 2012, from http://policy.nshealth.ca/Site_Published/ dha9/document_render.aspx?documentRender. IdType=5&documentRender.Id=29030

Paterson, G. I. (2008). *Boundary infostructures for chronic disease: Constructing infostructures to bridge communities of practice.* Saarbrücken, Germany: VDM Verlag Dr. Muller.

Phinney, J., MacDonald, J. M., & Spiteri, L. (2012). *A health policy language for Nova Scotia: A Dalhousie school of information management reading course project.* Paper presented at APLA 2012: Discovering Hidden Treasures. Wolfville, Canada.

Rogers, E. M. (1983). *Diffusion of innovations* (3rd ed.). New York: Free Press.

Simmons, R., & Shiffman, J. (2007). Scaling up health service inovations: A framework for action. In Simmons, R., Fajans, P., & Ghiron, L. (Eds.), *Scaling up health services delivery from pilot innovations to policies and programmes* (pp. 1–30). Geneva, Switzerland: World Health Organization.

Smith, R. (1996). What clinical information do doctors need? *British Medical Journal, 313*(7064), 1062–1068. doi:10.1136/bmj.313.7064.1062 PMID:8898602.

Stephanovich, P. L., & Uhrig, J. D. (1999). Decision making in high-velocity environments: Implications for healthcare. *Journal of Healthcare Management, 44*(3), 195–205.

Tengelin, E., Arman, R., Wikström, E., & Delive, L. (2011). Regulating time commitments in healthcare organizations: Managers' boundary approaches at work and in life. *Journal of Health Organization and Management, 25*(5), 578–599. PMID:22043654.

University of Arizona. (2011). *Administrative policy formulation.* Retrieved 12, 16, 2012, from http://policy.arizona.edu/policy-formulation

U.S. National Library of Medicine. (2012). *Unified medical language system (UMLS®).* Retrieved 12, 16, 2012, from http://www.nlm.nih.gov/ research/umls/

Walton, G., & Booth, A. (2004). *Exploiting knowledge in health services.* London: Facet Publishing.

Wedlake, S. (2012). *Law amendments bill 147 - An act respecting the Nova Scotia regulated health professions network.* Retrieved 12, 16, 2012, from http://nslegislature.ca/pdfs/committees/61_4_LAC-Submissions/20121129/20121129-147-03.pdf

Willis, C. D., Mitton, C., Gordon, J., & Best, A. (2012). System tools for system change. *BMJ Quality & Safety, 21*(3), 250–262. doi:10.1136/ bmjqs-2011-000482 PMID:22129934.

Zitner, D., Paterson, G. I., & Fay, D. F. (1998). Methods for identifying pertinent and superfluous activity. In Tan, J. (Ed.), *Health Decision Support Systems* (pp. 177–197). New York: Aspen Publishers, Inc..

KEY TERMS AND DEFINITIONS

Data Quality Framework: Aggregation of data from individual patient records to fulfill data requirements for measuring patient and population health and health system performance.

eHealth: Health care practice which is supported by electronic information and communication systems.

Health Data Standards: Standards developed by international standards organizations and adopted or adapted by Canada's Standards Collaborative to determine how health data is classified or grouped, and how it is encoded in machine-readable representation for electronic manipulation.

Health Informatics Policies: Explicit statements directing how to address issues that arise with the introduction of information technology into the health system, including topics such as ethics; information security and privacy; interoperability; health communication; social implications of computing; and, quality, risk and patient safety.

Health Organization Models: Health organization models of care delivery vary based on the philosophies of care and service as well as sites of care and use of multi-disciplinary care teams.

Health Policy Informatics: A subdiscipline of health informatics that addresses challenges experienced by health service managers and other policymakers and problems that arise from the multidimensional nature of information used for policy creation, dissemination, implementation and evaluation.

Knowledge Management: Aims to leverage the intellectual capital held in the skills and expertise of personnel so that the knowledge that is critical to them is made available in the most effective manner to those people who need it so that it can add value as a normal part of work.

Policy Implementation: Policy management across the lifecycle including release, communication, translation, compliance monitoring, effects evaluation and revision.

Policy Monitoring: Feedback loop that allows you to monitor for policy effects.

Shared Health Policy Development: Inter-organizational policy development, ideally using a framework that addresses capacity, authority and resourcing to achieve policy development, approval and distribution at the meso and macro levels.

APPENDIX

Table 2. Tasks in the Administrative Policy Process identified by the OP3 Working Group

Quadrant	Policy Process (Cog)		Task	Definition
Create	Initiate	1.	Identify Issue	Recognize policy need
Create	Initiate	2.	Consult	Consult with several colleagues to see what they think of an issue
Create	Initiate	3.	Compare Situations	Compare 2-3 similar incidents and decide whether a policy is needed
Create	Initiate	4.	Respond	Respond to provincial policy or legislation with DHA policy
Create	Initiate	5.	Acknowledge	Recognize policy gap and decide to create a policy
Create	Initiate	6.	Set Policy Level	Decide where admin or other type of policy is needed
Create	Initiate	7.	Stakeholders	Identify stakeholders & contributors & approvers, including legal, ethics
Create	Initiate	8.	Plan For Education	Decide whether education will be required
Create	Initiate	9.	Plan For Monitoring	Decide whether monitoring will be required
Create	Initiate	10.	Plan For Evaluation	Decide whether evaluation will be required
Create	Initiate	11.	Plan Timing	Decide when policy should go live (ideally)
Create	Develop	12.	Literature Search	Search for current research evidence and best practice
Create	Develop	13.	Environmental Scan	See who is doing what in similar organizations
Create	Develop	14.	FEMA (Failure Mode Effect Analysis)	Consider effect of policy failures and design policy for maximum success
Create	Develop	15.	Appraise	Appraise, synthesize and integrate information gathered
Create	Develop	16.	Review Rules	Ensure congruency with legislation and provincial health policy
Create	Develop	17.	SBAR	Create SBAR to communicate policy need
Create	Write	18.	Draft	Create first draft
Create	Write	19.	Define	Define less familiar terms
Create	Write	20.	Revise	In plain language and appropriate writing style
Create	Write	21.	Reference	Support text with references and reference list
Create	Write	22.	Procedure	Identify and draft associated procedures
Create	Write	23.	Forms	Identify form requirements and locate or create forms
Create	Write	24.	Appendix	Create required appendices
Create	Format	25.	Algorithms	Create decision tree
Create	Format	26.	Template	Format in appropriate template
Create	Format	27.	Toc	Add table of contents
Create	Write	28.	Input	Seek stakeholder input
Create	Write	29.	Revise	Synthesize, appraise and integrate stakeholder format
Create	Write	30.	Legal/ethical	Seek and integrate input from legal and ethical experts
Create	Write	31.	Review	Seek stakeholder input on revisions

continued on following page

Table 2. Continued

Quadrant	Policy Process (Cog)		Task	Definition
Create	Write	32.	Director	Seek input & approval from org unit director
Create	Write	33.	Committee	Seek input and approval from DHA policy committee
Create	Approve	34.	Approve	Have DHA authority approve policy
Disseminate	Communicate	35.	Communicate	Design and implement communication plan
Disseminate	Educate	36.	Educate	Design and deliver education
Disseminate	Publish	37.	Publish	Make policy available on op3 site
Implement	Pilot	38.	Pilot	Test policy in limited setting for limited period
Implement	Tweak	39.	Tweak	Revise pilot following user experience
Implement	Go Live	40.	Go Live	Release policy effective DHA wide
Evaluate	Evaluate	41.	Evaluate Employee Knowledge	Test to determine employee awareness of policy
Evaluate	Evaluate	42.	Evaluate Policy Content	Survey to determine if content meets needs
Evaluate	Evaluate	43.	Evaluate Policy Education	Survey to determine if education was effective
Evaluate	Evaluate	44.	Evaluate Policy Compliance	Monitor to establish DHA complies with policy
Evaluate	Evaluate	45.	Evaluate Policy Outcomes	Determine whether policy meets need

Chapter 9
Towards Healthy Public Policy:
GIS and Food Systems Analysis

Julie Yang
York University, Canada

ABSTRACT

As an issue that affects a significant portion of the Canadian population, food security must be addressed in public health policy and research. Decision-making for food security is a complex task that needs to take into account a diverse range of issues including production, processing, distribution, access, consumption, and waste management. This approach to policymaking for food security, known as food systems analysis, makes use of a large amount of geospatial data. Public health informatics can offer some potential answers to handling and using this large amount of information. The purpose of this chapter is to provide a brief introduction to Geographic Information Systems (GIS) and how they are used in public health, particularly for food systems analysis. A hypothetical scenario that envisions using a type of spatial analytic tool, called Spatial On-Line Analytic Processing (Spatial OLAP or SOLAP), for public health decision-making is also introduced. In describing both GIS and spatial OLAP, a case for incorporating food systems analysis into public health practices is made.

INTRODUCTION

Despite Canada's position as one of the wealthiest and most developed countries in the world, food security is still an issue of concern for many Canadians. The Food and Agriculture Organization of the United Nations (2010) defines food security as existing when "all people, at all times, have access to sufficient, safe, and nutritious food to meet their

dietary needs and food preferences for an active and healthy life." To achieve this vision, the full life cycle of food from production to consumption needs to be taken into account by policymakers. This is known as the food systems approach to food security. Planning for food systems requires a large amount of geospatial data. For example, it is important to know which neighbourhoods have a high prevalence of food insecurity, where healthy food sources are located, and whether people have access to healthy foods through public transit. To

DOI: 10.4018/978-1-4666-4321-5.ch009

this end, several public health informatics technologies can be useful for food systems analysis and research. This paper reviews some of the ways that geographic information systems have been used to analyze public health and food systems issues and explores the use of a newer geographic analytic technology, called spatial on-line analytic processing, to aid in decision-making.

BACKGROUND

In 2007-2008, 7.7 percent of Canadian households, equivalent to almost a million households in Canada, were food insecure (Health Canada, 2012). Food security is a matter of importance, not only because of the breadth of its reach, but also because it is significantly associated with other health conditions. The loss of food security can impact people physically, psychologically, and socially. The condition is associated with low self-rated health, nutritional inadequacy, higher rates of chronic disease, higher odds of suffering from major depression and distress, and less social support (Tarasuk, 2009). As food bank usage and global food prices continue to rise (Matern & Kim, 2012; World Bank, 2011), the food security of whole communities is being put at risk. Thus, addressing food security is a matter of public health. However, past attempts to respond to growing food insecurity has not been without problems.

Food banks were the first collective response at the local level to deal with food insecurity but it soon became clear that they were an inadequate solution to the issue. Food banks, after all, were first designed in the 1980s as emergency responses to what was seen as temporary economic recessionary times (Riches, 1997). These non-profit organizations collect, store and distribute donated food items to people who need to supplement what they can afford to buy. As a short-term, reactionary measure, food banks are not designed to address long-term livelihood issues, such as earning adequate income to ensure stable food supplies in the home.

The subsequent shift toward the community food security movement saw a change from a reliance on food banks to finding community-based, non-emergency solutions to the problem. These included using backyard and community gardens, community kitchens, farmers' markets, and community supported agriculture, among other alternative methods, to increase access to food supplies. However, critics of the community food security movement, such as Tarasuk (2001), believe it is ineffective because its strong focus on food production masks the issue of poverty and the lack of adequate income to buy food. While the food bank and community food security movements have very different roots, the common critique of both approaches is that they view the issue as the result of a single cause, whether it is a lack of income, as in the food bank movement, or problems of food production, as in the community food security movement.

Rather than stemming from a single cause, food security is a multi-dimensional issue, necessitating a multi-level, multi-sectorial approach to addressing the issue. Food security can be defined as comprising of five components: availability, accessibility, adequacy, acceptability, and agency (Ryerson University, 2010). These five 'A's identify the matter as related to issues of sufficient quantity, physical and economic access, safe and nutritious foods, environmentally sustainable food practices, cultural acceptability, producing and procuring foods in ways that do not compromise human dignity, and policies and practices to attain food security. To address this multi-dimensional issue, advocates for food security have begun to examine the whole food system, tackling problems that occur 'from farm to fork' and beyond. This approach entails accounting for the whole food cycle including production, processing, distribution, access, consumption, and waste management

(Mendes, 2008). Included within this definition are agricultural activities, food processing facilities, transportation and distribution networks, grocery stores and other food retail establishments, people and their consumption practices, and food composting and disposal. Many of these areas are affected by public policy. The sectors and disciplines involved in these activities are numerous and include agriculture, industry, transportation, retail, economics, public health, and city planning, among others.

The analysis of food systems has only recently become a major policy endeavor. Writing in relation to the planning profession, Pothukuchi and Kaufman, in 2000, note that the food system "is notable by its absence from the writing of planning scholars, from the plans prepared by planning practitioners, and from the classrooms in which planning students are taught" (p. 113). This is changing in significant ways. Food systems analysis is now accepted as a legitimate planning activity by the American Planning Association with the release of the "Policy guide on community and regional food planning" (2007). In Canada, the Ontario Professional Planners Institute (2011) put out a call to action to make food systems planning a priority. City governments are also starting to take notice. Major cities such as London, England and Toronto, Canada have recently put out comprehensive food strategies that seek to address the entire food system (London Development Agency, 2006; Toronto Public Health, 2010). Shifts in attitude toward food systems are accompanied by the growing recognition of the social, economic and environmental impacts of food.

The food system has major consequences for multiple sectors and touches on many aspects of people's lives:

- The food and beverage sector is a major driving force of the local economy. Food sector establishments include grocery stores, supermarkets, restaurants, fast food places, bars and pubs, wholesale food establishments, specialty food stores, food processing plants, and farmers' markets. In Toronto, Canada, the food and beverage sector generates $20 billion annually in sales and is the second largest employment sector (Blackwell, 2012; Ajayi, Denson, Health, & Wilmot, 2010).

- Depending on income levels, households spend 10 to 40 percent of their income on food, with lower income households spending larger proportions of their income (Pothukuchi & Kaufman, 1999).

- Food banks in the Greater Toronto Area in Canada received over a million client visits in 2010-2011 (Matern & Kim, 2012).

- The food sector has significant impacts on the environment. In Canada, the agricultural sector is the largest consumer of fresh water, accounting for 25.9 percent of the total (Statistics Canada, 2009). In 2007, 38 percent of food available for retail sale was wasted (Statistics Canada, 2009). Additionally, the food sector accounts for 20 to 30 percent of the total environmental impact of human consumption (Tukker, et al., 2006).

- Marketing practices of large food retailers and the envelopment of planning activities for food retailers under general retail planning have led to the formation of 'food deserts', which is a term used to describe urban areas where residents do not have a food retailer within walking distance (Sonnino, 2009; Pothukuchi & Kaufman, 2000).

For some of these issues, place and space play a significant role, whether it is the physical space of food establishments, distances to supermarkets or water consumption patterns. As such, geospatial analytic techniques can be used to greatly enhance food systems analysis. To this end, the field of public health informatics can offer many tools for geospatial analysis. The remainder of this paper will describe how geographic information systems and spatial on-line analytical processing can be used to support public health and food systems policymaking.

GEOSPATIAL ANALYSIS FOR PUBLIC HEALTH AND FOOD SYSTEMS DECISION-MAKING

Public Health Informatics

Public health informatics is defined as "the systematic application of information and computer science and technology to public health practice, research, and learning" (Yasnoff, O'Carroll, Koo, Linkins, & Kilbourne, 2000, p. 68). Yasnoff et al. identify four features that set public health informatics apart from other sub-disciplines of health informatics: 1) information science and technology is used to advance the health of populations instead of focusing on individuals; 2) aligning with the goals of public health, public health informatics is used for health promotion and disease and injury prevention; 3) public health informatics is not limited to working within the medical model but instead, should take into account all possible causal factors including social, behavioural and environmental contexts; and 4) public health informatics is applied within a government context, which brings with it a different set of priorities and constraints compared to a health care setting. Public health informatics goes beyond simply automating existing public health activities. Notably, Yasnoff et al. remark that informatics have been instrumental in transforming public health practices by allowing for the targeted allocation of resources and by improving upon surveillance practices. A defining characteristic of both of these activities is the importance of geographic information to their practice. Targeting resources requires knowledge of where need is greatest and identifying disease clusters requires the identification of incidences of illness. It is no surprise,

then, that a large portion of the public health informatics literature concentrates on examining geographic information systems and other spatial analytic tools.

The Role of Geospatial Information and GIS in Public Health and Food Systems Research

The recognition that geography plays a part in determining the health of communities is an old concept dating back to the times of ancient Greece. However, perhaps the most well-known incidence where geography was recognized as playing a major role in public health was when Dr. John Snow, in 1854, identified the source of a cholera outbreak (Cameron & Jones, 1983). By plotting the known cases of cholera on a map of the Soho district of London, England, Dr. Snow was able to ascertain the source of the outbreak as a water pump located on Broad Street. The absence of new cases following the removal of the water pump handle confirmed that contaminated water caused the cholera outbreak.

The use and analysis of geospatial information plays a key role in the work of policymakers and city planners to develop public policy. According to Boulos (2004), 80-90 percent of all government data in the United States feature geographic location, with this spatial reference becoming the 'main key' in transforming these data into information. This statistic can be generalized to other similar countries, including Canada. Indeed, a number of recommendations made by the American Planning Association (2007) in their policy on food systems planning include retrieving geospatial information of some sort. These include mapping the availability of healthy and unhealthy food options in low-income neighbourhoods, mapping the incidence of food insecurity, and mapping the location of diverse food assets such as community gardens, farmers' markets, and urban farms in addition to the conventional supermarkets and restaurants.

Geographic information systems are tools that can be used for the analysis of geospatial data for public health purposes. They have been described as an "enabling technology" (Nykiforuk & Flaman, 2008, p. vii) because they allow public health professionals to use and analyze spatial data in ways that are meaningful to their practice. According to Nykiforuk and Flaman (2008), "a GIS combines cartography and multivariate statistical analysis to allow for the investigation of sophisticated relationships (i.e., linking 'people' to 'place') while presenting the information in a vivid, visual manner. This technique can be applied at a range of aggregation" (p. 1). A GIS can be characterized as a collection of six components: 1) computer hardware; 2) computer software; 3) data; 4) spatial analysis techniques and methods; 5) people; and 6) policies and procedures (Boulos, 2004; Nykiforuk & Flaman, 2008). The first four components may seem intuitive to include in a definition of GIS but the last two components, people and policies and procedures, are just as important to include as they play an important role in determining the use of GIS in public health.

As the users of GIS, people need to be properly trained and be given sufficient work time to use the computer systems. This ensures that proper analytical methods are employed and that GIS use is incorporated into everyday practice. Concurrently, policies and procedures need to be in place to guide the use of GIS for public health purposes. The absence of a GIS use policy can have significant legal and privacy-related consequences, such as when the improper use of the technology results in the accidental release of highly sensitive information to the public. It is for these reasons that GIS is sometimes referred to as a science, in recognition of its use as determined by more than just the system itself.

GIS as a discipline falls under the scope of geomatics, which is defined as "the science and technology of gathering, storing, analyzing, interpreting, modeling, distributing and using georeferenced information" (Boulos, Roudsari, & Carson, 2001, p. 197). The term geographic information systems was not added to the Medical Subject Headings, or MeSH, a controlled vocabulary thesaurus maintained by the United States National Library of Medicine, until 2003 (Boulos, 2004). While indicating the relative newness of GIS to the field of health and health care analysis, it also indicates its importance and growing use within the field.

GIS is a valuable tool for policy analysis because it can bring to attention all three components of the person/time/place triad that underlies public health epidemiology and surveillance (Green, 2012). That is, GIS can summarize a large amount of data into a form that can be easily interpreted by decision makers. Most intuitively, it highlights the place dimension since geospatial analysis is the main purpose behind GIS tools. However, temporal relationships can also be demonstrated using GIS such as when a series of maps of the same area, called lag maps, are used to show changes in disease patterns over time. Finally, GIS can help enhance the person dimension by adding important details about a person's socioeconomic status, educational attainment and other social determinants of health to epidemiological and surveillance data.

A literature review conducted by Nykiforuk and Flaman (2008) found that most uses of GIS for health promotion and public health fell under four categories: disease surveillance, risk analysis, health access and planning, and community profiling. Nykiforuk and Flaman also note that these categories are not entirely distinct from each other and often overlap.

Disease surveillance, defined as the "compilation and tracking of information on the incidence, prevalence, and spread of disease" (Nykiforuk & Flaman, 2008, p. 9), was the most common theme to emerge in the literature and has been a longstanding use of GIS for public health. This is not surprising considering that public health informatics became popular around the same time as the September 11, 2001 terrorist attacks in the United States and the subsequent anthrax attacks (Kukafka & Yasnoff, 2007). Kukafka and Yasnoff note that the United States' investment into public health after the September 11 attacks was the single largest investment into this sector since the Second World War, with much of the funding allocated exclusively toward bioterrorism and preparedness. Surveillance activities fall under two sub-categories: disease mapping, which is used to understand the past or present geographic distribution or spread of disease, and disease modeling, which is used to understand the future distribution or spread of disease. John Snow's work to uncover the source of a cholera outbreak in 1850's London is an example of disease mapping. In a more recent example, the Public Health Agency of Canada maintains a Website that provides surveillance on notifiable diseases and injury (Public Health Agency of Canada, 2012). In a unique example of modeling, Ballas and colleagues (2006) used a spatial microsimulation approach to analyze the role of socio-economic characteristics in determining health inequalities in Britain.

Risk analysis is related to disease modeling and involves examining at least one aspect of risk, such as assessment, management, communication or monitoring. The purpose of carrying out this analysis is to identify urgent need, increase the effectiveness of control efforts and prevent outbreaks and epidemics (Nykiforuk & Flaman, 2008). Risk analysis studies are usually related to ecological or environmental factors such as examining environmental exposure to water, soil or air contaminants, exposure to hazardous materials, or virus transmission. Some studies also analyze the link of environmental exposure to certain health outcomes. For example, Rull, Ritz and Shaw (2006) examined the effects of maternal residential proximity to agricultural pesticides and the development of neural tube defects in their infants. Hashemi Beni et al. (2012) note that, while the use of GIS for risk analysis in public health is relatively well-established, there

are comparatively fewer examples of their application to assessments of risk in food distribution systems. Their study adds to this small but growing body of literature by examining the use of GIS for spatio-temporal analysis of food distribution systems at a national scale, especially in relation to food contamination incidents. This spatial distribution of food contamination over time is then quantified into a risk index to demonstrate its public health impact. The ability to model and predict risk events can impact upon response capacity during actual public health incidents.

Health access and planning is concerned with examining the multiple aspects of supply and demand for health services. Studies generally fall under two sub-categories, network analysis and health care utilization and market segmentation. Network analysis is used to answer questions related to access such as the route, distance and proximity of health services. For example, Fulcher and Kaukinen (2005) used GIS technology to map and examine the geographic distribution of HIV services in Toronto, finding that some HIV-related services such as emergency and preventive resources are inaccessible in some parts of the city. In food systems research, Russell and Keidkamp (2011) used road network analysis to examine how the loss of a supermarket affected a community's food system in New Haven, Connecticut. Health care utilization and market segmentation is concerned with analyzing actual use of services and profiling the users of health services in order to better allocate resources and plan health promotion activities. Morrison, Nelson and Ostry (2011), for example, were able to link population-level, aspatial data on food consumption trends to demographic information in order to map and analyze spatial variations in eating habits. This information can be applied to promote local food consumption activities.

Finally, community health profiling is concerned with examining the relationships between variables that may influence health and health outcomes in order to better understand the link between people and their communities. Many applications of GIS toward food systems research fall under this category. Some examples include: Peters, Bills, Lembo, Wilkins and Fick (2009) examined the spatial relationship between food production capacity and the food needs of New York State population centres; Eckerty and Shetty (2011) used GIS to plan for food retail; Kremer and DeLiberty (2011) used GIS to estimate the land potential of Philadelphia for urban food production; and Hallet and McDermott (2011) quantitatively determined the costs of distance imposed on consumers living in food deserts. Of significance, the United States Department of Agriculture (2012) developed a publicly available Food Environment Atlas that assembles various food environment indicators and visually presents this information as maps. This Atlas was developed for the purposes of stimulating research on the determinants of food choices and diet quality and to provide a visual overview of a community's access to healthy foods.

Despite the growing popularity and use of public health informatics, Boulos (2004) notes that the greatest contribution GIS has made to public health so far has been to low-level tasks such as mapping variables, and that its use has been largely fragmented and uncoordinated. Likewise, Kremer and DeLiberty (2011) note that local food advocates have rarely applied advanced spatial analysis techniques to the examination of local food systems. Instead, they have relied upon basic mapping exercises. A methodological review by Charreire et al. (2010) recommends that future uses of GIS for defining food environments would benefit from using more sophisticated GIS methods that combine availability and proximity and by combining GIS methods with survey approaches to enrich study results with contextual information. While GIS offer many advantages (as noted below), there are also a number of challenges and limitations associated with their

use for public health purposes. These present a number of barriers that must be overcome in order to increase the uptake of GIS for public health and food systems analysis.

Advantages of Using GIS for Public Health Purposes

As a tool for public health decision-making, geographic information systems offer advantages over the use of hand-drawn or electronic map images for the visualization of geospatial data and the computation of multivariate spatial statistical analysis, and they are able to perform these tasks with speed and ease. GIS allows for the creation of customized and complex maps. For example, geographical boundaries can be modified, the scale can be manipulated, symbols and colours can be customized, and multiple map layers representing different variables can be overlaid and integrated (Boulos, 2004). They are also better at analyzing causal relationships that include a spatial component than traditional statistical methods. According to Boulos (2004), a number of spatial analytic techniques can be conducted using GIS. These include analyzing multivariate spatial statistics, calculating spatial weights, assessing spatial auto-correlation on predictor variables, and exploring probability scenarios of mapped variables based on modeled changes in regression coefficients over time. Rushton (1998) notes that without GIS, two types of spatial analysis for public health cannot be performed. First, GIS can identify statistically significant areas of high disease incidence that can benefit from further analysis and second, it can aid in the examination of the spatial relationship between two variables that are differently geo-referenced. Mullner, Chung, Croke and Mensah (2004) note that georeferenced data are able to provide context to an issue that traditional statistical methods cannot. This context is important for public health purposes. Despite the advantages of GIS over traditional mapping tools, they pose a number of challenges and possess a number of limitations when applied in a policy decision-making setting.

Challenges and Limitations of Using GIS for Public Health Decision-Making

Higgs and Gould (2001) point out that there is a gap between GIS use in academic settings versus the United Kingdom's National Health Service, noting that GIS use in the public health sector has been mostly for low-level operational tasks and further noting that there is little evidence of its use for strategic decision-making. Reasons for the limited uptake of GIS in the health sector can be categorized into issues of resource, data, organizational factors and policy and technology.

The implementation of GIS within organizations requires significant short- and long-term human, time, and financial resources. Specialized training is needed in order to effectively use and analyze geospatial information, making it inaccessible to individuals who lack expertise in using the tool. It is for this reason that some public health decision-makers perceive GIS as technocratic tools that concentrate expertise within a few individuals (Joyce, 2009). In order to build GIS and geospatial analytic expertise within organizations, resources are required to initially train staff and for continuing education. Furthermore, implementing GIS tools within an organization means that further constraints are put on the work time of public health decision-makers. Finally, significant financial and human resources will also be needed to run and maintain these systems.

The data issues limiting the uptake of GIS are numerous. As many service organizations are still paper-based in their record keeping, there is a paucity of digital data in the right formats. Data quality is also an issue such as when there are missing or incorrect values. Confidentiality,

privacy, and security are significant issues as geospatial data hold the risk of identifying marginalized individuals or groups based on their location. Lastly, there is a lack of data sharing agreements between different organizations and levels of government, and many organizations are unaware of the data held by other organizations.

Organizational and policy issues also form a major roadblock to GIS uptake. These include a limited awareness of the benefits of geospatial information, lack of demand for GIS within some organizations, and the absence of policies for GIS use and data exchange. In order to seamlessly integrate GIS use into regular practice in public health, customizations must be made. These include finding the right hardware and software, tailoring GIS systems to the needs of public health professionals and decision makers, and designing system interfaces that are user friendly and accessible. Political will is also needed. Significantly, Boulos (2004) notes that GIS are not mentioned in UK health information strategy documents. Without the political impetus to incorporate GIS into practice, public health organizations may lack the reason and the support to do so.

The final barrier to GIS uptake is a technological one. Proulx, Bernier and Bédard (2007) note that as transactional systems, GIS tools are not optimized for the type of analysis used in decision-making processes. Proulx and colleagues identify four main issues that limit the use of GIS for decision-making. First, as transactional systems, GIS are designed for "the storage of, access to and updating of data and its integrity management" (p. 22) and not for complex queries that require the processing of a large amount of data. Second, they are not optimized for temporal analysis as their content is composed of detailed and current data instead of the aggregated and summarized data needed for this type of comparison. Third, there are often a number of these systems dispersed within an organization, working independently from each other and thus requiring their integration to be queried. Finally, GIS are difficult to use, requiring specific querying language and a specialized interface.

As evidenced by the challenges and limitations related to the use of GIS for public health and food systems policymaking, there remain a number of issues related to the use of geospatial information for public health that have yet to be studied. The next section introduces a relatively new software, called spatial on-line analytic processing, that some supporters (e.g. Proulx et al., 2007; Bédard et al., 2007) believe are better equipped than GIS for decision-making duties related to public health.

Spatial OLAP for Public Health and Food Systems Analysis

Ideally, to increase the uptake and use of geospatial analysis tools in public health, they should be accessible to mainstream practitioners who may not have specialized expertise, be seamlessly incorporated into everyday work flows, and integrated into the existing work environment (Boulos, 2004). As discussed above, some GIS technologies can be cumbersome to use and require specialized knowledge on the part of the user. Spatial OLAP, another tool for geospatial analysis, may be able to overcome some of the barriers that are preventing the seamless integration of GIS into public health units.

Food systems analysis is a complex task because the subject is multi-faceted, multi-scalar, and evolves over time. Since a large amount of government data are geospatial in nature, there is a need for a decision support tool that takes into account this type of information. Yet, geographic information systems are not ideally built to handle complex decision-making processes as they are complex to use and require a lot of time to run analyses. A recent innovation deriving from the Business Intelligence field has shown promise in supporting public health decision-making. Having already been applied to environmental health decision-making (Bédard, et al., 2003)

and community health assessments (Scotch & Parmanto, 2006), spatial on-line analytical processing technologies show promise for application to food systems analysis for public health policymaking purposes. Bédard et al. (2007) define spatial OLAP as "a type of software that allows rapid and easy navigation within spatial databases and that offers many levels of information granularity, many themes, many epochs and many display modes synchronized or not: maps, tables and diagrams" (p. 9). Compared to GIS, which have been described as slow, complex to use, and only able to handle one level of data that is non-aggregated, SOLAP has been characterized as fast, user friendly, and able to handle multiple levels of data in aggregated form (Proulx, et al., 2007). While not a replacement for GIS, SOLAP technologies are able to improve upon the decision support capacities of GIS.

Spatial OLAP technologies function differently from GIS since their foundations are in different paradigms. As the focus of this current endeavor is on the potential of SOLAP to support public health policy and not the technological details, Proulx et al. (2007) and Bédard et al. (2007) provide good comparisons of the technological differences between SOLAP and GIS. Stemming from their different paradigms, SOLAP technologies handle data and create information in ways that are different from GIS. For example, while allowing for the visualization of geospatial data, SOLAP also allows for the interactive exploration of data by providing 'drilling' capabilities in maps, charts, and tables. Without the need for specialized knowledge in using the software, users can drill down or up geographic levels and across geographic areas with a few clicks of the mouse (Proulx, et al., 2007). These drills can be synchronized across maps, charts and tables to create a collection of information that can be used to support analysis.

Furthermore, the multidimensional approach used by SOLAP technologies is found to be more in line with the mental models of data users

(Bédard, et al., 2003). With the multidimensional approach, users can ask questions that incorporate prevalence, geography and time such as 'what is the prevalence of food insecurity in Toronto, Ontario in the years 2002-2008 and how does it compare to the provincial and national prevalence rates?' SOLAP technologies also contain two conditions that are essential to allowing decision makers to maintain their train of thought, thus further assisting in analysis: they are easy to use and they work rapidly (Bédard, et al., 2003). SOLAP technologies typically use intuitive and interactive interfaces, allowing the user to concentrate on analyzing the data instead of spending time figuring out how to query the system. In addition, the SOLAP technology developed by Bédard et al. (2003) only took between three to 10 seconds to process queries on a notebook computer, regardless of the query complexity, allowing users to maintain their train of thought. As such, complex questions, such as the one posed above, can be queried in a short amount of time. Finally, SOLAP systems require very little training, allowing for sufficient use of the software with less than one hour of instruction (Bédard, et al., 2003). Thus, the speed of query and the ease of usability of these systems make SOLAP technologies a good option for providing food systems decision support within the public health setting.

A Hypothetical Application of a Food Systems Decision Support Tool within a Local Public Health Unit

This section provides a vision for the use of a spatial OLAP software within a local government in order to support food systems analysis. While the responsibility for various aspects of the food system is spread over all levels of government, as exemplified by London and Toronto (e.g., London Development Agency, 2006; Toronto Public Health, 2010), cities have been the frontrunners in taking the whole food system into account when developing policy. Ideally, the SOLAP will be housed in the local public health unit. However, as analyzing food systems is an activity that involves policymakers, planners and staff from all areas of government, a process should be implemented that opens up the use of the software to all government departments. Housing the system within the public health unit can serve several goals: it puts an entity in charge of maintaining the quality and integrity of the SOLAP, it allows for the central coordination of food systems analysis activities, and perhaps most importantly, it maintains the focus of food systems analysis on health and social equity. Opening up the use of the system to all government departments serves to emphasize that the food system is an issue that spans across multiple sectors and as such, requires inter-departmental and inter-sectorial collaboration. Developing, maintaining and evaluating a SOLAP for food systems analysis will likely involve a multi-disciplinary team including the users such as public policymakers and city planners, software developers, IT professionals, information systems and informatics specialists, and researchers with a range of backgrounds in health, geography and technology.

Different government departments will likely have different uses for a SOLAP for food systems analysis. While it can be useful for public health purposes, the technology can prove to be of value outside of this sector as well. To date and to the author's knowledge, a SOLAP tool for food systems analysis has not been developed for and used within any public health unit. The following scenarios, however, demonstrate that, with a proper tool developed and with the appropriate data available, a SOLAP can be of value to public health policymakers and city planners for different purposes related to the food system.

Scenarios for the Use of SOLAP for Food Systems Analysis

A policymaker within the public health unit may be interested in more overarching questions related to the food system that take a macro view of the problem. A question that may be of interest to a public health official is 'does income affect access to different food destinations (e.g. fast food restaurants or grocery stores selling healthy food options) in Toronto?' To answer this query, the policymaker will need to select a number of data including the region to be studied (Toronto), income (derived from census data), and types of food retailers (derived from business databases). The SOLAP software can map income and types of food retailers onto the map of Toronto and at the same time, can produce charts and tables of the same data. Using this information, relationships between income and access to certain food destinations can be determined.

A city planner, on the other hand, may be interested in more practical questions such as 'do low income neighbourhoods in Toronto have sufficient public transit access to grocery stores selling healthy foods?' To query this question, data will be needed on income, public transit routes, and grocery stores. All three of these dimensions can be plotted onto a map of Toronto. From this information, city planners can decide to add a new bus route that will increase access to a grocery store that was previously underserved by public transit.

While the decision-making needs of policymakers and city planners may be different, it is evident that a SOLAP for food systems analysis will be beneficial to both groups. More work is needed to determine what such a system will look like and what data is needed to fully support food systems analysis. While there is no question that geospatial information is important for public health research and analysis, there still remain issues related to the incorporation of geospatial analysis and spatial analytic tools into the public health field.

FUTURE RESEARCH DIRECTIONS

Integrating Geospatial Analysis into Public Health and Food Policy

A number of areas will need to be addressed in order to make full use of geospatial information in public health and food policy. As described earlier, GIS may not be adequately designed to support complex decision-making. Therefore, methods to better use geospatial information, including exploring the use of other tools or improving the usability of GIS, to support decision-making need to be explored. Furthermore, Boulos (2004) makes the claim that GIS are "usually applied to time-limited, single, isolated aetiological research or surveillance issues" (p. 2). Supporting this, Kukafka and Yasnoff (2007) state that the major focus of public health informatics has been on syndromic surveillance and outbreak detection for infectious diseases. This points to the need for efforts to implement wide-scale use of informatics and GIS in public health, especially related to the social determinants of health. Boulos (2004) also calls for a critical review of the evidence to determine "which method(s) specifically should be used by practitioners for each specific health condition of interest, and whether the proposed methods are cost-effective and scalable" (p. 42). Thus, more knowledge of geospatial analysis is needed within public health practice in order to understand what the proper statistical techniques are for analyzing issues at the individual or ecological levels. Finally, the integration of public health into the whole of government will also need to be considered. As the responsibility for food systems does not fall within one government department but is instead dispersed among many departments and levels of government, cooperation and integration is needed in order to acquire the necessary data for analyses and for coordinated planning and action. This ensures that not only are public health policies developed but so too are healthy public policies.

Important Data Considerations

In order for geospatial analysis to be truly integrated into public health policies and practices, whether through the implementation of GIS, SOLAP or another spatial analytic tool, there remains the issue of data. The ability to conduct population-level geospatial analysis hinges on the data that is available. Therefore, a significant amount of work must be put into attaining and maintaining the data. Acquiring the data itself can present as a challenge as there is little information about what data are available and who owns them. Once data are found, there must be agreements in place for the sharing and use of it, which can pose a considerable bureaucratic and legal challenge. Once data are acquired, a number of issues must be resolved before they can be integrated for use. These include cleaning the data, performing quality checks, validating the data, determining how to deal with missing values, and determining methods to link the data from different databases. Finally, a process needs to be in place to maintain the data. There is also the issue of where to house the data. In addition to being a matter of finding sufficient physical space to house the hardware, it is also a political concern as the physical data holdings can become symbolic of ownership.

In order to develop a spatial analytic system to support public health and food policy, methods of acquiring and holding the data must be taken into consideration. Some jurisdictions in Canada have taken to developing central repositories that contain linked data from a number of sectors. For example, the Manitoba Centre for Health Policy houses the Population Health Research Data Re-

pository (University of Manitoba, 2009). Used to support health policy research, this repository contains databases grouped under the domains of health, education, social, justice, registries, and database support files. The databases in the repository are linked at the record level, meaning that unique identifiers are used to identify the same individual in multiple databases but in a way that still ensures the anonymity of the individual. Similarly, the Alberta Centre for Child, Family and Community Research is developing the Child and Youth Data Laboratory (CYDL), a repository of information that is dedicated to examining the issues, policies and practices that affect the children and youth of Alberta (Alberta Centre for Child, Family, and Community Research, 2012). The CYDL is also a multi-sectorial effort and receives support from the Alberta Ministries of Human Services, Aboriginal Relations, Education, Enterprise and Advanced Education, Health, and Justice and Solicitor General. A data repository dedicated to food system issues will similarly need to be multi-sectorial, requiring data about demographics, agriculture, the environment, health, transportation, businesses, and education.

Integration and Interoperability

While central data repositories may provide one solution to integrating data from multiple sources, there remains the issue of optimizing the sharing of geospatial information. Many geospatial analysis tools are proprietary or closed systems that do not allow for the integration of information outputs from other systems. This makes collaboration between different agencies, levels of government, and governments of different countries very difficult as each may have implemented their own tools for use. In this age of globalization, where food and disease can travel great distances in short amounts of time, the ability to transmit information quickly is essential to preventing public health disasters. Interoperability of systems, whereby different systems are able to work together, is essential to ensuring that information outputs of one system can be read by another. Web-based tools may provide one solution to the issue of integration (Boulos, 2004) but more research is needed into the area of interoperability.

Privacy, Confidentiality and Security

Privacy, confidentiality, and security are issues that will continuously need to be addressed as these systems evolve. The confidentiality of information and the privacy of individuals are of utmost importance when it comes to the handling of data by governments. Similarly important is maintaining the security of the data, ensuring that there are access and integrity controls in place. As stated by Croner (2003), "public trust is essential to the conduct of government-supported data collection, analysis, and dissemination" (p. 60) and maintaining privacy, confidentiality, and security are integral to preserving this trust. When using geospatial data, there is the risk that an individual's identity may be revealed through location and with increasingly sophisticated technology, possessing the power to analyze multiple variables, dis-aggregate data, and zoom into the smallest scale, the risk of breaching privacy is all the greater. At the same time, aggregating data and using data-masking techniques can limit the ability to effectively analyze data. The challenge that lies ahead is to find the right balance between protecting the privacy of people while simultaneously allowing for detailed analysis of the data.

CONCLUSION

Food security is an issue that has significant implications for population health and social equity. As a complex issue comprised of a number of dimensions, a systems approach is needed in order to fully understand the issue. Geospatial technologies, especially GIS and spatial OLAP, can facilitate public health decision-making by providing policymakers with the tools to analyze space and place. A case was made here for using SOLAP to support public health and food policy within a local public health unit. Even though there still exists numerous challenges to the development of geospatial analysis tools that are capable of analyzing food systems while remaining usable by policymakers without specialized geospatial analytic skills, GIS and SOLAP hold promise in helping to build a health focused food system.

REFERENCES

Ajayi, J., Denson, C., Health, B., & Wilmot, K. (2010). *2010 Toronto food sector update*. Toronto, Canada: City of Toronto Economic Development & Culture.

Alberta Centre for Child, Family and Community Research. (2012). *Child and youth data laboratory so innovative, it's the first of its kind in the world*. Retrieved September 13, 2012, from http://www.research4children.com/admin/contentx/default.cfm?h=9999996&grp=1&PageId=9999996

American Planning Association. (2007). *Policy guide on community and regional food planning*. Retrieved June 25, 2011, from http://www.planning.org/policy/guides/pdf/foodplanning.pdf

Ballas, D., Clarke, G., Dorling, D., Rigby, J., & Wheeler, B. (2006). Using geographical information systems and spatial microsimulation for the analysis of health inequalities. *Health Informatics Journal*, *12*(1), 65–79. doi:10.1177/1460458206061217 PMID:17023399.

Bédard, Y., Gosselin, P., Rivest, S., Proulx, M.-J., Nadeau, M., & Lebel, G. et al. (2003). Integrating GIS components with knowledge discovery technology for environmental health decision support. *International Journal of Medical Informatics*, *70*, 79–94. doi:10.1016/S1386-5056(02)00126-0 PMID:12706184.

Bédard, Y., Rivest, S., & Proulx, M.-J. (2007). *Spatial on-line analytical processing (SOLAP): Concepts, architectures and solutions from a geomatics engineering perspective.* Quebec City, Canada: Centre for Research in Geomatics.

Blackwell, R. (2012, April 10). Toronto's economy marches on its stomach. *The Globe and Mail.*

Boulos, M., Roudsari, A., & Carson, E. (2001). Health geomatics: An enabling suite of technologies in health and healthcare. *Journal of Biomedical Informatics, 34,* 195–219. doi:10.1006/jbin.2001.1015 PMID:11723701.

Boulos, M. N. (2004). Towards evidence-based, GIS-driven national spatial health information infrastructure and surveillance services in the United Kingdom. *International Journal of Health Geographics, 3*(1). PMID:14748927.

Charreire, H., Casey, R., Salze, P., Simon, C., Chaix, B., & Banos, A. et al. (2010). Measuring the food environment using geographical information systems: A methodological review. *Public Health Nutrition, 13*(11), 1773–1785. doi:10.1017/S1368980010000753 PMID:20409354.

City of Toronto. (n.d.). *Key industry sector: Food & beverage.* Retrieved September 10, 2012, from http://www.toronto.ca/invest-in-toronto/food.htm

Croner, C. M. (2003). Public health, GIS, and the internet. *Annual Review of Public Health, 24,* 57–82. PMID:12543872.

Eckert, J., & Shetty, S. (2011). Food systems, planning and quantifying access: Using GIS to plan for food retailing. *Applied Geography (Sevenoaks, England), 31*(4), 1216–1223. doi:10.1016/j.apgeog.2011.01.011.

Food and Agriculture Organization of the United Nations. (2010). *Special programme for food security.* Retrieved October 9, 2010, from http://www.fao.org/spfs/en/

Fulcher, C., & Kaukinen, C. (2005). Mapping and visualizing the location HIV service providers: An exploratory spatial analysis of Toronto neighborhoods. *AIDS Care, 17*(3), 386–396. doi:10.1080/09540120512331314312 PMID:15832887.

Green, C. (2012). *Geographic information systems and public health: Benefits and challenges.* Winnipeg, Canada: National Collaobrating Centre for Infectious Diseases.

Hallett, L. F., & McDermott, D. (2011). Quantifying the extent and cost of food deserts in Lawrence, Kansas, USA. *Applied Geography (Sevenoaks, England), 31*(4), 1210–1215. doi:10.1016/j.apgeog.2010.09.006.

Hashemi Beni, L., Villeneuve, S., LeBlanc, D. I., Côté, K., Fazil, A., & Otten, A. et al. (2012). Spatio-temporal assessment of food safety risks in Canadian food distribution systems using GIS. *Spatial and Spatia-temporal Epidemiology, 3,* 215–223. doi:10.1016/j.sste.2012.02.009 PMID:22749207.

Health Canada. (2012). *Household food insecurity in Canada in 2007-2008: Key statistics and graphics.* Retrieved September 10, 2012, from http://www.hc-sc.gc.ca/fn-an/surveill/nutrition/commun/insecurit/key-stats-cles-2007-2008-eng.php

Higgs, G., & Gould, M. (2001). Is there a role for GIS in the 'new NHS'? *Health & Place, 7,* 247–259. doi:10.1016/S1353-8292(01)00014-4 PMID:11439259.

Joyce, K. (2009). To me it's just another tool to help understand the evidence: Public health decision-makers' perceptions of the value of geographical information systems (GIS). *Health & Place, 15*, 831–840. doi:10.1016/j.healthplace.2009.01.004.

Kremer, P., & DeLiberty, T. L. (2011). Local food practices and growing potential: Mapping the case of Philadelphia. *Applied Geography (Sevenoaks, England), 31*(4), 1252–1261. doi:10.1016/j.apgeog.2011.01.007.

Kukafka, R., & Yasnoff, W. A. (2007). Public health informatics. *Journal of Biomedical Informatics, 40*, 365–369. doi:10.1016/j.jbi.2007.07.005 PMID:17656158.

London Development Agency. (2006). *Healthy and sustainable food for London: The mayor's food strategy.* London: London Development Agency.

Matern, R., & Kim, S. (2012). *Who's hungry faces of hunger: 2012 profile of hunger in the GTA.* Toronto, Canada: Daily Bread Food Bank.

Mendes, W. (2008). Implementing social and environmental policies in cities: The case of food policy in Vancouver, Canada. *International Journal of Urban and Regional Research, 32*(4), 942–967. doi:10.1111/j.1468-2427.2008.00814.x.

Morrison, K. T., Nelson, T. A., & Ostry, A. S. (2011). Mapping spatial variation in food consumption. *Applied Geography (Sevenoaks, England), 31*, 1262–1267. doi:10.1016/j.apgeog.2010.11.020.

Mullner, R. M., Chung, K., Croke, K. G., & Mensah, E. K. (2004). Geographic information systems in public health and medicine. *Journal of Medical Systems, 28*(3), 215–221. doi:10.1023/B:JOMS.0000032972.29060.dd PMID:15446613.

Nykiforuk, C. I., & Flaman, L. M. (2008). *Exploring the utilization of geographic information systems in health promotion and public health.* Edmonton, Canada: Centre for Health Promotion Studies, School of Public Health, University of Alberta.

Ontario Ministry of Agriculture & City of Toronto Economic Development. (2002). *Food industry outlook: A study of food industry growth trends in Toronto.* Toronto, Canada: City of Toronto.

Ontario Professional Planners Institute. (2011). *Planning for food systems in Ontario: A call to action.* Retrieved June 27, 2011, from http://www.ontarioplanners.on.ca/pdf/a_call_to_action_from_oppi_june_24_2011.pdf

Peters, C. J., Bills, N. L., Lembo, A. J., Wilkins, J. L., & Fick, G. W. (2009). Mapping potential foodsheds in New York state: A spatial model for evaluating the capacity to localize food production. *Renewable Agriculture and Food Systems, 24*(1), 72–84. doi:10.1017/S1742170508002457.

Pothukuchi, K., & Kaufman, J. L. (1999). Placing the food system on the urban agenda: The role of municipal institutions in food systems planning. *Agriculture and Human Values, 16*, 213–224. doi:10.1023/A:1007558805953.

Pothukuchi, K., & Kaufman, J. L. (2000). The food system: A stranger to the planning field. *Journal of the American Planning Association. American Planning Association, 66*(2), 113–124. doi:10.1080/01944360008976093.

Proulx, M.-J., Bernier, E., & Bédard, Y. (2007). *Environmental health systemic review: How the new analytical geomatics technologies can help environmental health professionals and decision-makers to make further use of mapping than what is offered traditionally by geographic information systems (GIS) a.* Quebec City, Canada: Centre de recherche en géomatique, Université Laval.

Public Health Agency of Canada. (2012, February 1). *Disease surveillance on-line - Surveillance des maladies en direct.* Retrieved September 11, 2012, from http://dsol-smed.hc-sc.gc.ca/dsol-smed/

Riches, G. (1997). Hunger in Canada: Abandoning the right to food. In Riches, G. (Ed.), *First world hunger: Food security and welfare politics* (pp. 46–77). Toronto, Canada: Garamond Press.

Rull, R. P., Ritz, B., & Shaw, G. M. (2006). Neural tube defects and maternal residential proximity to agricultural pesticide applications. *American Journal of Epidemiology, 163*(8), 743–753. doi:10.1093/aje/kwj101 PMID:16495467.

Rushton, G. (1998). Improving the geographic basis of health surveillance using GIS. In Gatrell, A., & Loytonen, M. (Eds.), *GIS and Health* (pp. 63–80). Philadelphia: Taylor and Francis.

Russell, S. E., & Keidkamp, P. (2011). Food desertification: The loss of a major supermarket in New Haven, Connecticut. *Applied Geography (Sevenoaks, England), 31*(4), 1197–1209. doi:10.1016/j.apgeog.2011.01.010.

Ryerson University. (2010). *Food security defined.* Retrieved October 9, 2010, from http://www.ryerson.ca/foodsecurity/definition/

Scotch, M., & Parmanto, B. (2006). Development of SOVAT: A numerical-spatial decision support system for community health assessment research. *International Journal of Medical Informatics, 75,* 771–784. doi:10.1016/j.ijmedinf.2005.10.008 PMID:16359916.

Sonnino, R. (2009). Feeding the city: Towards a new research and planning agenda. *International Planning Studies, 14*(4), 425–435. doi:10.1080/13563471003642795.

Statistics Canada. (2009). *Human activity and the environment: Annual statistics.* Ottawa, Canada: Statistics Canada.

Tarasuk, V. (2001). A critical examination of community-based responses to household food insecurity in Canada. *Health Education & Behavior, 28*(4), 487–499. doi:10.1177/109019810102800408 PMID:11465158.

Tarasuk, V. (2003). Low income, welfare and nutritional vulnerability. *Canadian Medical Association Journal, 168*(6), 709–710. PMID:12642427.

Tarasuk, V. (2009). Health implications of food insecurity. In Raphael, D. (Ed.), *Social Determinants of Health* (2nd ed., pp. 205–220). Toronto, Canada: Canadian Scholars Press.

Toronto Public Health. (2008). *The state of Toronto's food.* Toronto, Canada: Toronto Public Health.

Toronto Public Health. (2010). *Cultivating food connections: Towards a healthy and sustainable food system for Toronto.* Toronto, Canada: Toronto Public Health.

Tukker, A., Huppes, G., Guinée, J., Heijungs, R., de Koning, A., & van Oers, L. et al. (2006). *Environmental impact of products (EIPRO): Analysis of the life-cycle environmental impacts related to the final consumption of the EU-25.* Seville, Spain: European Commission.

United States Department of Agriculture. (2012, December 11). *Food environment atlas.* Retrieved December 28, 2012, from http://www.ers.usda.gov/data-products/food-environment-atlas.aspx

University of Manitoba. (2009, December 18). *Population health research data repository*. Retrieved September 13, 2012, from http://umanitoba.ca/faculties/medicine/units/community_health_sciences/departmental_units/mchp/resources/repository/index.html

World Bank. (2011, April 14). *High and volatile food prices continue to threaten the world's poor*. Retrieved April 20, 2011, from http://go.worldbank.org/DGNYAFM0Y0

Yasnoff, W. A., O'Carroll, P. W., Koo, D., Linkins, R. W., & Kilbourne, E. M. (2000). Public health informatics: Improving and transforming public health in the information age. *Journal of Public Health Management and Practice*, 6(6), 67–75. PMID:18019962.

ADDITIONAL READING

American Planning Association. (2007). *Policy guide on community and regional food planning*. Retrieved June 25, 2011, from http://www.planning.org/policy/guides/pdf/foodplanning.pdf

Bédard, Y., Rivest, S., & Proulx, M.-J. (2007). *Spatial on-line analytical processing (SOLAP): Concepts, architectures and solutions from a geomatics engineering perspective*. Quebec City, Canada: Centre for Research in Geomatics.

Bernier, E., Gosselin, P., Badard, T., & Bédard, Y. (2009). Easier surveillance of climate-related health vulnerabilities through a web-based spatial OLAP application. *International Journal of Health Geographics*, 8(18). PMID:19344512.

Boulos, M. N. (2004). Towards evidence-based, GIS-driven national spatial health information infrastructure and surveillance services in the United Kingdom. *International Journal of Health Geographics*, 3(1). PMID:14748927.

Cameron, D., & Jones, I. G. (1983). John Snow, the broad street pump and modern epidemiology. *International Journal of Epidemiology*, 12(4), 393–396. doi:10.1093/ije/12.4.393 PMID:6360920.

Charreire, H., Casey, R., Salze, P., Simon, C., Chaix, B., & Banos, A. et al. (2010). Measuring the food environment using geographical information systems: A methodological review. *Public Health Nutrition*, 13(11), 1773–1785. doi:10.1017/S1368980010000753 PMID:20409354.

Cromley, E., & McLafferty, S. (2002). *GIS and public health*. New York: The Guilford Press.

Green, C. (2012). *Geographic information systems and public health: Benefits and challenges*. Winnipeg, Canada: National Collaobrating Centre for Infectious Diseases.

London Development Agency. (2006). *Healthy and sustainable food for London: The mayor's food strategy*. London: London Development Agency.

Maheswaran, R., & Craglia, M. (2004). *GIS in public health practice*. Boca Raton, FL: CRC Press. doi:10.1201/9780203720349.

Nykiforuk, C. I., & Flaman, L. M. (2008). *Exploring the utilization of geographic information systems in health promotion and public health*. Edmonton, Canada: Centre for Health Promotion Studies, School of Public Health, University of Alberta.

Olvingson, C., Hallberg, J., Timpka, T., & Lindqvist, K. (2003). Ethical issues in public health informatics: Implications for system design when sharing geographic information. *Journal of Biomedical Informatics*, 35, 178–185. doi:10.1016/S1532-0464(02)00527-0 PMID:12669981.

Ontario Professional Planners Institute. (2011, June 24). *Planning for food systems in Ontario: A call to action*. Retrieved June 27, 2011, from http://www.ontarioplanners.on.ca/pdf/a_call_to_action_from_oppi_june_24_2011.pdf

Pothukuchi, K., & Kaufman, J. L. (1999). Placing the food system on the urban agenda: The role of municipal institutions in food systems planning. *Agriculture and Human Values*, *16*, 213–224. doi:10.1023/A:1007558805953.

Pothukuchi, K., & Kaufman, J. L. (2000). The food system: A stranger to the planning field. *Journal of the American Planning Association. American Planning Association*, *66*(2), 113–124. doi:10.1080/01944360008976093.

Proulx, M.-J., Bernier, E., & Bédard, Y. (2007). *Environmental health systemic review: How the new analytical geomatics technologies can help environmental health professionals and decision-makers to make further use of mapping than what is offered traditionally by geographic information systems (GIS) a*. Quebec City, Canada: Centre de recherche en géomatique, Université Laval.

Rivest, S., Bédard, Y., & Marchand, P. (2001). Toward better support for spatial decision making: Defining the characteristics of spatical on-line analytical processing. *Geomatica*, *55*(4), 539–555.

Toronto Public Health. (2010). *Cultivating food connections: Towards a healthy and sustainable food system for Toronto*. Toronto, Canada: Toronto Public Health.

Université Laval. (2009). *Spatial OLAP*. Retrieved June 27, 2011, from http://www.spatialbi.com/

KEY TERMS AND DEFINITIONS

Food Security: The physical and economic means to access sufficient, safe, and nutritious food to meet one's food preferences in a way that does not compromise dignity.

Food System: The complex set of interrelationships between food production, processing, distribution, access, consumption, and waste management.

Geospatial Information: Data that features the geographic or geospatial aspect as the main component.

Geographic Information System: A tool used for the storage, management, analysis and presentation of geospatial information.

Public Health Informatics: A sub-discipline of health informatics, public health informatics uses information and computer science techniques to support public health research and practice.

Spatial On-Line Analytic Processing: Stemming from the business intelligence field, spatial on-line analytic processing is a type of software that allows for the easy and rapid manipulation of geospatial data to support decision-making.

Chapter 10

Caring for our Aging Population:
Using CPOE and Telehomecare Systems as a Response to Health Policy Concerns

Sama Al-Khudairy
York University, Canada

ABSTRACT

An increasing senior population and national fiscal challenges affect the provision of healthcare in many ways. Keeping this in mind, the Ontario Ministry of Health and Long-Term Care's recent release of the Ontario Action Plan for Health Care (2012) aims to manage scarce resources and healthcare dollars to improve the health of Ontarians while making care available to seniors closer to home. One highly viable approach to attaining such goals is through the adoption of various healthcare technologies. Computerized Physician Order Entry Systems and Telehomecare are two examples presented in this chapter that describes how health informatics can be used as a solution to policy concerns.

INTRODUCTION

Health studies, at times, tend to be divided into separate categories, namely Health Informatics, Health Management, and Health Policy. These three areas of study, however, are highly intertwined and evidently so. For a clear indication of this link, one needs to simply examine the government's recently released *Ontario Action Plan for Health Care* (Ontario Ministry of Health and Long-Term Care, 2012). This document highlights

DOI: 10.4018/978-1-4666-4321-5.ch010

problem areas to be tackled in order to ensure a more patient-centered system that considers the province's aging population and fiscal challenges which both effect the ways in which health care is delivered. Among other things, the plan indicates issues of hospital readmissions, misuse of the system, and the increased strain brought upon by an aging population.

In its simplest form, this chapter aims to answer the question of how health informatics relates to health policy, if it does at all. Through the use of secondary resources (i.e., journal articles, government documents and reports), I will attempt to validate what I hypothesize to be a positive correlation between health informatics and health policy and management. This will be accomplished through the use of two forms of health informatics (i.e., Computerized Physician Order Entry Systems [CPOEs], and Telehomecare). More specifically, the examination of various studies on the subject will guide this chapter and assist in describing how informatics in the field of health is capable of responding to healthcare management issues (including quality improvement, cost cutting, and wait time reduction) as well as health policy concerns (more specifically, health promotion and prevention strategies). Following a brief background on the subject, the chapter transitions into the identification of the current healthcare situation as per the needs of the elderly population. By examining issues present within the system and government initiatives in response to the situation at hand, one can begin to understand the needs and ways in which healthcare technologies can help transition Ontario's healthcare system into a better one that provides optimal care.

BACKGROUND

In February of 2012, Ontario's Health Minister Deb Matthews held a conference to discuss the recently release Ontario Action Plan for Health Care with three priorities in mind. That is, to keep Ontarians healthy, speed up their access to family health care and ensure the right care is delivered at the right time and in the right place (Ontario Ministry of Health and Long-Term Care, 2012). With that in mind, the plan sets out a number of goals to be accomplished in the years to come which bear in mind Canada's aging population and fiscal changes. This document is highly influential as it reiterates the various problem areas to be tackled from the view of key health policy players. As such, it will be the main document used in this chapter to describe ways by which health informatics can relate and respond to health policy priorities and concerns.

Among the future goals listed within the action plan is to reduce the cost of healthcare, 25% of which are attributed to preventable illnesses (Ontario Ministry of Health and Long-Term Care, 2012). Furthermore, the issue of patient safety is also, indirectly, touched on through the realization that 140,000 accounts of hospital readmissions in 2009 were made within a month of initial discharge due to a lack of appropriate home care.

A vital indicator of patient safety may be incidents of adverse events. Plainly defined, adverse events are unintentional harm or complications resulting in disability at the time of discharge, death, or prolonged hospital stays, which are a result of health care management rather than the patient's underlying illness (Baker et al., 2004). In particular, adverse drug events (ADEs), involving the unintended and harmful effects of medications on patients, account for a large percentage of adverse events in hospitals (Cadario, 2005; Casey, Moscovice & Davidson, 2006).

In 2000, a study of adverse events in 20 selected acute care hospitals across Canada, estimated that 1.6% of admitted patients experienced serious ADEs (Cadario, 2005). This translates into an approximate 40,000 such incidences each year in acute care hospitals alone. Though a number of these cases may have been unavoidable, the study also found that almost half the cases were considered to be preventable. That is, over 80% of ADEs are categorized as 'type A' in nature, which is dose-related, and is therefore predictable and avoidable. This is enough reason to ensure that ADEs have been recognized as a major healthcare issue requiring immediate attention and intervention.

Another prominent issue that continuously presented itself within this Action Plan, which is also highly related to the former issue presented, was that concerning the health and care of the senior population within Ontario. With the aging of Canada's 'baby-boomers', Ontario will exhibit a doubling of its senior citizens within the next 20 years and it is no secret that as people get older, they become more dependent on the system (Ontario Ministry of Health and Long-Term Care, 2012). Seniors generally tend to present unique challenges to the healthcare system (Laurent, 2002). For one, due to the fact that they are more prone to disabilities and illnesses, this population is considered to be the largest consumers of healthcare services and resources. More specifically, their cost of care tend to be approximately three times that of any average person (Laurent, 2002; CIHI, 2011; Ontario Ministry of Health and Long-Term Care, 2012).

Firstly, in terms of resources, drugs commonly found on the lists of medications most likely to be used by the elderly (including antibiotics, anticoagulants, digoxin, diuretics, hypoglycemic agents, antineoplastic agents and non-steroidal anti-inflammatory drugs) are the same drugs most likely to be associated with ADEs and are also responsible for 70% of ADEs occurring within hospitals (Routledge, O'Mahony & Woodhouse, 2003).

In fact, studies have found that ADEs increase with age, making the elderly population most at risk for experiencing such events (Baker et al., 2004; Routledge, O'Mahony & Woodhouse, 2003). Some reasoning cited within various studies have included a greater intake of numerous medication, which has been said to be exponentially related to the risk of ADEs; the failure of physicians to consider the patient's age and frailty on the disposition of drugs; or the failure to consider the increased pharmacodynamic sensitivity of the elderly to several commonly used drugs when prescribing dosages (Routledge, O'Mahony & Woodhouse, 2003).

Secondly, when examining the use of healthcare services, it is important to stress the fact that the senior population is most dependent and in need of health services since sensory memory and cognitive physiological capacities do deteriorate with age making them more prone to disability and chronic illnesses (Laurent, 2002; Nourizadeh et al., 2009). Additionally, in terms of physical health,

Canada's elderly population is more susceptible to osteoporosis, and other physical impairments, that may have severe consequences on their mobility (Laurent, 2002; Nourizadeh et al., 2009).

To make matters worse, in Canada, rural populations tend to be older than urban populations and generally have a much lower health status in comparison to other Canadians (Hay, Varga-Toth & Hines, 2006). In other words, seniors are often over-represented in rural regions of Canada. Generally, the delivery of healthcare services in rural and northern communities is especially difficult (Ministry of Health and Long Term Care, 1998). This may be due to the fact that healthcare facilities in these areas are fewer and tend to be farther apart than those in urban areas. Hence, travel distances to and from these service providers, especially during the winter season, makes 'around-the-clock' access to healthcare, and emergency facilities very difficult. In any case, getting to a healthcare provider proves to be a challenge for frail seniors (Ontario Ministry of Health and Long- Term Care, 2012). As such, numerous seniors only enter the healthcare system once admitted to the Emergency Department once their health condition becomes acute.

Overall, the document presented by Deb Matthews successfully recognizes that the senior population requires much needed attention and a system that will guarantee they are continuously connected to the healthcare system while ensuring they become key players in their own health (Ontario Ministry of Health and Long-Term Care, 2012).

These policy concerns may be tackled by the application of various health care technologies; software and/or hardware considered to fall under the category of health informatics. For one, CPOEs are the most commonly cited solution for reducing ADEs relating to medication errors or various errors in transcribing or executing physician orders during hospital stays (Ohseldt et al., 2004; Cutler et al., 2005; Campbell et al., 2006; Doolan et al., 2002; Poon et al., 2004). More specifically, these systems are said to reduce the incidence of serious medication errors by approximately 55% to 80% (Poon et al., 2004; Cutler et al., 2005). Along the same lines, telehealth has previously been suggested as a response to the lack of appropriate care received closer to home (Liddy et al., 2008; Botsis & Hartvigsen, 2008; Nourizadeh et al., 2009; Bowles & Baugh, 2008). However, there are a number of applications and devices that may be considered a function of telehealth, this chapter will focus on Telehomecare. Simply defined, telehomecare is known to be the use of information technologies and electronic communication to make possible the delivery of health services and expertise to patients in their own home (Liddy et al., 2008; Hsu et al., 2011).

MAIN FOCUS OF CHAPTER

Issues

As a society, we have been bombarded by news reports, magazine articles, and television screens displaying government funded advertisements encouraging healthy lifestyle behaviors by means of increasing physical activities in schools, campaigns and resources to assist in smoking cessation, and food labels supporting healthier food choices. However, our aging population, which is believed to rapidly increase within the next 20 years, are already facing more complex issues namely chronic illnesses that do not only require interventions but medication, self-management, and maintenance.

In a leap towards improving the quality of care and overall health of our aging population, the Canadian Institute for Health Information's annual report on healthcare in Canada has focused on seniors and aging (2011). With a close examination on the subject, the report revealed issues of sustainability, access to primary care,

and medication while identifying current practices across the nation that governments have and/or plan to implement in the years to come.

Generally, primary health care, involving treatment, health promotion and prevention, tends to be the main source of care for seniors (CIHI, 2011). Primary healthcare may also be seen as an important aspect of senior care as providers here also assist patients in navigating through the 'continuum of care'. The most common point of initial contact with this form of care is the family physician, whom the senior population are more familiar with when compared to the remaining Canadian population. Still, not all seniors have access to family physicians (5% as estimated in 2010) (CIHI, 2011). Studies carried out in 2009 indicate that of those seniors without family physicians, 61% received care through clinics, while 17% sought out care from emergency departments. In Ontario, this issue was recognized and prompted the establishment of 200 family healthcare teams, which provide various services according to the surrounding community (CIHI, 2011). Though, this initiative proved to be successful in improving access with 24/7 response and a patient-centered model, it does not align with the need to provide care closer to home.

In terms of sustainability, it should be indicated that hospitals, of all the different components of healthcare, receive the largest share of public healthcare dollars- 37.3% (CIHI, 2011). Although seniors, currently, make up only 14% of the Canadian population, they make up the largest population of hospital service users. Not only may this be attributed to the use of hospital care for conditions treatable in other settings, but also due to the fact that the rates of chronic illnesses among this population remain high (i.e., a 2008 survey showed 76% of seniors in Canada reported being diagnosed with at least one chronic illness while 24% reported being diagnosed with three or more) (CIHI, 2011). Treating these chronic illnesses is undertaken by the prescription of various medications, each one treating a different chronic illness. This leads to the previously explained issue of adverse drug events (Routledge, O'Mahony & Woodhouse, 2003).

CIHI (2011) examined this topic closely, reporting on three different strategies carried out across the nation with the aim of promoting safe and appropriate use of medications. Firstly, education assessment reviews, as implemented in Saskatchewan, Quebec, British Colombia, Ontario, New Brunswick and Nova Scotia, require prescribing physician(s) and pharmacist(s) to review the list of medications taken by their patient with the aim of identifying any possible drug interactions (Health Council of Canada, 2011). Though this has seen some success in the reduction of inappropriate prescribing, it remains problematic in the sense that the providers must rely on the patients to provide such information (CIHI, 2011). This could be difficult for seniors who are prescribed large quantities of medication. Secondly, academic detailing programs are another government-funded strategy where by trained educators visit physicians on site to share the most up to date information on treatment guidelines (CIHI, 2011; Sketris et al., 2007). Though adopted in Alberta, Manitoba, Nova Scotia, British Colombia, and Saskatchewan, there are limited studies on this topic (Sketris et al., 2007). Findings fluctuate from 1-2% improvements to 24-25% improvements in other studies, while not all physicians are open to the approach and the limited information available point to its high cost (Sketris et al., 2007). Finally, nearly one third of community pharmacists and approximately half the hospital pharmacies and emergency departments across Canada have access to a drug information system (Health Council of Canada, 2011). However, British Colombia, Saskatchewan, Prince Edward Island, Alberta and Manitoba all have these systems in place, the remaining provinces and territories are currently in different stages of planning or implementation. This approach to tackling the issue proves

to be most beneficial as will be explained in the following section. The big problem, however, is the fact that Ontario lags behind other provinces, with only 20% of all its hospitals having access to such systems while there have yet to be any community pharmacists to report its use.

87% of Canadians over the age of 55 hope to live at home for as long as possible (CIHI, 2011). With chronic illnesses increasing with age, and adverse drug events being a possible outcome from such diagnoses, one great approach to ensuring quality care for our aging population is providing care closer to home. At any given moment, one million Canadians across the nation are receiving some form of homecare (CIHI, 2011). The definition of what homecare involves remains somewhat vague and changes according to the needs of the individual receiving care. For the most part, it is recognized as involving a broad range of services from health to home support services and is provided by a vast array of providers including nurses, allied health professionals and physicians (CIHI, 2011). As this form of care is not covered under the Canada Health Act, the onus of its implementation lies in the hands of provincial and territorial governments who have made no formal obligations to encourage its use, despite the benefits, as will be outline in the following section (Seggewiss, 2009). As such, legislations concerning homecare differ from one province and territory to another and patients interested in such services must worry about whether or not these services exist within their vicinity and what they may consist of (Seggewiss, 2009). Overall, critics point to policy neglect in the subject of homecare resulting in a 'patchwork' of programs across the country (Seggewiss, 2009, pp. 90).

Solutions and Recommendations

This section will detail the two aforementioned technologies, providing a detailed description of their functions and benefits. In doing so, the CPOE and Tele-homecare are basically examples of how health informatics helps manage the health of elderly patients and responds to the concerns outlined by the Minister of health (linking informatics to policy).

E-prescribing is the method of transmitting prescriptions from an authorized prescriber to a patient's pharmacy of choice through the use of a secure electronic software (Health Council of Canada, 2011). In 2010, Canada Health Infoway anticipated that such software would generate $436 million in cost savings and efficiencies by streamlining pharmacists' work, in turn, improving medication compliance, reducing ADEs, and medication abuse. In general, Canada falls behind other countries in implementing such systems with only 11% of primary healthcare physicians practicing its use (Netherlands 85%, New Zealand 78%, UK 55%, and Australia 81%) (Sketris et al., 2007).

CPOEs are one form of e-prescribing and, in its basic form, refers to the process in which physicians or other eligible healthcare professionals directly enter medical orders into a computer application by the use of voice entry, mouse, keyboard, or other device (Campbell et al., 2006; Ash et al., 2004). Typically, CPOEs exist as one of numerous integrated clinical applications in larger information systems for ordering medications (Campbell et al., 2006; Teufel et al., 2009). They generally work to ensure standardized and legible orders by accepting only typed orders; however, a more complex system allows for the integration of order entry with other patient information, while allowing physicians to access real-time clinical decision support and guidelines, cost information, and electronic message transmissions (Cutler et al., 2005; Campbell et al., 2006; Teufel et al., 2009). In all, these applications complement one another and provide physicians the ability to process hospital orders to pharmacies and create timely, legible prescriptions (Cutler et al., 2005).

Through various functions and methods, the primary benefit of CPOEs is the decrease in medication errors such as incorrect dosages and prescribing which are the main sources for 58% of ADEs; prescribing medications that patients are allergic to; and, prescribing incorrect medications (Goldzweig et al., 2009; Kuperman et al., 2003; Sibbald, 2001). CPOEs have also been proven to increase the quality of care, through more appropriate prescribing methods (Subramanian et al., 2007). In addition, although there has been quite a debate on the feasibility of adopting such a system and the implications of spending large sums of money on its implementation, some researchers have cited cost savings as a major advantage.

As CPOEs are intended for electronic prescribing, at a minimum, healthcare professionals benefit from the elimination of handwritten, illegible prescriptions, which have previously been known to take up extra time due to the need for clarification of orders with pharmacists before they are filled (Subramanian et al., 2007). As such, the electronic ordering component of the CPOE makes for faster delivery of medication orders to the pharmacy and provides other healthcare professional with more time to cater to other needs of the patients, hence increasing the quality of care (Subramanian et al., 2007). This not only assists in achieving the goal of improving the speed at which patients can access care as outlined in Ontario's Action Plan, but also allows healthcare professionals to act sooner to manage their patients' health which in turn leads to a decrease in unnecessary hospital visits and improves their quality of life (Ontario Ministry of Health and Long- Term Care, 2012).

Another adamant point made in Ontario's Action Plan stresses the concept of patient centered care that is easily made possible through the use of electronic health records (Ontario Ministry of Health and Long- Term Care, 2012). The CPOEs are similarly capable of considering the needs of each individual patient as it incorporates their health records and personal information (e.g.: demographics, medication list, and laboratory results) to strengthen its clinical decision support function (Metzger & Turisco, 2001). Firstly, incorporating such personalized information makes checking for therapeutic overlaps and drug interactions possible since the physician is able to evaluate a current medication order alongside other active medication orders as well as medication reference knowledge. Secondly, the CPOE uses such information in its surveillance function. That is, it connects orders and newly reported information regarding the patient (whether it be renal function or vital signs) while extending the application of logic to times between ordering sessions. The system then looks for changes in patient condition and follows up by initiating an alert that requests the physician to reconsider a particular order. This can especially increase practice efficiency when dealing with senior patients, of whom 75% with complex needs receive care from six or more physicians following hospital discharge with another 30% receiving medications from three or more pharmacies (Ontario Ministry of Health and Long- Term Care, 2012).

Finally, cost savings can be recognized in relation to every other benefit that the CPOEs provide. In other words, the elimination of handwritten prescriptions, the quickening of the ordering phase, the increase in quality of care and most of all the reduction of ADEs all lead to cost savings (Park et al., 2003, Sibbald, 2001). In fact, Sibbald (2001) estimated that such a system could save hospitals up to US$500,000 each year in direct costs alone, excluding liability costs or that of injuries to patients. Laboratories and pharmacies lower their future costs as they eliminate paper based orders while streamlining the process of ordering tests and medications, leading to the reduction of any errors that may have once occurred in transmission. Patients may also see cost savings as the CPOEs' alert functions suggest alternative medicines, generics or lower-tiered drugs whenever applicable. However, most notable would be the cost savings that may arise due to the clinical decision support function of the CPOEs as previously described. This function ensures the reduction of dosing errors, ordering of incorrect medication or medications that may induce allergic reactions or adverse drug reactions. As such out-

comes tend to prolong hospital stays and at times lead to complications, disability or death, there is sure to be a saving in cost to all stakeholders. For example, ADEs lead patients to prolong their hospital stay by an additional 8-12 days (Sibbald, 2001). This translates into a per-patient cost of US $16,000- 24,000; or, an annual US $5.6 million per hospital. More recently, a study on the return on investment for a CPOEs at Bringham and Women's Hospital (BWH) found that over a decade, the CPOEs lead BWH to a cumulative net saving of $16.7 million and a net operating budget saving of $9.5 million (Kaushal et al., 2006). With Ontario's fiscal changes, this benefit would surely impress policy makers who could re-inject these cost savings back into the system and improve other areas within the healthcare system.

Though some may argue that the implementation of such a system may be too costly, and require more healthcare professionals, Ontario's Action Plan hints that the main concern is rather to create seamless delivery of care (Ontario Ministry of Health and Long- Term Care, 2012). That being said, the CPOE will function better when connected with some form of telehealth. Telehomecare ensures a seamless transition and access to care and responds perfectly to the concept of right care, right time, and right place as prioritized by the Minister of Health (Ontario Ministry of Health and Long- Term Care, 2012). Not only will the adoption of Telehomecare improve the efficiency of service delivery, it is also capable of tackling the barriers to accessing primary healthcare providers (i.e., the issue of distance).

Telehomecare systems can be installed in patients' homes and be as simple or complex as necessary, given the specific patient's health requirements (Liddy et al., 2008). As previously mentioned, this can be especially beneficial to the senior population as the need for care increases with age (Botsis & Hartvigsen, 2008). Botsis and Hartvigsen (2008) point out that the scarcity of nurses and facilities to accommodate the aging population may prove to be problematic in the future. Furthermore, this problem may be amplified when considering the fact that individuals aged 85 and above are four times as likely to require daily care in comparison to individuals aged 65-74. Hence, the aging population, along with cost reduction, plays a major role in developing Telehomecare.

The system in question is composed of a simple unit that is capable of connecting to one or more peripheral devices (Liddy et al., 2008). This may include items such as a weight scale, blood pressure monitor, glucometer and the like. Via regular phone lines, this clinical information and communication system also allows patients to carry out voice and video conferences with their healthcare professionals in addition to relaying data related to their personal health (Bowels & Baugh, 2007). The patients must either manually enter data concerning vital signs and other health related issues, or upload it automatically by use of the supplied peripherals (Liddy et al., 2008). Following its transfer to the manufacturer's data center, the data is uploaded to a Web application accessible to healthcare providers to review their patients' information from any Internet accessible location (Liddy et al., 2008; Nourizadeh et al., 2009).

The benefits derived from such a system are twofold. First, as intended, Telehomecare increases patients' independence and quality of life (Bowels & Baugh, 2007; Liddy et al., 2008; Hsu et al., 2011). Having the ability to communicate with physicians and nurses, in addition to tracking their vitals, ensures chronically ill patients and the elderly are able to manage their own health while minimizing the hassle and stress of traveling to and from healthcare centers (Botsis & Hartvigsen, 2008; Bowels & Baugh, 2007; Liddy et al., 2008; Nourizadeh et al., 2009; Hsu et al., 2011). The daily assessments derived from inputting personal health data leads to a better understanding of their health status and disease, which in turn translates into improved self-care (Botsis & Hartvigsen, 2008). In this sense, Telehomecare can be seen

as a response to the Minister's hopes to ensure all individuals play an active, participatory role in their own health (Ontario Ministry of Health and Long- Term Care, 2012). Patients' increased involvement and determination is also in line with the document's advocacy for a patient centered system (Bowels & Baugh, 2007; Ontario Ministry of Health and Long-Term Care, 2012).

A great function of the Telehomecare system gives healthcare professionals the capability of setting suitable limit values specific to their patient (Liddy et al., 2008). Since the system identifies trends, overdue and abnormal data sets, the healthcare professional can receive e-mail alerts once deviations are detected, prompting them to alter medications or plans for action. Not only does this create a sense of security for patients as it improves preventative measures, but they also receive the right care at the right time in the convenience of their own home as the province's new Action Plan hopes to achieve.

Contrary to popular beliefs that older patients suffering from chronic illnesses may be more hesitant to adopt this new, virtual form of care, many studies have found them to be positively receptive (Bowels & Baugh, 2007; Botsis & Hartvigsen, 2008; Liddy et al., 2008). Keeping in mind that levels of satisfaction differ among studies, there have been reports outlining COPD (Chronic Obstructive Pulmonary Disease) patients' comfort in utilizing the Telehomecare's conference tool, with some patients preferring this to in-person consultations, while other patients boast its ease of use (Botsis & Hartvigsen, 2008; Bowels & Baugh, 2007). Similarly, some studies found diabetic patients to feel technologically empowered, while having the Telehomecare system in their daily presence acted as a reminder to prepare for nurse visits (Bowels & Baugh, 2007). So, although the elderly may not be too familiar with the newest technologies, many studies combine to prove that there is hope and reason to believe that they, willingly, will be in the near future especially given the rapid increase in communication technology at lower prices

(Botsis & Hartvigsen, 2008; Bujnowska-Fedak et al., 2011). Similarly, though research concerning telehomecare is limited, there is hope to abolish concerns over the difficulty to utilize new and unfamiliar technologies. As per a pilot study in Ottawa, just over a third of telehomecare patients required technical support (Liddy et al., 2008). Of these, the majority of cases were combated over the phone with troubleshooting mainly involving the unplugging and re-plugging of the unit. The same study also found that no technical issues persisted longer than a 24-hour period.

The second benefit resulting from the adoption of Telehomecare is the indirect cost savings that arise from the reduction of unnecessary re-hospitalization (Liddy et al., 2008; Botsis & Hartvigsen, 2008; Bowles & Baugh, 2008; Hsu et al., 2011). A grand review of Telehomecare studies done by Bowles and Baugh (2008) reveals that this system can reduce in-person visits by 45%. Such programs focus on self-management by allowing patients to track their vitals, keep up to date on their health status, and use video conferencing tools to contact healthcare professionals and become more educated on their illness and health status (Bujnowska-Fedak et al., 2011). As such, Kobb et al. (2008) find that patients tend to make better choices concerning the care and services they consume and are more likely to adhere to the treatment process. They also shared more specific findings citing a study carried out by Chumlber et al. who focused on the effects of Telehomecare on diabetic patients. In their examination of 297 diabetic patients, the group exposed to less intensive daily monitoring were found to have 52% less 'all-cause' hospitalization in comparison to the group exposed to intensive weekly interventions. Similarly, the former group had 53% less diabetes- related hospitalization and 8 days less of bed care over a 12 month period (Bowles & Baugh, 2008). Such findings are also mimicked by studies completed in Poland (Bujnowska-Fedak et al., 2011). The key is outlined within *Ontario's Action Plan for Healthcare*: receiving the proper

care necessary reduces the likelihood for hospital treatment thus creating less strain on the system (Ontario Ministry of Health and Long- Term Care, 2012). The alert function, for example, allows for the monitoring of patients' long-term trends and emerging issues (Liddy et al., 2008). Such information assists health professionals in making more timely medical decisions, reducing the possibility of error, and unnecessarily prolonging health issues. As such, clinical and/or office visits may be minimized, if not eliminated completely; saving both time and cost of resources and travel (Liddy et al., 2008; Botsis & Hartvigsen, 2008; Nourizadeh et al., 2009).

The Ontario Action Plan also calls for evidence- based decision making when considering the allocation and investment of scarce resources and healthcare dollars while ensuring that seniors continuously receive the proper care required closer to home (Ontario Ministry of Health and Long-Term Care, 2012). Telehomecare is the appropriate response in this situation. Though the start up costs of Telehomecare tend to be high, Bowels and Baugh (2008) identified a study carried out by Dansky et al. which points out that such a system creates considerable savings from decreased rates of re-hospitalizations with no concession to the quality of care provided. Furthermore, "the financial benefit increases exponentially as the duration and number of patient care episode increases" (Bowels & Baugh, 2008, p. 5). Furthermore, although implemented in most provinces on different levels, homecare does not exhibit as many cost saving benefits as telehomecare (Britton et al., 2000). The difference of having the ability to carry out video and phone conferencing eliminates unnecessary home visits, not only does this save time and money on transportation but it also allows nurses to cater to more patients, saving costs on human resources that could be more beneficial in other areas of the healthcare system (15 a day using telehomecare as opposed to 6 visits a day when using traditional homecare).

FUTURE RESEARCH DIRECTIONS

E-prescribing has begun to pick up though skepticism surrounding the more new telehomecare make the journey to its implementation much slower. These health technologies are fairly new, and have yet to be wholly embraced as concerns of start up costs and resistance to change and technology continue to create some apprehension (Goldzweig et al., 2009; Campbell et al, 2006). Hence, future research and planning must be invested within the area of health informatics to have a comprehensive understanding of its benefits, downfalls and ways to improve and fund the systems. For one, much research is needed on telehomecare, especially as it relates to primary healthcare as well as accessibility and communication between health practitioners and patients (Bujnowska-Fedak et al., 2011; Nilsson et al., 2008). With an aging population, most of whom make use of primary healthcare, this area of study would be beneficial to examine more in depth. Additionally, as it stands, policy makers' main concerns with telehomecare systems are that of financing (CIHI, 2011). Though Ontario's demographics, population needs and availability of resources may be different than other countries or provinces, research into their funding schemes may provide a better insight into how the system may be successfully adopted. This may include research into the public versus private funding schemes exhibited across Canada (Seggewiss, 2009) or division of telehomecare provision by the social versus healthcare systems as exhibited in France, Spain, and the United Kingdom (CIHI, 2011).

In the end, as Kobb et al. (2008) makes evident, the question then becomes how much data is enough to prove such technologies are beneficial in cost saving, improving quality care and efficiency, decreasing hospitalization and providing care that is patient-centered that empowers individuals? There should be a plan set forth so as to move forward rather than continue to discuss the topic. Hence, a closer examination of various international implementation processes concerning such healthcare technologies may provide some important lessons on the next steps to be taken by Canadian governments in order to successfully attain the health goals initially outlined in this chapter.

CONCLUSION

Slowly, along with healthcare providers, leaders within the field of health policy are beginning to recognize the importance of maintaining a technologically savvy approach to tackling healthcare issues in a society driven by the virtual world in which technology is highly influential and dependent upon (Ontario Ministry of Health and Long-Term Care, 2012; Nilsson et al., 2008). More importantly, the opportunity to take advantage of such systems is ever present and should be embraced in order to improve the health of Ontarians (Speedie et al., 2008; Ontario Ministry of Health and Long-Term Care, 2012).

Seniors, being the population of focus in this chapter, are more open to adopting information technology than one may initially have thought. To boot, the trend towards the adoption of such systems in healthcare is on the rise as there are already evident forms of telehealth currently in place, whether it be the beginning of EHRs, use of hand held devices by health educators and pharmaceutical representatives, of telehealth phone lines. In particular, through the examination of various reports on the topic, it seems as though the telehomecare trend is picking up and receiving more attention within the past couple of years. If the benefits found in various international studies are any indication of the future, this 'trend' will continue to gain popularity and will be the best response to the needs of an aging population.

As this chapter shows, CPOEs and Telehomecare are two examples of how healthcare technologies that can be used to respond to health policy and management issues. They work to assist healthcare professionals in medical decision making through prompts and alerts while ensuring patients have a comprehensive understanding of their health status, allowing them to be more empowered and involved in managing their own health. Combined, these systems have the capabilities to ensure patients receive the right care (specific to the individual patient, given their most up to date information), at the right time (through alerts and notifications, Internet connections and phone lines), in the right place (at the point of care as well as in the comfort of their own home).

Overall, policy makers must realize the fact that we are living in a hi-tech society and in order to be successful, one must adapt. Any change comes with a risk but the reality of a rapidly growing senior population in conjunction with limited resources should be enough reason for policy makers to gain courage and assume the risk, adopting health technologies that ensure greater care for all. The standardization of an electronic health record connected to both CPOEs and telehealth systems would only ease the ability to create a truly patient centered system characterized by seamless care. As such, policy makers may want to begin by ensuring that the aim of implementing EHRs on a national scale is finally met.

REFERENCES

Ash, J. S., Gorman, P. N., Seshadri, V., & Hersh, W. R. (2004). Computerized physician order entry in U.S. hospitals: Results of a 2002 survey. *Journal of the American Medical Informatics Association*, *11*(2), 95–99. doi:10.1197/jamia. M1427 PMID:14633935.

Baker, G. R., Norton, P. G., Flintoft, V., Blais, R., Brown, A., & Cox, J. et al. (2004). The Canadian adverse events study: the incidence of adverse events among hospital patients in Canada. *Journal of the Canadian Medical Association*, *170*(11), 1678–1686. doi:10.1503/cmaj.1040498 PMID:15159366.

Botsis, T., & Hartvigsen, G. (2008). Current status and future perspectives in telecare for elderly people suffering from chronic diseases. *Journal of Telemedicine and Telecare*, *14*, 194–203. doi:10.1258/jtt.2008.070905 PMID:18534954.

Bowles, K. H., & Baugh, A. C. (2007). Applying research evidence to optimize telehomecare. *The Journal of Cardiovascular Nursing*, *22*(1), 5–15. PMID:17224692.

Britton, B. P., Engelke, M. K., Rains, D. B., & Mahmud, K. (2000). Measuring costs and quality of telehomecare. *Home Health Care Management & Practice*, *12*(4), 27–32. doi:10.1177/108482230001200409.

Bujnowska-Fedak, M.M., Puchala, E., & Steciwko, A. (2011). The impact of telehome care status and quality of life among patients with diabetes in primary care setting in Poland. *Telemedicine and e-Health Journal*, *17*(3), 153-163.

Cadario, B. (2005). New appreciation of serious adverse drug reactions. *British Columbia Medical Journal*, *47*(1), 14.

Campbell, E. M., Sittig, D. F., Ash, J. S., Guappone, K. P., & Dykstra, R. H. (2006). Types of unintended consequences related to computerized provider order entry. *Journal of the American Medical Informatics Association*, *13*(5), 547–554. doi:10.1197/jamia.M2042 PMID:16799128.

Canadian Institute for Health Information. (2011). [*A focus on seniors and aging*. Ottawa, Canada: CIHI.]. *Health Care in Canada*, 2011.

Casey, M. M., Moscovice, I. S., & Davidson, G. (2006). Pharmacist staffing, technology use, and implementation of medication safety practices in rural hospitals. *Journal of National Rural Health Association*, *22*(4), 321–330. doi:10.1111/j.1748-0361.2006.00053.x PMID:17010029.

Cutler, D. M., Feldman, N. E., & Horwitz, J. R. (2005). US adoption of computerized physician order entry system. *Journal of Health Affairs*, *24*(6), 1654–1664. doi:10.1377/hlthaff.24.6.1654.

Doolan, D. F., & Bates, D. W. (2002). Computerized physician order entry systems in hospitals: Mandates and incentives. *Journal of Health Affairs, 21*(4), 180–185. doi:10.1377/hlthaff.21.4.180 PMID:12117128.

Goldzweig, C. L., Towfigh, A., Maglione, M., & Shekelle, P. G. (2009). Cost and benefit of health information technology: New trends from the literature. *Journal of Health Affairs, 28*(2), 282–293. doi:10.1377/hlthaff.28.2.w282.

Hay, D., Varga-Toth, J., & Hines, E. (2006). Frontline health care in Canada: Innovations in delivering services to vulnerable populations. *Canadian Policy Research Networks.* Retrieved from http://www.frontlinehealth.ca/pdfs/CPRN-ResearchReport.pdf

Health Council of Canada. (2011). *Progress report 2011: Health care renewal in Canada.* Toronto, Canada: HCC.

Hsu, C., Tseng, K. C., & Chuang, Y. (2011). Predictors of future use of telehomecare health services by middle-aged people in Taiwan. *Journal of Social Behavior and Personality, 39*(9), 1252–1262. doi:10.2224/sbp.2011.39.9.1251.

Kaushal, R., Jha, A. K., Franz, C., Glaser, J., Shetty, K. D., & Jaggi, T. et al. (2006). Return on investment for a computerized physician order entry system. *Journal of the American Medical Informatics Association, 13*(3), 261–266. doi:10.1197/jamia.M1984 PMID:16501178.

Kobb, R., Chumber, N.R., Brennan, D.M., & Robinowitz, T. (2008). Home telehealth: Mainstreaming what we do well. *Telemedicine and e-Health Journal, 14*(90), 977-981.

Laurent, S. (2002). Rural Canada: Access to health care. *Government of Canada Economics Division.* Retrieved from http://dsp-psd.pwgsc.gc.ca/Collection-R/LoPBdP/BP/prb0245-e.htm#2Age

Liddy, C., Dusseault, J. J., Dahrouge, S., Hogg, W., Lemelin, J., & Humbert, J. (2008). Telehomecare for patients with multiple chronic illnesses. *Canadian Family Physician Medecin de Famille Canadien, 54*, 58–65. PMID:18208957.

Metzger, J., & Turisco, F. (2001). Computerized physician order entry: A look at the vendor marketplace and getting started. *The Leapfrog Group.* Retrieved from http://www.leapfroggroup.org/media/file/Leapfrog-CPO_Guide.pdf

Ministry of Health and Long Term Care. (1998). *Access to quality health care in rural and northern Ontario.* Retrieved from https://ospace.scholarsportal.info/bitstream/1873/7175/1/10276872.pdf

Nourizadeh, S., Deroussent, C., Song, Y. Q., & Thomesse, J. P. (2009). A distributed elderly healthcare system. *Inria.* Retrieved from http://hal.inria.fr/docs/00/43/12/02/PDF/A_Distributed_Elderly_healthcare_System.pdf

Ontario Ministry of Health and Long-Term Care. (2012). *Ontario's action plan for health care.* Retrieved from http://www.health.gov.on.ca/en/ms/ecfa/healthy_change/docs/rep_healthychange.pdf

Park, W., Kim, J. S., Chae, Y. M., Yu, S., Kim, C., Kim, S., & Jung, S. H. (2003). Does the physician order-entry system increase the revenue of a general hospital? *Journal of Medical Informatics, 71*, 25–32. doi:10.1016/S1386-5056(03)00056-X PMID:12909155.

Poon, E. G., Blumenthal, D., Jaggi, T., & Honour, M. M. (2004). Overcoming barriers to adopting and implementing computerized physician order entry systems in U.S. hospitals. *Journal of Health Affairs, 23*(4), 184–190. doi:10.1377/hlthaff.23.4.184 PMID:15318579.

Routledge, P. A., Mahony, M. S., & Woodhouse, K. W. (2003). Adverse drug reactions in elderly patients. *British Journal of Clinical Pharmacology, 57*(2), 121–126. doi:10.1046/j.1365-2125.2003.01875.x PMID:14748810.

Seggewiss, K. (2009). Variations in home care programs across Canada demonstrate need for national standards and pan-Canadian program. *Canadian Medical Association Journal, 180*(2), E90–E92. doi:10.1503/cmaj.090819 PMID:19506265.

Sibbald, B. (2001). Use computerized systems to cut adverse drug events: Report. *Canadian Medical Association Journal, 164*(13), 1878.

Sketris, I., Ingram, E. L., & Lummis, H. (2007). *Optimal prescribing and medication use in Canada: Challenges and opportunities.* Ottawa, Canada: Health Council of Canada.

Speedie, S.M., Ferguson, A.S., Sanders, J., & Doarn, C.R. (2008). Telehealth: The promise of new care delivery models. *Telemedicine and e-Health Journal, 14*(9), 964-967.

Subramanian, S., Hoover, S., Gilman, B., Field, T. S., Mutter, R., & Gurwitz, J. H. (2007). Computerized physician order entry with clinical decision support in long-term care facilities: Costs and benefits to stakeholders. *Journal of the American Geriatrics Society, 55*(9), 1451–1457. doi:10.1111/j.1532-5415.2007.01304.x PMID:17915344.

Teufel, R. J., Kazley, A. S., & Basco, W. T. Jr. (2009). Early adopters of computerized physician order entry in hospitals that care for children: A picture of US health care shortly after the institute of medicine reports on quality. *Journal of Clinical Pediatrics, 48*(4), 389–396. doi:10.1177/0009922809331801 PMID:19224864.

ADDITIONAL READING

Canadian Health Services Research Foundation. (2011). *Better with age: Health systems planning for the aging population (synthesis report).* Ottawa, Canada: CHSRF.

Chan, M., Campo, E., Esteve, D., & Fourniols, J. Y. (2009). Smart homes—Current features and future perspectives. *Maturitas, 64*(2), 90–97. doi:10.1016/j.maturitas.2009.07.014 PMID:19729255.

Finkelstein, S. M., Speedie, S. M., Demiris, G., Veen, M., Lundgren, J. M., & Potthoff, S. (2004). Telehomecare: Quality, perception, satisfaction. *Telemedicine Journal and e-Health, 10*(2), 122–128. doi:10.1089/tmj.2004.10.122 PMID:15319041.

Kaushal, R., & Bates, D.W. (2001). Computerized physician order entry (CPOE) with decision support systems (CDSSs). *Making Health Care Safer: A Critical Analysis of Patient Safety Practices,* (43), 59-69.

Lamothe, L., Fortin, J. P., Labbe, F., Gagnon, M. P., & Messikh, D. (2006). Impacts of telehomecare on patients, providers, and organizations. *Telemedicine Journal and e-Health, 12*(3), 363–369. doi:10.1089/tmj.2006.12.363 PMID:16796505.

Ludwig, W., Worlf, K. H., Duwenkamp, C., Gusew, N., Hellrung, N., & Marschollek, M. et al. (2012). Health-enabling technologies for the elderly- An overview of servies based on a literature review. *The Journal of the Korea Contents Association, 12*(2), 349–357.

Ohsfeldt, R. L., Ward, M. M., Schneider, J. E., Jaana, M., Miller, T. R., Lei, Y., & Wakefield, D. S. (2005). Implementation of hospital computerized physician order entry systems in rural state: Feasibility and financial impact. *Journal of the American Medical Informatics Association, 12,* 20–27. doi:10.1197/jamia.M1553 PMID:15492033.

KEY TERMS AND DEFINITIONS

Adverse Events: Unintended harm or complications resulting from the management of a patient's health rather than the patient's underlying illness. This typically leads to death, disability following hospital discharge, or extended hospital stays.

Computerized Physician Order Entry System (CPOEs): A hand-held device that allows physicians to enter patient's prescriptions and forward them to pharmacists in real time. Various functions in the software alert physicians of allergies and drug-drug reactions, helping reduce adverse drug events.

Health Informatics: A discipline that combines information science and technology to the field of healthcare.

Ontario's Action Plan for Health Care: A document put out by the Minister of Health in February of 2012, outlining the future objectives to improve healthcare for Ontarians. This includes the assurance that all Ontarians have the needed support to become healthier, have faster access to care, and receive the proper care at the right time and place.

Seniors: The elder individual. A senior citizen typically aged 65 or older.

Telecare: Healthcare provided to patients by means other than in-person visits.

Telehomecare: A form of telecare installed in the patient's home, that uses phone lines and the Internet to connect patients to healthcare professional. The system allows for phone and video conferencing while relaying data on vital signs, etc. through the use of peripheral medical devices.

Section 3
Informatics Challenges

Chapter 11
Normalizing Cross-Border Healthcare in Europe via New E-Prescription Paradigms

Alexander Berler
National School of Public Health, Greece & epSOS, Greece

Ioannis Apostolakis
National School of Public Health, Greece

ABSTRACT

The 21ˢᵗ century started with some significant efforts globally in the e-health sector. This was mainly pushed as a generic strategy from many nations and international organizations in order to cope with issues such as ageing population, demographic shift, social security limitations, and financial instability. A second reason was the introduction of new technologies such as cloud computing, Web interoperability standards, mobile health, and social media that are steadily changing the way healthcare has been seen in the last decades. In addition to that, globalization, commuting, immigration, and increased mobility raised the issue of cross-border healthcare and the right to access normalized healthcare services anywhere, anytime. In that context, the authors analyze the technological offerings and result of the epSOS (European Patient Smart Open Services) framework and how it has affected strategic decisions in electronic prescription in Greece, thus creating a new useful e-health national application. They prove that by rethinking healthcare, reusing established standards such as HL7 CDA (Health Level Seven Clinical Document Architecture) and IHE (Integrating the Healthcare Enterprise) profiles, it is possible to propose a new innovative system that is in fact based upon new technological propositions such as REST (Representational State Transfer) architecture and cloud computing.

INTRODUCTION

The healthcare delivery landscape will change significantly in the future to master changes of society, such as constant population ageing and demographic rise (Mirkin, 2001). Those changes have already started and demand that e-health plays a significant role within a reformed healthcare system (European Commission, 2012). It is commonly agreed that e-health is a benefit for the patients, the healthcare practitioners, the healthcare provider organizations and the nations as a whole.

DOI: 10.4018/978-1-4666-4321-5.ch011

Eysenbach states that:

E-health is an emerging field in the intersection of medical informatics, public health and business, referring to health services and information delivered or enhanced through the Internet and related technologies. In a broader sense, the term characterizes not only a technical development, but also a state-of-mind, a way of thinking, an attitude, and a commitment for networked, global thinking, to improve health care locally, regionally, and worldwide by using information and communication technology. (Eysenbach, 2001)

The future of healthcare is to be patient-centric and with a focus on health promotion and health maintenance. Patient centred healthcare implies that patients and their relatives have a more active role in the design and enforcement of new healthcare treatments. So, patient should be the centre of care and all related information and decisions should incorporate each patient's individual options for better treatment. Patients and practitioners should operate in partnership so that medical decisions respect patient's need, beliefs and preferences. Practitioners should focus on making sure that patients have substantial information and support so that they can make appropriate decisions and participate in their own care (Institute of Medicine, 2001). New e-health services with the use of ICT (Information and Communication Technologies) such as Internet, cloud computing, social media are reshaping day by day the healthcare delivery systems (Apostolakis et al, 2012; Gwee, 2011; Cambria et al, 2010).

Appropriate and viable use of interoperable e-Health solutions has already demonstrated its ability to propose a strategy for reshaping the system towards a patient centred system. In other words, e-health seems to have the ability to enable and establish patient centred healthcare systems, where information systems interoperate and exchange patient information seamlessly on behalf of patient's welfare and social rights. However, the more complex and the more fragmented the

healthcare provision and the insurance systems are the more complex and fragmented will the e-Health services be. Both positive as negative lessons learned from the past should influence future decisions (Calliope, 2010b).

On the demand side, citizens and patients want to be empowered and are increasingly well informed with the use of social media. Life expectancy steadily rises (Leon, 2011) and so is the prevalence of chronic conditions that are more often diagnosed at early stages. At the moment, the vast majority of national healthcare budgets concerns chronic disease management (Kaiser, 2012). Medical treatments, diagnostics tools and procedures, as well as the extensive use of new technologies in equipment and pharmaceutical industry increase the cost of healthcare. The use of new ICT technologies can and should automate and optimize healthcare delivery and related costs to the extent possible. Patient societies and other stakeholders demand and expect that no geographical borders exist in healthcare delivery, that seamless and adequate continuum of care prevails. Today's citizens are far more mobile for leisure or work than before, and this is well studied and documented (Rosenmöller et al, 2006; Glinos, 2012). Early epidemiological surveillance via warning and alert systems (WHO, 2005), as well as research and continuous professional training will require enhanced secondary use of aggregated health data of individuals to support the effectiveness, efficiency and sustainability of the health systems.

On the supply side, the demographic shift and population ageing has puts increased pressure on healthcare delivery systems (Mirkin, 2001, Bloom, 2011). In addition, the increase of patients' numbers creates a shortage of skilled healthcare labour resources and medical expertise. As a consequence healthcare systems and process should be re-invented to deal with those pressures. In addition, the increased complexity of healthcare delivery and the need for increasingly shared information demand new working procedures and workflows.

The World Health Organization (WHO) has issued an important report in 2002 (WHO, 2002), that focused on that year, on the amount of disease, disability and death in the world that is attributed to a specific selection of the most significant risks to human health. The same document also calculates how much of this burden could be avoided in the upcoming decades, if the same risk factors are reduced from now and onwards. One way to reduce risk is to establish monitoring facilities (AHRQ, 2003; NHMRC, 2010). They would then control, benchmark and assess risk factors at a national and a global level. In that sense, Health cannot be restricted within national borders. In the way the planet, with the significant intervention of technology, has moved towards globalized structures, people, goods and services are constantly moving between regions and nations. As health is concerned, it is obvious that cross border healthcare has become an inevitable matter to deal with in all its instances: legal, social, technical, medical. Extensive information exist in the reference section of this chapter (WHO 2002b; WHO 2008b; Salgado, 2010, Samb et al, 2009). Globalization is putting the social cohesion of many countries under stress, and health systems, as key constituents of contemporary societies, are not performing as well as they should (WHO, 2008).

European Union has foreseen the aforementioned needs and open issues and has created policy papers and directives to respond to them (European Commission, 2004 & 2012), especially noting the need for standardization and cross border healthcare regulations in an attempt to provide adequate care for all citizens independently of their location within a unified Europe. As a consequence, the Large Scale Pilot Project on cross border e-Health interoperability, epSOS (European Patient Smart Open Services), and the thematic network of CALLIOPE (CALL for InterOPErability) until 2011 and now the e-Health Governance Initiative are the new drivers for creating, initially, new working paradigms in e-Prescription and Patient Summary use cases across Europe (eHGI, 2012).

EpSOS has created a series of new technical and functional requirements that enable the safe routing of medical information across regional and national healthcare systems, based on the efficient reuse of existing standards and integration profiles. After more than three years of hard work to develop feasible cross-border e-Health services, the efforts of the epSOS project team have now culminated in the large scale pilot entering into operational mode on the 13th of April 2012. In this piloting phase, the developed solutions are tested in a real-life environment during a one-year period (epSOS, 2008).

The technical and functional requirements already have a significant acceptance within EU member states (20 of which participate in epSOS) and not only (Norway, Switzerland and Turkey have Joined epSOS). In that sense, a significant, common ground has been introduced, assessed, disseminated and openly accepted concerning interoperability issues, codification and nomenclature reuse, transcoding, security, data privacy and many more.

EpSOS has introduced concepts such as the National Contact Point (NCP) which is, in fact, an enterprise information bus that securely, seamlessly transport medical information across healthcare systems of any type and complexity. This enables a democratic regulation of health IT market allowing common testing procedures (by reusing profiles and test tools provided by IHE), common interoperability frameworks (by accepting common HL7 CDA r2 type documents for the electronic prescription) and certification procedures (by deploying national certification and accreditation bodies and reusing IHE, EuroRec Institute or HL7 EHR-FS (Electronic Healthcare Record Functional System) standards and methods).

In this chapter we propose to demonstrate the flexibility and reuse of the epSOS framework at a national and regional level by depicting the Greek e-Prescription case. It will explain how new and innovative e-services were introduced, in order to shape the new paradigm shift in e-Health in the 21st Century. From a methodological point of view, the chapter will follow a top down approach starting from presenting in the Background section; the high level European strategic decisions and mandates will then proceed to a thorough presentation and analysis of the epSOS case and analyze the current situation regarding e-Prescription. The next paragraphs present a detailed analysis of specific adoption of the EU approach at a country level with emphasis on the New Greek e-Prescription case, which introduces a new business paradigm in e-Prescription. In the "future research direction" section, we will propose the relative areas where future research is dominant in relation with the topics of this chapter. Finally, the author with deploy a synthesis of the chapter and state their opinions and beliefs in the conclusion section.

BACKGROUND

The Need for Cross Border Healthcare

WHO in its 2010 report (WHO, 2010) states the need for finding financial tools to achieve universal health coverage for patients and citizens. The literature on universal health coverage mostly focuses on five main themes such as accessibility to healthcare resources, population coverage capacity, point of care geography, rights to healthcare access and population protection from social and economic consequences of the lack of health. In that sense WHO is seeking ways to find ways to make universal health coverage financially sustainable especially in more underserved countries (Stuckler et al, 2010)

People are increasingly impatient with the inability of health systems to deliver services that meet stated demands and new needs. So many European patients, for example, seek healthcare services on the global scale, either because their country is, unfortunately, unable to serve them,

or because they seek high expertise and skills at the point of delivery. In the latter case, information and communication technologies (ICT) have proven again to be a driver for fast information dissemination via the Internet and social media (Biermann et al, 2006; DeVries, 2012; Chou et al, 2009; Eysenbach 2002; Eysenbach, 2008).

As a consequence, Europe for many years know has focused on the subject and tried to find ways to include the need for cross border healthcare and adequate quality of healthcare delivery for all European citizens. Cross-border health care has simply become a more prominent phenomenon in the European Union (E.U.). When in need of medical treatment, patients supported by social media, for example, act as informed consumers who claim the right to choose their own provider beyond their national borders. Cross-border health care is also not restricted to patients. Medical doctors and nurses go abroad for training, to provide services temporarily or to establish them in another Member State. Increasingly, individual doctors and hospitals in different Member States cooperate with each other (Wismar et al, 2011). The above mentioned relations between actors and tools for cross border healthcare are depicted in Figure 1.

In order to deal with the cross border issue Europe has envisaged three alternatives to reduce legal burden. The first alternative focuses on the law of each country. So, when an action or service is performed in a different country that the country of establishment, then the applicable law is the one of the country of establishment. This is a basic principle taken focusing of the free movement of services and goods. The second alternative is the introduction of specific ruling in the framework of coordination of social systems, which resulted in the establishment of the council regulation No 1408/71 of 14 June 1971 that focused in building a common European labor market. The third alternative was the most complex and time consuming that ended recently with the adoption of the new "Directive 2011/24/EU of the European parliament and the council of 9

Figure 1. Cross border healthcare actors and new tools

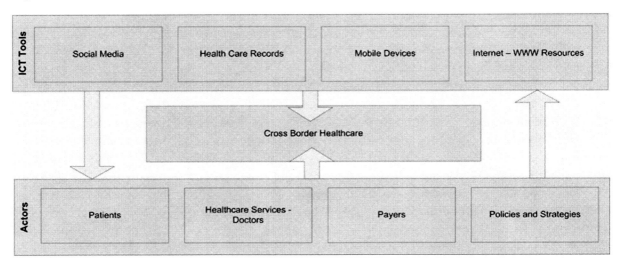

March 2011on the application of patients' rights in cross-border healthcare" (OJEU, 2011). In fact, this was an open discussion and need noted more than a decade ago (Busse & Wismar, 2002).

European Strategy for E-Health

The European Union provides a common framework, policies, and service across all Member States. In many areas, there are common policies, but healthcare remains a national prerogative. There are substantial variations between the respective national healthcare systems, although, many similar issues exist – i.e. ageing population, chronic diseases prevalence, financial pressures. However, the capital right for mobility, both for patients and healthcare workers, has intensified the need for sharing of health records across national boundaries and the use of standards, processes and technologies to support them. In this ambiguous environment, most Member State Governments assume that they have full responsibility and control over their own health services, on the basis of Article 152 of the Amsterdam Treaty, but in fact, it is apparent that the Single European Market (SEM) has a substantial impact on health services (Busse & Wismar, 2002). The SEM relies on a set of principles such as free movement of goods and services and freedom of establishment. Those influence health services since patient often move for business, leisure of better care selection, thus demanding to receive equal care with Europe based upon SEM principles (Wismar et al, 2011).

The "Bolkestein Directive on services in the internal market", introduced in December 2006 (OJEU, 2006), kept the delivery of healthcare out of scope. A number of official rulings of the European Court of Justice (ECJ), regarding the application of the internal market principles to health, clearly state, that internal market regulation have an influence on the delivery of health services. Consequently, a legal document was called for, to settle the ECJ's open issues, concerning patients' rights to get reimbursement for healthcare services done in another Member State. This resulted in the directive 2011/24/EU as a response to the raised concerns, in the context of cross-border healthcare, with a focus on e-Prescription.

This Directive states that patients are allowed to receive healthcare in another Member State and get reimbursement up to the costs accepted in the country of origin, as if this treatment had been provided inland. For reasons of general interest, a country may restrain the application of cross-border healthcare rules on reimbursement. In order to monitor incoming flows of patients and to ensure efficient access to healthcare, the country of delivery of care is allowed to adopt measures concerning access to treatment where this is justified. This means that the Directive targets European citizens and protect their rights to equal care within E.U. borders, but it is not effective for other foreigners where other official documents and bilateral agreements are legally binding healthcare processes. Finally, Member States need to establish national contact points in order to provide patients with information concerning their rights and practical aspects of getting cross border healthcare.

In parallel, the EU has also matured in terms of introducing ICT in the healthcare sector in order to deal with issues such as those aforementioned. In the past decades a series of important studies, reports and communications, issued by the European Commission, urge Member States to take immediate action in that domain. Willing not to make extensive description of EU strategic goals and decisions, it is nevertheless important to state at least the most important steps that lead us to today's situation and future promising prospects. Those are duly noted and analyzed in CALLIOPE project documentation (Calliope, 2010a, 2010b) with the focus on e-Health.

The vision for health is for a smart, citizen-centered health system paradigm in which each citizen's needs are at the centre of redesigned health and social care services, but there are a number of challenges to address. Some of those issues have been technically addressed at a regional level (Berler, 2009). Europe's Member States are continually attempting to respond to demand for quality, safety and access. They are also fighting for healthcare systems sustainability in an unfriendly environment led by of demographic changes, ageing population reactions, increasing incidence of chronic diseases, rising demand for personalized healthcare and financial pressures.

The 2010 OECD (Organisation for Economic Co-operation and Development) report (OECD, 2010) provides clear evidence of the benefits that can result from ICT implementation into four domains: increasing quality of care and efficiency, reducing operating costs of clinical services, reducing administrative costs and enabling new care modalities. European Union's current initiatives focus on implementing the Europe 2020 strategy (European Commission, 2010a), while keeping up on the recommendation made in the Communication of the European Commission in 2004 (European Commission, 2004). This chapter is also proposing an analytical listing of further reading in this subject.

In short, "Europe 2020" proposes three priorities: Smart growth, Sustainable growth and Inclusive growth. The Digital Agenda (European Commission, 2010b), as part of the Europe 2020 strategy, places e-Health in a cross-sectoral framework with the following action points:

- **Key Action 13:** Undertake pilot actions to provide Europeans with secure online access to their personal health data by 2015 and to achieve by 2020 extensive deployment of telemedicine and telecare services.
- **Key Action 14:** Define a minimum common data set for interoperability of healthcare records to be accessed or exchanged electronically by 2025.

Major reports and studies (Stroetmann et al, 2011; Valeri, 2010; Warden, 2012) conclude that there is a significant healthcare improvement potential using e-Health as a catalyst. Examples of quantified potentials include (Gartner, 2009):

- 5 million outpatient prescription errors per year could be avoided through e-Prescriptions.
- 100,000 inpatient adverse drug events per year could be avoided through Clinical Decision Support and Computerized

Physician Order Entry Systems. This would free up 700,000 bed-days per year, corresponding to a value of almost €300 million.

- 9 million bed-days per year could be released, through the use of Electronic Patient Records, thus increasing output or decreasing waiting times, corresponding to a value of approximately €3,7 billion.

Project epSOS

In order to support health policies at a European Level, standardization effort in healthcare, e-health, to promote and to establish the enforcement of the new EU Directive on cross border healthcare, the European Commission, via the Information and Communication Technologies Policy Support Program (ICT PSP) as part of the Competitiveness and Innovation Framework Program, is co-funding the Large Scale Pilot (LSP) "European Patient Smart Open Service" or epSOS in short.

EpSOS mandate is to design, build and evaluate a service oriented infrastructure that demonstrates cross-border interoperability between electronic health record systems in Europe (epSOS, 2008). EpSOS is a large scale pilot involving more than 105 healthcare provider point of care (Hospitals / General Practitioner / Medical Specialist offices) and 168 Pharmacies all spread across 23 countries in Europe. The whole extend and description of

the pilot settings can be reached electronically via epSOS central access point at www.epsos.eu. The project features are shortly described in Table 1.

EpSOS goal is to offer seamless healthcare to European citizens and a technical and functional framework for cross border healthcare. Key goals are to enhance the quality and safety of healthcare services for people travelling or commuting to another country. Moreover in Europe, it concentrates on developing a practical e-Health framework and ICT infrastructure that enables secure access to patient health information among different European healthcare systems. EpSOS aspiration is to makes a significant contribution to patient safety by reducing the frequency of medical errors when providing quick access to patient summary documentation. In emergency situations, this documentation may provide the medical personnel with important life-saving information and minimize the repetition of diagnostic procedures that are both costly and unnecessary (Abba, 2009; Forni, 2010).

The project also tests for more than one full year the technical, legal and organizational concepts developed during the project. EpSOS today tests cross-border services in the following areas concerning patient summary and cross-border use of e-prescriptions. In a later phase (epSOS has been extended until end of 2013) the project envisions the following new scenarios: Integration of the 112 emergency services at each nation, Integration of the European Health Insurance Card

Table 1. epSOS in figures

Time period	1st July 2008 - 31st December 2013
Duration	66 months (5 1/2 years)
Volume	€ 36,5 Million: co-funded by the European Commission Competitiveness and Innovation Programme (CIP) within the ICT Policy Support Programme
Number of Beneficiaries	47 Beneficiaries (national ministries of health, national/regional competence centers, a consortium of industry and the Project Management Team):
Number of countries	23 different European countries: 20 EU member states and 3 non-EU member states.

(EHIC), patient access to their own data, the latter being the most important for all as noted in the new e-health action plan released by the European Commission in December 2012 (European Commission 2012).

epSOS intention is to prove that cross-border healthcare services are possible within Europe. Patients will have the opportunity when seeking healthcare in participating epSOS pilot countries to have access to epSOS cross border healthcare services in many different scenarios whether as tourists, business travelers, commuters or exchange students. All epSOS material is freely available to reuse and distribute via its Web portal.

Rethinking E-Health and Reusing What's Worth

Eysenbach described the term e-health as emerging in 2001. This is not the case anymore. As described in previous paragraphs, designing e-health services is not new, almost two decades have passed at a global level with extensive business planning, business process reorganization activities, brainstorming, piloting, standardization activities, and many more (Eder, 2000; Harmoni, 2002; Shortliffe et al, 2001; Stegwee, 2001; Black, 2011). We are now on the process of rethinking e-health's definition, focusing more on issue such as patient centered healthcare (Finkelstein, 2012), patient empowerment (Wald, 2011) and social media in healthcare (Neuhauser, 2003; Gwee, 2011; DeVries, 2012).

During this process, a lot of effort was dedicated to consensus building and stakeholder's managements. In fact, this is the right thing to do since in healthcare everyone is a stakeholder (Yasnoff, 2004). One of the most crucial issues that all involved technocrats learned is that what is essential is the user satisfaction, where a user is practically anybody. In that sense, building successful application is not about using the best technology nor the more innovative one, it is

about understanding what is needed to be done (Iakovidis 1998; Iakovidis, 2000).

So, what is actually needed to make the e-health story a success? After many years of globally successful and unsuccessful projects, the most noteworthy thing relies in the three pillars of quality in healthcare as described by Avedis Donabedian many years ago (Donabedian, 1980, 1982, 1985, 1993, 2003): a healthcare organization is a system formed by the interaction of structures, processes, and outcomes. Structures establish processes that create healthcare outcomes. Those have a back effect on structures which then need to change or adjust new processes to meet the new required outcomes. Healthcare outcomes should be more influential than financial outcomes in any healthcare system. As such, intangible assets are more valuable than tangible assets. (Cleverley, 2007; Berler 2005; Berler, 2008). Redirecting the Donabedian approach to the case of creating sustainable e-health systems since outcomes are mostly located in the Medical domain, we need to focus on the processes (thus functional specifications) and structures (thus standards and semantics).

It becomes then quite clear that what is needed is to focus on semantics and interoperability. In fact, the epSOS project did exactly that. This multi-million international co-investment spent most of its financial and human resources on decrypting those two sides of the Donabedian triangle by building cross border consensus, by focusing on semantic interoperability and by sticking to existing and viable international healthcare standards.

Using ICT for Health Policy and Management

Nations face similar challenges of meeting the increased need for care that are caused by the rapid aging of populations and the respective increase in patients with chronic and expensive diseases. In publicly financed health systems such as the ones existing in Europe (each one with its variations), these challenges are transformed into demand for care and a strain on shrinking healthcare budgets (OECD, 2011). The historical origins of national healthcare systems across the EU often vary. This is reflected in all aspects of a healthcare system: the structure, the manpower and its skills, the financing models. Nevertheless, all systems converge towards common future visions concerning healthcare delivery models and reforms needed to manage common epidemiological and financial pressures. ICT technologies can help in addressing key health policy and management issues (Calliope, 2010b) such as:

- **Patient Centered Care and Personalized Care:** The individual—patient, citizen—is a fundamental part of the care group who cooperates with healthcare practitioners to reach safe health related decisions. A healthcare system must respect cultural traditions, personal preferences and values, family situations, and lifestyles. The empowered individual is thus an active participant in the regional, national, and possibly international health system network, a trend that is highly supported by social media and their related applications. Healthcare in the near future will be a personalized care totally independent and focused to each one of us, driven by our own biological markers. DNA analysis will make possible new feature of personalized care such as health promotion, disease prediction, prevention, and individualized therapy

- **Continuity of Care Integration:** Patient-centered care demands that providers, departments, and healthcare settings are coordinated and operate efficiently. Care integration provides an effective means to re-

ducing waste and to balancing health needs against demands for care. It aims to realize a new model of cross-sectoral, person-centered service delivery that will break down boundaries between different organizations' missions and resources. Semantics and Interoperability are the cornerstones of care integration. Languages and processes must be ported to each stakeholder individually. The seamless care environment should be one where the ratio of effectiveness to cost reaches its highest value while avoiding duplicating information.

- **Information Management:** As stated earlier the seamless interchange of information is key to the success of any electronic service in the healthcare sector. Information management means to know what the needed information are, at what time, and whom to address it to. In fact, it is all about semantic interoperability.

- **Rethinking Health Policy:** Generally, much of the health of populations is dependent on social and environmental factors. Thus, healthcare systems have a remarkable opportunity to control costs by extending influence outside their borders, supporting WHO policies for international health regulations with the support of new technologies for early epidemiology warning and crisis management.

- **Open Collaboration of Stakeholders:** Consensus building and strategic partnerships for healthcare restructuring can manage healthcare complex processes, foresee different type of risks and establish common values. Open and transparent collaboration between major stakeholders is of tremendous importance to set up a viable mechanism that will handle the needed changes.

- **Incentives:** creating effective and operable e-health processes must be rewarded at all levels. As a consequence, regulatory bodies at a national and international level need to establish adequate incentives.
- **Legal Aspects:** Legislation should be a facilitator by legally supporting innovation and its change dynamics by means of full protection and legal certainly, rather than inserting constant burden and insecurity as it is often, unfortunately, the case. This can be achieved in synergy with other enablers including standardization bodies, clinical governance and through fostering security and quality cultures under an integrated framework of trust that is enforced and protected by law.

E-Services for the Healthcare Sector: It's an Interoperability Issue

Taking into account all the above issues, a successful electronic service, e-Prescription, for example, should focus on solving, or at least propose a series of tools of dealing with semantic sustainability and interoperability. In fact, semantic sustainability is an interoperability issue; it is one of the pillars of an interoperability framework that historically had three distinct dimensions: organizational, semantic, and technical. The European Interoperability Framework—EIF (ISA 2011)—extends this by adding political and legal dimension, resulting in Political – Legal – Organizational – Semantic –Technical (see Table 2).

All the dimensions of the proposed EIF model interact with each other. Each dimension though is extremely valuable to achieve an end to end interoperability. Especially in healthcare the Political and Legal dimension are of extreme importance due to the domain's complexity (eHGI, 2012). The other three dimensions are somehow known and dealt with many years ago, unfortunately, in a separate manner and from different stakeholders. In 2009, the United States' branch of the Institute of Electrical and Electronic Engineers (IEEE) revised its initial definition of interoperability for the healthcare sector stated in 1990 as being too vague:

In healthcare, the ability "to use the information that has been exchanged" means not only that healthcare systems must be able to communicate with one another, but also that they must employ shared terminology and definitions. This latter emphasis places a much greater burden upon system designers and electronic engineers to make the information truly usable in the distributed clinical setting of our healthcare environment" (IEEE-USA, 2009, p 1).

Table 2. European interoperability framework dimensions

Political Context	Legal Interoperability	Organisational Interoperability	Semantic Interoperability	Technical Interoperability
Political mandates and statements	Legal foundations	Business process alignment	Ability to share information	Apply Open International Standards
Policies	Data privacy	Organisational interconnectivity	Reuse of coded data and International Standards and Nomenclatures	Ability of Systems to exchange information
Business needs - Social Needs	Access to information	Interaction between two or more distinct organisations	Use commonly agreed data sets	Collaborative data processing and transaction synchronizations

Historically, technical interoperability in the healthcare started in the mid 80s via a group of visionaries under the umbrella of what is today known as Health Level Seven – HL7 (Datta, 2010). Semantic interoperability and the creation of commonly understood data set started way behind the era of computing since the need for medical practitioners to interact existed before with the use of nomenclature and codifications such as the International Classification for Diseases – ICD, Systematized Nomenclature of Medicine – SNOMED, and many others (Stroetmann, 2009). Organizational Interoperability is also often seen as process interoperability, where the correct organization and management of processes and workflows between distinct and independent organization is the key issue (Gibbons, 2007). In healthcare, for example, the creation and maintenance of a master patient index is such an issue, the exchange of medical information as part of a nationwide healthcare record is another. It is clear that coded data and data exchange in not enough to achieve interoperability, processes need to be there to integrate and orchestrate the information (Ducrou 2009).

The European Commission introduced the concepts of Political Context and Legal interoperability in order to reach a consensus and manage business and legal complexity amongst the European nations. The classical three-dimension model for interoperability did not result in to practical success since legal constraints and the associated policies tampered the good technical and scientific results.

This "five dimension model" for interoperability is now the key for the successful completion of large scale implementation projects in the healthcare sector. It is the basis for an Interoperability Framework (Berler, 2004; Mykkänen, 2006; Grilo, 2010) that is necessary to achieve consistent and interoperable healthcare scenarios, such as needed for cross border healthcare. As a consequence, project epSOS embraced this approach and created its own interoperability Framework. This docu-ment analyses all the steps taken in each of the five aforementioned interoperability dimensions (epSOS, 2010).

Europe (and epSOS) decided to opt for the reuse of existing standards in the fields, the collaboration with existing standard organization bodies and interaction with industry vendors and communities to enhance sustainability of the final result. Project epSOS collaborated with official standardization bodies such as International Standards Organization (ISO), International Electro-technical Commission (IEC) and International Telecommunication Union (ITU). It also collaborated with the United Nations Centre for Trade Facilitation and Electronic Business (UN/CEFACT), the European Telecommunications Standards Institute (ETSI), Health Level Seven (HL7), the European Committee for standardization (CEN) and the International Health Terminology Standards Development (IHTSD). The established interoperability framework also included standards and processes from the Organization for the Advancement of Structured Information Standards (OASIS), and the World Wide Web Consortium (W3C). This framework has also references to the Internet Engineering Task Force (IETF), the European Computer Manufacturers Association (ECMA), the Object Management Group (OMG), the Web Services Interoperability Organization (WS-I) and Integrating the Healthcare Enterprise (IHE).

From all the above HL7 and IHE do have a leading role. HL7 is the Standards Development Organizations that has created the CDA (Clinical Document Architecture) Release 2.0 used to create and semantically exchange documents in the form of XML (eXtensible Markup Language) documents while IHE is the Profile Enforcement Organization that have created the needed analytical technical frameworks and integration profiles. Those XML Medical documents must be valid according to CDA.xds schema. A CDA document has in two sections a "header" and a "body". The aim of this chapter is not to expand on technical analysis of both standards that can be located in their respective Web portals (www.hl7.org and www.ihe.net) and further readings of this chapter. It is necessary though to understand that epSOS specifications substantially reuse concepts and processes from those two principal international independent organizations.

Of course, other standards need to be used to create the adequate interoperability framework with all its pillars. SAML 2.0 (Security Assertion Markup Language), for example is an adequate choice for encoding security tokens (OASIS, 2005b). Legal interoperability usually is about handling data privacy and confidentiality issues, thus creating a need for a strong security and legal framework. XACML (eXtensible Access Control Markup Language) deals with identity management issues and handles complex rules and policies related to patient consent mechanisms needed to give or revoke access to personal and sensitive medical information (OASIS, 2005a). Other standards such as WS-security and WS-Trust from the World Wide Web Consortium (W3C) complete a full security framework related to Web Services technologies. Since the goal of Web service technology is to provide an interoperable platform that facilitates distributed computing based on the messaging paradigm, a standardized messaging platform is an essential requirement. The foundation for the standards is the SOAP (Simple Object Access Protocol) Messaging Framework which defines an XML based message format and rules for message processing. IPSec (Internet Protocol Security) and SSL (Secure Sockets Layer) provide additional security by networking protocols in order to secure the communication channel based on encryption and public key infrastructure technologies.

Semantic interoperability is of foremost importance. Data elements should be coded, for example, with UCUM (Unified Code for Units of Measures) and HL7 code system. Adequate terminology must be used to control, transcode and translate the vocabulary. The most dominant terminology standards are EDQM (Standard Terms of European

Directorate of Quality in Medicine), LOINC (Logical Observation Identifiers names and codes), ATC (Anatomical Therapeutic Chemical classification system), ICD (International Statistical Classification of Diseases and Related Health Problems) and SNOMED CT (Systematized Nomenclature of Medicine-Clinical Terms).

E-Prescription

E- Prescribing is the use of computing devices to create, modify, review, and/or transmit medication prescriptions from a healthcare provider to a pharmacy (Center for Health Transformation 2008). The Institute of Medicine published a report on medication errors, revealing startling statistics on the dangers patients face in the healthcare system in the US, where 1.5 million medication errors happened every year, up to 98,000 Americans are killed every year by preventable medical errors, and more than 7,000 Americans are killed every year from preventable medication errors (Kohn, 2000).

In general, an electronic Prescription Service (e-Prescription) consists of electronic prescribing and electronic dispensing. e Prescribing is defined as the electronic prescribing of medicine with the use of software by a legally authorized health professional and the electronic transmission of said prescription data to a pharmacy where the medicine can then be dispensed (Hider, 2002; Hale, 2007). E-Dispensing is defined as the electronic retrieval of a prescription and the dispensing of medicine to the patient as indicated in the corresponding e-Prescription. Once the medicine has been dispensed, the dispenser is to report the dispensation information using the e-Prescription software (epSOS, 2008).

E- Prescribing has been the subject of extensive discussions, white papers, policy papers, strategic plan and e-Health Roadmap (Center for Health Transformation, 2008; Teich, 2004). By itself, it should be a simple process: the use of ICT to make a medicine prescription at a healthcare provider organization and dispense this prescription at a pharmacy. In reality it is a complex service that encompasses many stakeholders, involve fully or partially a lot of people with conflicting interests, thus making process story boarding a puzzle in multiple dimensions. This complexity can be explored in the literature where many nations, profiling and standardization bodies has released extensive functional and technical documentation. To the Authors' knowledge, the most complete sets of specification can be reached, most of them as open data (creative commons rules or similar), via the Web. Table 3 is a non-exhaustive list of similar specifications.

In the United States, e-Prescription started as pilots and standardization activities in 1995 and became an increasing necessity due to the Medicare modernization act established in 2003 (Hale, 2007). As stated in the national progress report on e-prescribing and interoperable Healthcare for 2011, (Surecripts, 2011), the number of e-prescription issued increased from 54 Million in 2008 up to 789 Million in 2011 which an incremental

increase of 15 times in four years time. In the same period, the active prescribers have risen from 74.000 to 390.000 users. Certified software systems were 43 in 2008 and are 157 in 2011. By the end of 2011, 58 percent of office based physicians in the United States had adopted electronic prescribing. This figure was 10 percent in 2008.

Nowadays, only some European countries have managed to create an operational National e-Prescription service for the primary care sector. Nevertheless, most of the EU Member States mention e-Prescription in their e-Health strategy and implementation plan since 2006 (European Commission 2007), a number which reached 22 in 2010 (Stroetmann et al, 2011). Denmark, England, Estonia, Iceland, Scotland, Croatia, Greece, Belgium, and Sweden are nations that have implemented or are in the process of implementing nationwide e-Prescription systems. The Netherlands have established and are using e-Prescription in some regions, with different maturity levels, depending on the GP or hospital environment. In Spain, the region of Andalucía has implemented

Table 3. Freely available eprescription documentation

epSOS D3.1.2 Final definition of functional service requirements – ePrescription	http://www.epsos.eu/uploads/tx_epsosfileshare/D3.1.2_Final_Definition_of_Functional_Service_Requirements_ePrescription_01.pdf
IHE Common Parts Document	http://www.ihe.net/Technical_Framework/upload/IHE_Pharmacy_Suppl_Common_Rev1-1_TI_2010-12-30.pdf
IHE Community Medication Prescription and Dispense (CMPD)	http://www.ihe.net/Technical_Framework/upload/IHE_Pharmacy_Suppl_CMPD_Rev1-2_TI_2011-12-31.pdf
IHE Hospital Medication Workflow (HMW)	http://www.ihe.net/Technical_Framework/upload/IHE_Pharmacy_Suppl_HMW_Rev1-2_TI_2011-12-31.pdf
IHE Pharmacy Dispense (DIS)	http://www.ihe.net/Technical_Framework/upload/IHE_Pharmacy_Suppl_DIS_Rev1-2_TI_2011-12-31.pdf
IHE Pharmacy Pharmaceutical Advice (PADV)	http://www.ihe.net/Technical_Framework/upload/IHE_Pharmacy_Suppl_PADV_Rev1-2_TI_2011-12-31.pdf
IHE Pharmacy Prescription (PRE)	http://www.ihe.net/Technical_Framework/upload/IHE_Pharmacy_Suppl_PRE_Rev1-2_TI_2011-12-31.pdf
Healthcare Information Technology Standards Panel (HITSP) IS 07 - Medication Management	http://www.hitsp.org/Handlers/HitspFileServer.aspx?FileGuid=ffc182f4-2e73-44dc-b00d-810f2f9e86de
NEHTA - National E-Health Transition Authority e-Medication Management	http://www.nehta.gov.au/e-communications-in-practice/emedication-management
HL7 version 3 & CDA	http://www.hl7.org/implement/standards/index.cfm?ref=nav

a fully functional regional e-Prescription service. However, this services in not applicable for the other Spanish regions, which are engaged in different regional strategies. Norway, the Czech Republic, Austria, Finland, Italy, France, Portugal and Poland are currently piloting different solution at a regional or national level.

In Estonia, the digital prescription (e-prescribing) was launched in 2010. This countrywide project lasted 5 years and its aim was to make e-prescribing of drugs possible in every doctors' office and filling in digital prescriptions in every pharmacy of Estonia. In May 2011, just 15 months after the launch, 84% of prescriptions are issued digitally. More than 95% of pharmacies are ready to process e-prescriptions. According to a survey "Citizens' satisfaction with health and healthcare" 91%, of users of digital prescription are satisfied with the service (EIPA, 2011).

In Denmark (Purves 2002) reported ten years ago that Medcom has effectively rolled out e-Prescription in Denmark with on average 63% of all prescriptions items transferred electronically in 2002—this varies across Counties. It has taken 8 years to get to this point, where 3500 GP's in about 2000 general practice with 14 different IT-systems—85% of the GP's are able to send electronic prescriptions and 332 pharmacies with 4 different IT-systems—100% are able to receive electronic prescriptions. Today 85% of Danish prescriptions are electronically transferred (MEDCOM, 2012).

After Denmark, Sweden is the most e-health oriented nation in Europe. In December 2007, 68% of all new prescriptions were transferred electronically in Sweden (Åstrand, 2009). In another study, most respondent physicians believed they were able to provide the patients better service by e-Prescribing (92%), and regarded e-Prescriptions to be time saving (91%) and to be safer (83%), compared to handwritten prescriptions (Hellström, 2009). Finally, a nationwide survey showed that a vast majority of Swedish patients had positive attitudes towards e-prescriptions and electronic storing of prescriptions (Hammar, 2011).

Iceland has a national e-Prescription system, is based on one technical solution and it has the approval of the Data Protection Ombudsman. Medical Practitioners enter the prescription through a portal which is part of the national Healthnet framework. All healthcare facilities are connected to a single administrative entity and make use of special data sets (Doupi, 2010). In England, the program "connecting for Health" responsible for computerizing the National Healthcare System (NHS), started designing the Electronic Prescribing System (EPS) in the 1990s. The EPS project has been divided into two "releases": In Release One (R1) (which has now been completed), a mechanism was developed whereby General Practitioners (GP) systems can download drug data automatically from the core network, but the system still uses a paper prescription infrastructure. In Release Two (R2), the main feature is the switch to an electronic encrypted signature instead of the traditional paper signature. The only physical item remaining will be a numeric or barcode token, which the patient can present to the pharmacist when picking up his or her prescription. Currently R2 is in the deployment phase with only 1.5 Millions of prescriptions have been dispensed via this system (Van Dijk, 2011).

In the Netherlands, the first computer at a Dutch GP office was installed in 1978. By 1990, 23 percent of GPs were using a computer. Today, 97 percent of GPs use a computer-based GP Information System (Van Dijk, 2011). The electronic prescribing procedure through e-Prescription between GPs and pharmacists has been regional routine in the Netherlands for many years now via the regional OZIS network, a regionally accessible electronic medication record communication protocol layer responsible for medication data exchange. Up till now, no national standard has been defined yet. The take up for the regional transmission of e-Prescription lies between 20 and 50%, whereas a distinction has to be made between general GPs and specialists: GPs have an estimated take up of 50% and specialists below 10% (Flim, 2010).

There are multiple reports and documents on how different nations are coping with the introduction of e-Prescription systems and related electronic services. The authors provide a short list of further readings where extensive information can be extracted. The Greek case and its innovative approach are described in more details in the next sections of this chapter.

DESIGNING A NATIONAL E-HEALTH INFRASTRUCTURE THAT IS CROSS BORDER HEALTHCARE READY: A PARADIGM SHIFT AND A SUCCESS STORY

Creating Sustainability with ICT in Healthcare

EpSOS has introduced concepts such as the National Contact Point (NCP) which is, in fact, an enterprise information bus that securely, seamlessly transport medical information across healthcare systems of any type and complexity. This enables a democratic regulation of the health IT market allowing common testing procedures (by reusing profiles and test tools provided by IHE), common interoperability frameworks (by accepting common HL7 CDA r2 type documents for the electronic prescription) and certification procedures (by deploying national certification and accreditation bodies and reusing IHE, Eurorec or HL7 EHR-FS standards and methods).

Semantic interoperability is one of the keys towards sustainable and interoperable information systems. EpSOS invested a lot on securing the semantic interoperability layer, due to its dramatic importance and enhanced by the cultural

and linguistic puzzle that comprises the European Union. As a consequence, across epSOS participating nations, there are different languages, different standards and different coding schemes, and so the challenge was how to address this. The solution was to produce two master files: the Master Value Sets Catalogue (MVC), which applies across all members and the epSOS Master Translation / Transcoding Catalogue (MTC). The content of the MVC is in English; the terms are based on criteria defined by the use-cases identified by the Participating Nations. Each nation has then translated the terms into their language and transcoded into them in their national coding system, thus creating the epSOS Master Translation / Transcoding Catalogue (MTC). The value sets in the MVC have been selected from many Standards Development Organizations (SDOs) as noted earlier in this chapter. The MVC and MTC are supported by the epSOS Central Reference Terminology Server; each nation has its own Local Terminology Repository as a copy of its MTC. If an update is made to the epSOS Central Reference Terminology Server, the Local Terminology Repositories are notified and updated.

At a European Level, the European Commission is preparing itself for the large scale deployment of e-Health services under the Connecting Europe Facility (CEF) which will run in the timeframe between 2014 and 2020. The need for ensuring cross-border connectivity through optimizing functional, semantic and technical interoperability is necessary, including enabling cross-organizational & cross-border information flows to support further clinical needs such as chronic disease management. This leads to the second fundamental need for sustainability: create the Market. Thus, in addition to semantic interoperability, which requires institutions and procedures from the buyer side, the provider side need to adhere, support and enhance the needed technical viable solutions that encompass all technical and functional specifications needed additionally for cross border healthcare. In order to support that the European Commission via its EIF program is supporting the establishment of open source reference implementations to boost the economic market and reduce investment risks for the Market. EpSOS also focused a lot on this instance, by initially creating a reference implementation of the needed components that all together create the aforementioned NCP. This reference implementation is to be strategically created and ported into open source software built, supported by participating nations, as well as the industry team of the project, OpenNCP as it is named, should be ready by the end of the project in 2013. All material is and will be made publicly available on the EU open source repository at the Join-up (www.joinup.eu) portal.

Use of epSOS Specifications: The Case of Greece

Project epSOS selected W3C SOAP as a top level messaging protocol considering the project's tight time frame for implementation and piloting, the strong demand for well known security measures and the existing experiences in industry (epSOS, 2010). An alternative is to use the REST (Representational State Transfer) architectural style, which relies on HTTP (Hypertext Transfer Protocol) commands and URIs (Uniform Resource Identifier). IHE and HL7 experts, task forces and working groups commonly agree on those technological approaches, and define healthcare actors as Web services and actions as REST commands.

Finally, coming to the Greek case, Greece is participating in epSOS from the beginning of the project with significant participation at all levels. Recent development in Greece and the introduction of a new central e-Prescription system that operated for the first time in October 2010 changed the importance of the epSOS project at a National level. The Greek pilot in epSOS focuses only in a simple scenario of dispensing EU citizen existing prescription in a number of pharmacies in Greece.

At the design phase of the project, Greece had no existing e-Health infrastructure in place. This lead to a paradigm shift: while all countries organised themselves in order to connect existing systems with the proposed NCP structure of epSOS, Greece decided to do the opposite and expand its initial small pilot system so that it can be immediately "epSOS ready", thus being able to handle both national and cross border prescriptions. This has been depicted in the official tender documents of the National e-Prescription system initially released in August 2011 and heavily supported by the European Commission (IDIKA, 2011). The aforementioned issues are the reasons that are positioning the Greek case as a different approach in e-prescription implementation at a global scale.

In parallel the initial pilot system, which is a Web-based system, grew substantially covering basic prescription scenarios, solving initial user interface issues, creating and training the user community. In August 2012, the system is able to handle more than 590.000 prescription transactions per day (IDIKA 2012a). The pilot Web system is able to cover classic prescription transactions but was unable to provide the rich environment needed by the end users both at the pharmacies (dispensing the prescriptions) and at the physicians (creators of the prescriptions), creating an ongoing debate on the quality and capabilities of the system as a whole. It is at that point that it was decided to invest in the epSOS specification and mostly in its interoperability framework. This resulted in the creation of an Enterprise Service Bus, a simplified approach of the epSOS NCP than proposed to exchange all prescription (and future documents) in the CDA R2 format proposed by epSOS (IDIKA, 2012b).

The proposed overall architecture relies on the REST architectural style on the end user application layer for two main reasons: the existing system is based on Web technologies to which the REST architecture is faster to implement and secondly the existing system did not support CDA type documents nor had the ability to create such high level WS to implement a full WS SOAP approach. This architecture is depicted in Figure 2.

This architecture implies the creation of a RESTful API that is called by the third party end user applications. Information is transported via WS/Messaging services and an enterprise service bus to ensure and monitor document delivery to the main eP system. The use of additional IHE compliant tools enables the system to be compliant with epSOS scenarios and specifications while enabling the possibility of more enhanced cross border or cross enterprise scenarios between multiple data repositories

Figure 3 describes the Enterprise Information Bus (EIB) application layer from a functional point of view. In that sense, the Greek eP System has created a series of WS to handle information exchange. Those are connected to the IHE service components that transform and validate the information in HL7 CDA format. All messages are queued via a Java Messaging Service (JMS) and sent to the appropriate recipient ensuring safe delivery (will keep message history until safe delivery). The IHE client is the RESTful structure that via a set of commands makes the information available to the end users applications passing through a Load balancing mechanism to

Figure 2. REST type architecture of the Greek eP system

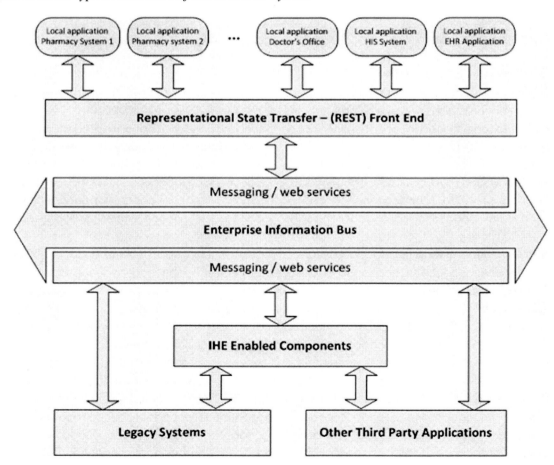

Figure 3. Enterprise information bus logical architecture

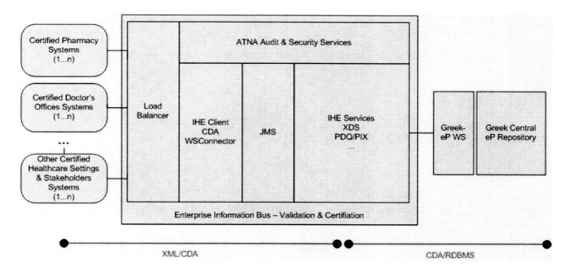

ensure timely delivery and workload distribution (a series of virtual machines). On top, the ATNA (Audit Trail and Node Authentication) Audit and security service logs and monitor the whole process ensuring data security and privacy according to the respective IHE ATNA integration profile. All messages are encrypted, and users are strongly authenticated (use of API KEY and hashtags conformant to RFC 2104 specifications). The whole system is epSOS compatible since it can handle SAML messaging and Public Key Infrastructure (PKI) tokens.

The propose architecture has a series of significant benefits and advantages, namely:

- The system is epSOS Ready and will allow the Greek Government to implement its obligations under the EU Directive 2011/24/EC on time before the deadline of October the 25th, 2013.
- The system is HL7 compliant allowing for efficient functional scalability and interoperability.
- The system can implement both cross border healthcare scenarios and national prescription scenarios.

- The system is technologically up to date with the current technological trends.
- The system is service oriented and compatible with both REST and WS/SOAP technology.
- The system is "cloudable" and thus can operate in various business scenarios in the future both as a governmental cloud or a private cloud or both.
- The system has a strong and internationally approved interoperability framework.
- The system is based on current profiling approached and profile standards (namely IHE) enabling a democratic involvement of the market and reducing the "vendor lock in effect."
- The system allows third party software to be certified to specific use cased and scenarios enhancing market competition and quality of services.

As shown in Figure 4 the system is high scalable at many levels. It can support the integration with multiple repositories (IHE Cross-Enterprise Document Sharing-XDS compliant structures), it is scalable on a physical architecture point of

Figure 4. Proposed system scalability and sustainability

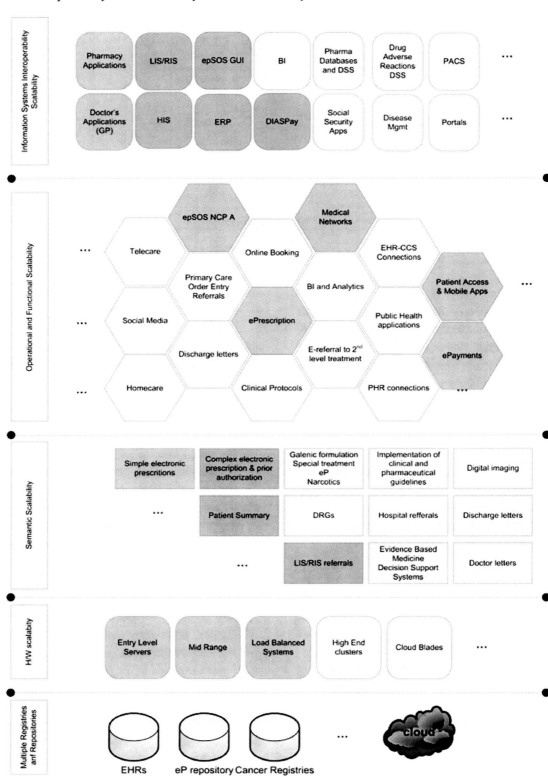

view enabling complex, and up to date virtualization techniques, and it is scalable at the semantic interoperability level, at the service provision level and the information systems interoperability.

Solutions and Recommendations

The case of Greece is in our opinion a good focal point were European strategies, cross border healthcare needs, e-prescription implementation and e-health standards all collide to create a new strategy that could be the mirror of Europe's future. Greece was for many years a lager in e-health issues and is probably still is in some features. This case proves that by focusing on European policy, major steps can be made in a quite reasonable time frame. Of course, Greece has the need and the opportunity to rely on Europe to restructure its entire government and national strategy, willing to come closer to Europe mindset. As a conclusion, one could say that in the e-prescription case the reuse of European standards and methods can conclude to success and a European best practice. Europe has vastly invested in e-health. Those investments seem to have quite good acceptance overseas and

reach out to decision makers in the United States, since the cross border scenarios used with epSOS for Europe present little discrepancy to be effectively implemented at a global scale. The recent Memorandum of Understanding that has been signed between Europe and the US clearly marks that success story (MoU, 2010).

Coming back to the proposed solution in Greece, one of the main benefits of the proposed architecture is its flexibility to operate in different business modalities. In Figures 5, 6, 7, and 8 we shortly present four different mode of operation.

Figure 5 describes the logic of a central EIB facility strongly bound to the existing eP system. This proposition has the fastest implementation time since the EIB is located in the same physical structure of the current eP system. By the use of virtualisation methods, one can efficiently use physical devices in the best possible manner. In this case since the eP system is operated as Governmental cloud setup, the EIB facility can only operate as a G-cloud structure. Otherwise, the whole system has to be given as managed service or business service provision in order to work in another business mode. In this case, providing

Figure 5. Central EIB facility

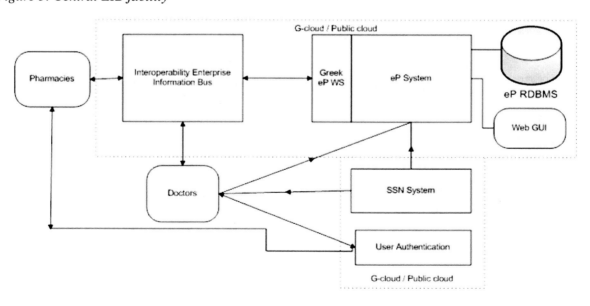

Figure 6. Software as a service EIB facility

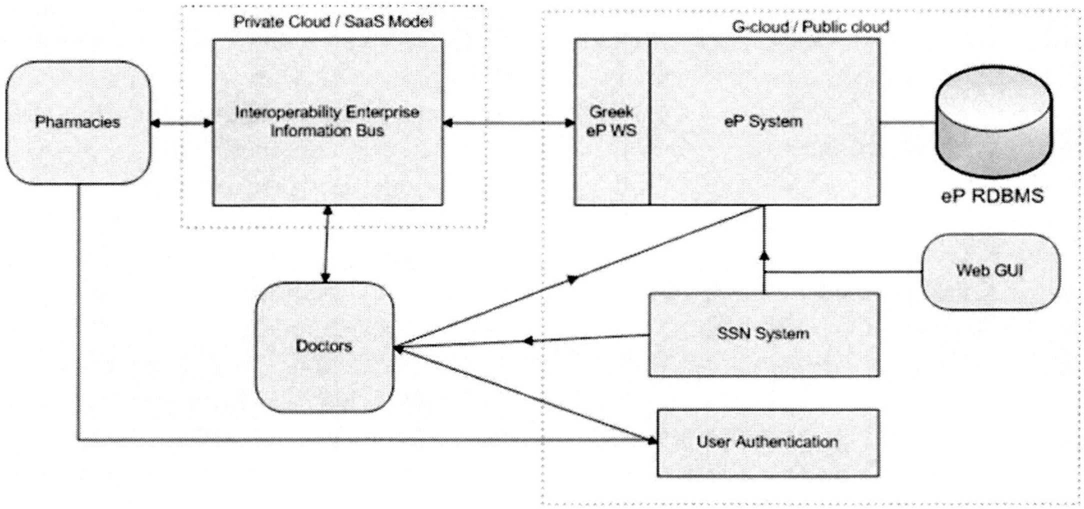

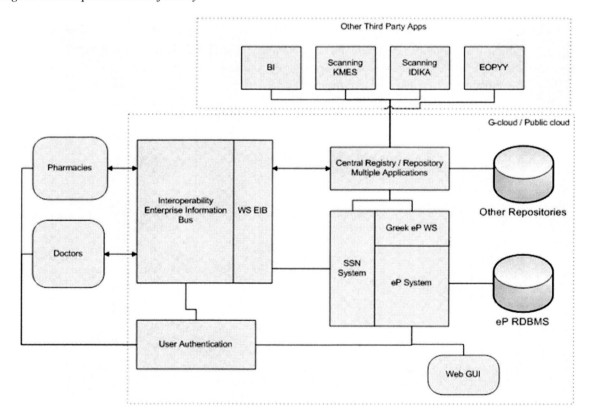

Figure 7. Independent EIB facility

Figure 8. Federated EIB facility

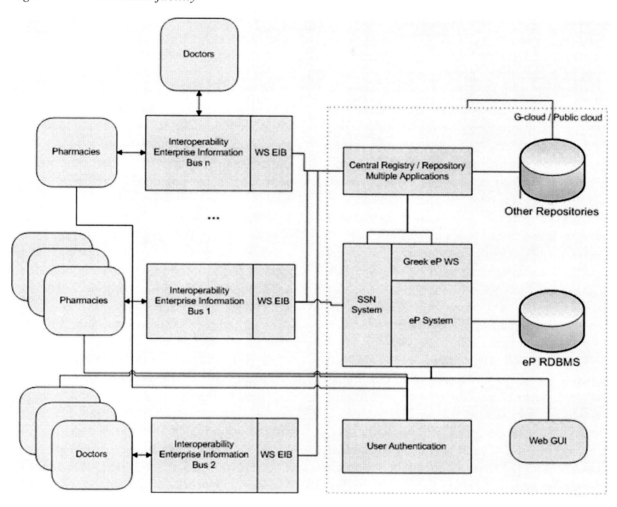

control of sensible data out of a public setting may under some circumstances created data protection related risks.

In Figure 6 we propose to operate the EIB service as a separate service that can be located in another physical location, other that the location of the eP system. This scenarios increases flexibility and enable to operate the EIB in a private cloud model in a Software as a Service mode enabling new and more viable financial models for sustainability.

Figure 7 correspond to an EIB that has the capacity of handling multiple repositories enabling in that sense the possibility to have more complex business scenarios. Such a setting can serve with the same infrastructure more than one e-health scenarios and multiple healthcare stakeholders. For example the same EIB could handle discharge letters and e-referral documents and link the primary and secondary healthcare facilities. The system can both operate in a G-cloud or a private cloud setting, and thus does not create any business barriers. In fact, both operation modes could be combined in a hybrid cloud approach where the EIB could run in a SaaS mode in a private cloud while the eP system and/or any other system can be in the G-cloud.

Finally, Figure 8 points out a variation of the system where we can have multiple, federated EIB structures connected to the central eP system (or other systems and repositories) by enhancing the reuse of IHE enabled components that are XDS compliant (multiple repositories). This scenario is extremely flexible allowing, for example, the EIB structure to be managed by relevant stakeholder group and collectively connect their software system uniformly to central government systems. This would allow for faster implementation of regional settings and architecture versus a more rigid and inflexible central system. This scenario has of course to be compliant with national strategies concerning healthcare data handling. It has though the advantages that there is no single point of failure and in case of unexpected events the system can partially operated serving specific geographical locations or specific stakeholders groups (i.e. pharmacy associations, etc).

The State Authority that manages the e-Prescription (IDIKA) system decided to implement the architecture of the independent EIB mostly because of its increasing role in Greece as a de facto e-health competence authority and the need to incorporate and reuse IEB components as much as possible for the seamless integration of other information systems in place. Other systems that need to be integrated for example are existing legacy systems such as the prescription antifraud and control system (KMES) located at the National organization for the provision of healthcare services (EOPYY in Greek). Up to the date of finalization of this chapter, the EIB structure is handling transaction for the community pharmacies, whose stakeholder's organization (pan-Hellenic society of pharmacies) heavily supported the integration of the existing pharmacy information systems with the e-Prescription system. All 12 software providers have been able to interoperate via the EIB and certify their respective products. IDIKA has setup a thorough roadmap to complete the integration process of all interested stakeholders and existing public information systems that need to

transparently interoperate with the e-Prescription system. A significant next step of the system is to allow physicians to electronically prescribe not only medicines but also send referrals and order entries for examinations and treatments.

In order for the above to happen, some fundamental issues need to be strongly kept in mind and continuously dealt with. It is essential to always keep in mind that e-Health can only grow and expand if all stakeholders are informed and participate in decision making process via a well established consensus building mechanism. Such a mechanism can be installed with the assistance of organizations that have built their success and results based upon consensus. HL7 and its affiliates as well as IHE are organization capable of supporting central e-Health competence centre in deploying such mechanisms.

A second point of importance is certification. There is no serious and robust interoperability framework without rules and code of ethics. This is a point that was immediately foreseen by the European Commission which has established the necessary structures in all interoperability related project. In epSOS, this role has been dedicated to IHE. IHE Europe is a member of the consortium and is providing testing and certification services to the Commission. As a consequence, epSOS has periodically undergone the so called "projectathons" that are exact replicas of the connectathon process that certifies adherence of software products to IHE integration profiles. We believe that is in the best interest of the Greek government to incorporate such practices as soon as possible. The exact process of IHE is well described on its international Web portal.

A third point is installing an open mechanism for data privacy and security. All European countries have to adhere to particularly strong framework that protects personal data for misuse or abuse. The fundamental rights and the principles recognized in particular by the European Convention of Human Rights and Fundamental Freedoms (1950) have to be respected and duly protected.

The fundamental right of privacy is of key importance (Art 8). Also, rights to healthcare have been recognised in the Charter of Fundamental Rights of the EU in 2000. The right to healthcare during a temporary stay in another member state (MS) was foreseen in Regulation 1408/71, for all persons insured under the legislation of a MS. The common EU framework on data protection is provided by "Directive 95/46/EC of the European Parliament and of the Council of 24 October 1995 on the protection of individuals with regard to the processing of personal data and on the free movement of such data". It is the most prestigious European legally binding document governing protection of personal data. The EU Article 29 Working Party (hereinafter "the WP29") has played a key role promoting harmonization of data protection in order to achieve a high level of data protection in the EU, fostering compliance with the data protection standards set up by Directive 95/46/EC and providing guidance and advice to the different actors in the data protection arena (WP29, 2004). Its Working document on the processing of personal data relating to health in electronic health records (WP 131) provides guidance on a uniform interpretation of the Directive 95/46/EC. Although documents of WP29 are not legally binding this document is one of those which must be taken into consideration. We recommend that the Greek e-Prescription system adhere to the strong policies for data privacy of epSOS (epSOS, 2009).

A fourth point of recommendation is to always keep in mind the patient itself. The European Directive on data protection and its Greek exact translation (Law 2472/1997) clearly states that all personal and sensitive data belong to the patient, and as a consequence he has a right to know on how his personal information is processed. He has the right to revoke access to his data (totally or partially) and can grant access to specific third parties. For this to happen, a series of processes and regulations must be in place. In addition, this is a must as cross border healthcare is concerned since in the country of treatment the rules that are valid are the rules and policies of the country of establishment. EpSOS has established extremely strict rules for handling patient consent and is now moving to the next step which is to grant direct patient access. We recommend that the Greek e-Prescription systems incorporate those rules. From a technical point of view XACML, is an open protocol that enable to handle direct rules based upon central e-Identity structure, thus personalising access rights to information.

FUTURE RESEARCH DIRECTIONS

Cross border healthcare is an issue that has been foreseen from a public health point of view from the World Health Organization at least since 2002 in order to reduce health risks and cross border dissemination of diseases. Information technology is now being seen a key driver to this. EpSOS is as such by itself a living proof of the importance of normalizing healthcare processes across nations. Another fact is the newly installed collaboration at a high level on this issue between the United States and the European Union. In fact, a Memorandum of Understanding (MoU, 2010) has been signed in mid December 2010. This MoU opens the agenda for joint working groups in creating commonly accepted policies in the region of health IT. Thus, this is an area of research that surpasses the health IT domain and promotes research in areas such as health economics, interoperability, health policy and many more. In that sense, cross border healthcare is not a European term but a global one. The same concepts that apply to Europe certainly apply to the borders between states and provinces in the United States, Canada and elsewhere. The recent MoU between the US and the European Commission clearly mark the interest of the American policy makers to import from Europe all the best practices that are possible.

Another important area of research is the direct implication of the end user. At a global level, it is already proven that new technologies such as mobile health and social media are already altering the patient – physician equation (Apostolakis et al, 2012). Social media in healthcare have introduced the term Social Health. Gwee (2011) describes the 6 Ps' of social health which reflect the leading role of social media in health as being personalization, participatory (online patient communities and e-Patients), preventative medicine, Peer-to-Peer patients, portability and passion. As a consequence, in a world of constant changes where social media and mobile applications are changing the way we know the delivery of healthcare services, it obvious to say that those two areas by themselves or combined are valid area of research. E-Health services are already hugely improved and will be even more affected in the near future. Patients are already demanding to have direct access to their information that is being handled via national or international e-health settings. For example epSOS has foreseen this need adding a patient access feature to the epSOS services (epSOS, 2010). On the same path in the United States, the Blue Button Project is expanding, giving the opportunity to the end user to control and manage the access to his medical information created during the various episodes of care (Chopra, 2010).

When expanding the end user involvement one cannot omit the Patient oriented outcomes domain which is our third relevant discussion and future research direction. It seems that information technology do have some impact on healthcare outcomes by reducing medical errors and empowering the patient (Mitchell, 2010). Clinical outcome measures examine discrete, patient-focused endpoints such as readmission, length of stay, morbidity and mortality. Those are easily monitored by information systems (ACEP, 2010). An alternative approach is to start from the patient's needs and select a goal oriented approach to monitor healthcare outcomes for each individual alone (Reuben, 2012). Going a few steps further patient oriented outcomes are often monitored easily by patients via the support of patient advocates and patient societies. Both are

handling extremely well the new social media and tools on behalf of the patients. Thanks to social media, patient advocacy is moving from focusing on lobbying government officials towards working more with individuals online to create local change in communities (Brandt, 2011).

A fourth relevant area of discussion a continuous improvement that will not leave the healthcare sector unaffected is cloud computing. We already described an architecture that enables both cross border healthcare and allow establishing different cloud computing scenarios. One thing is certain, in an era of global financial instability where healthcare costs are redesigned and restructured cloud computing and its different business model will play a key role. This has been clearly depicted in a recent study for the Greek market (Danchev, 2011). Cloud computing is becoming a trend of the IT landscape. Each year, millions of users add up and remotely use data centers and Web-based applications in order to exchange various types of information.

Finally, the domain of interoperability itself is a driver for further research. For example, HL7 International has done, within 2012, two extremely significant announcements that will change once again the shape of interoperability. Initially, it has officially announced its decision to make much of its intellectual property (IP), including standards, freely available under licensing terms. This landmark decision represents HL7's commitment to the betterment of healthcare worldwide by ensuring that all stakeholders have equal access to its healthcare information technology standards. The new policy is expected to take effect in the first quarter of 2013 (HL7, 2012a). The second turning point is the release of Fast Healthcare Interoperability Resources (FHIR) Initiative (http://HL7.org/fhir). FHIR is a new HL7 draft standard for data exchange in healthcare that is based on current industry principles, including the cloud, Web 2.0 and RESTful principles. It defines a set of "resources" representing granular clinical concepts that can be managed in isolation, or aggregated into complex documents (HL7, 2012b). This flexibility offers coherent solutions for a range of interoperability problems. As described in this chapter, the proposed architecture is a RESTful implementation, and as such, is already in line with upcoming future developments.

In parallel, IHE has focused a lot in the integration process of devices and mobile devices. It has created a new technical framework called IHE Patient Care Device and has also implemented a new integration profile for Mobile Health Devices (MHD) that also reuses RESTful approaches. This is a booming area of research and innovation not so much in the technical background but mostly in creating, new innovative, healthcare scenarios that implicate the use of connected medical devices and mobile applications. It is thus not surprising that high tech evangelist envision a world of 50 billion interconnected devices by 2020 in a machine to machine (M2M) mode (Ericsson, 2011).

CONCLUSION: DISCUSSION

In this chapter we made an attempt to analyze as thoroughly as possible the need of cross border healthcare and how the European Union, which indeed needs to solve existing issues in that domain, is proposing to deal this theme. As stated earlier, people are increasingly impatient with the inability of health services to deliver services that meet stated demands and new needs. So many patients seek healthcare services on the global scale, either because their country is, unfortunately, unable to serve them, or because they seek high expertise and skills at the point of delivery. As a consequence, Europe for many years know has focused on the subject and tried to find ways to include the need for cross border healthcare and adequate quality of healthcare delivery for all European citizens. Cross-border health care has simply become a more prominent phenomenon in the European Union (E.U.). Those issues have been taken into account in the directive 2011/24/EU with a focus

on the need for e-health. As a consequence, the European Commission has established an e-health network (article 14 of the Directive).

Part of the solution relies on creating ICT facilities that will enable to interchange medical information between nations is a seamless and secure fashion. The epSOS project is operating since 2008 as a facilitator and a test bed to gradually get to the needed result. All participating nations gave their best of themselves in this endeavor and have manager to reach consensus in many issues. As it is stressed many times in this chapter, e-Health success does not rely solely on technological excellence but mostly on the way consensus and common decision are made. Until now the results are promising since for the initially designated scenarios of cross border healthcare an extensive set of technical and functional specification focusing on e-prescription and patient summary, were openly and publicly released.

This effort is closely monitored both by the EU Commission which expects to reach to a solution that will make the implementation of the new Directive on cross border healthcare a reality, and by the nation themselves. Each nation seems to act differently to the new prospect. In general, smaller countries such as Greece, Slovakia, and Portugal for example tend to seek a way to transfer this knowledge back home and do the best possible action with the local stakeholders to adhere and implement the new technologies. Other countries, the more mature ones in the e-health domain, such as Sweden, Denmark, Finland, Norway do their best to connect their existing infrastructure to the new need pointed out at a European level. All the other rely in between and act in various flavors according to stakeholders needs and taking into account that ongoing strategic plan are in the process of deployment.

It is important to distinguish the policy layer from the technological layer when trying to introduce new paradigms in a domain so complex as healthcare. The policy layer is needed in order to set the goals and agree on actions and plans.

The technological layer has its complexities but the recent developments in healthcare interoperability have made the solutions to look more feasible. HL7 is a global leader in this domain and will grant free access to its standards starting from 2013. IHE is another key driver in this domain, having cleared out successfully an important series of barriers by proposing and continuously improving its technical frameworks and integration profiles.

The case of Greece, has proven until now that efficient reuse of best practices and adherence to new technological solutions of the 21st century, namely interoperability standard reuse, cloud computing business models, and semantic clarity via CDA document, can make the deployment of user friendly new e-services in the healthcare sector. The Greek e-Prescription case has incorporated epSOS specifications and other innovative technological features. The final success remains to be seen, analyzed and assessed in the forthcoming years. Until now though one cannot deny the huge success it already has since a nonexistent application in October 2010 is now able to handle almost 600.000 transactions per day. Of course many steps have still to be made and many battles to be won.

From the technical point of view, CDA specifications seem to work fine and cope with the complexity of the healthcare sector. The proposed introduction of RESTful technologies has proven to operate correctly. The recent trend toward this technology both by HL7 with the FHIR Initiative and IHE with its new integration profiles prove the validity and technical excellence of the proposed solution. In fact a recent connectathon in Baltimore, US was conducted by 16 large IT companies under the supervision of HL7 International proved that FHIR will very soon be the new version of the HL7 family of standards. From our side we feel lucky to have had the opportunity to monitor closely those new developments and participate in their application and test beds in the European Health IT world. A lot has still to be done and all hope for a soon adoption of e-Health technologies so that we deal more efficiently with global issues such as cross border healthcare, ageing population, healthcare systems restructuring, financial difficulties and many more.

REFERENCES

ACEP. (n.d.). Quality of care and the outcomes management movement. *American College of Emergency Physicians*. Retrieved 30 December 2012 from http://www.acep.org/content.aspx?id=30166

Agrawal, A. (2009). Medication errors: Prevention using information technology systems. *British Journal of Clinical Pharmacology*, 67(6), 681–686. doi:10.1111/j.1365-2125.2009.03427.x PMID:19594538.

AHRQ. (2003). *AHRQ's patient safety initiative, building foundations, reducing risk*. Interim Report to the Senate Committee on Appropriations. Retrieved 28 December from http://www.ahrq.gov/qual/pscongrpt/

Apostolakis, I., Koulierakis, G., Berler, A., Chryssanthou, A., & Varlamis, I. (2012). Use of social media by healthcare professionals in Greece: An exploratory study. *International Journal of Electronic Healthcare*, 7(2). doi:10.1504/IJEH.2012.049873 PMID:23079026.

Åstrand, B., Montelius, E., Petersson, G., & Ekedahl, A. (2009). Assessment of e-prescription quality: An observational study at three mail-order pharmacies. *BMC Medical Informatics and Decision Making*, 9(8). doi: doi:10.1186/1472-6947-9-8 PMID:19171038.

Berler, A. (2009). *Service oriented information management model in a citizen centred regional healthcare network.* (Doctoral dissertation). National Technical University of Athens and the Medical School of the University of Patras, Patras, Greece. Retrieved 30 August 2012 from http://nemertes.lis.upatras.gr/dspace/handle/123456789/2489

Berler, A., Pavlopoulos, S., & Koutsouris, D. (2004). Design of an interoperability framework in a regional healthcare system. In *Proceedings of Engineering in Medicine and Biology Society* (*Vol. 2*, pp. 3093–3096). IEEE. doi:10.1109/IEMBS.2004.1403874.

Berler, A., Pavlopoulos, S., & Koutsouris, D. (2005). Using key performance indicators as knowledge-management tools at a regional health-care authority level. *IEEE Transactions on Information Technology in Biomedicine, 9*(2), 184–192. doi:10.1109/TITB.2005.847196 PMID:16138535.

Berler, A., Pavlopoulos, S., & Koutsouris, D. (2008). Key performance, indicators and information flow: The cornerstones of effective knowledge management for managed care. In Jennex, M. E. (Ed.), *Knowledge Management: Concepts, Methodologies, Tools, and Applications* (pp. 2808–2828). San Diego, CA: San Diego State University. doi:10.4018/978-1-60566-050-9.ch022.

Biermann, J. S., Golladay, G. J., & Peterson, R. N. (2006). Using the internet to enhance physician-patient communication. *The Journal of the American Academy of Orthopaedic Surgeons, 14,* 136–144. PMID:16520364.

Black, A. D., Car, J., Pagliari, C., Anandan, C., & Cresswell, K. et al. (2011). The impact of ehealth on the quality and safety of health care: A systematic overview. *PLoS Medicine, 8*(1), e1000387. doi:10.1371/journal.pmed.1000387 PMID:21267058.

Bloom, D. E., Canning, D., & Fink, G. (2011). *Implications of population aging for economic growth* (Working Paper 64). Boston: Harvard. Retrieved 30 December 2012 from http://www.hsph.harvard.edu/pgda/WorkingPapers/2011/PGDA_WP_64.pdf

Brandt, J. (2011). *The changing world of patient advocacy.* Retrieved 30 December 2012 from http://pixelsandpills.com/2011/04/04/changing-world-patient-advocacy/

Busse, R., & Wismar, M. (2002). Scenarios on the development of consumer choice for healthcare services. In Busse, R., Wismar, M., & Berman, P. C. (Eds.), *The European Union and Health Services* (pp. 249–258). Amsterdam: IOS Press.

Calliope. (2010a). *CALLIOPE D4.3 standardisation status report.* Retrieved 29 August 2012 from http://www.calliope-network.eu/Portals/11/assets/documents/CALLIOPE_D4_3_Standardisation_Status_ReportN.pdf

Calliope. (2010b). *EU ehealth interoperability roadmap.* Retrieved 29 August 2012 from http://www.calliope-network.eu/Consultation/tabid/439/Default.aspx

Cambria, E., Hussain, A., Durrani, T., Havasi, C., Eckl, C., & Munro, J. (2010). Sentic computing for patient centered applications. In *Proceedings of the 2010 IEEE 10th International Conference on Signal Processing (ICSP),* (pp. 1279-1282). IEEE.

Castillo-Salgado, C. (2010). Trends and directions of global public health surveillance. *Epidemiologic Reviews, 32*(1), 93–109. doi:10.1093/epirev/mxq008 PMID:20534776.

Center for Health Transformation. (2008). *Electronic prescribing: building, deploying and using e-prescribing to save lives and save money.* Retrieved 6 September 2012 from http://www.surescripts.com/media/660347/cht_eprescribing_paper_06.10.2008.pdf

Chopra, A., Park, T., & Levin, P. L. (2010). *Blue button provides access to downloadable personal health data*. Retrieved 30 December 2012 from http://www.whitehouse.gov/blog/2010/10/07/blue-button-provides-access-downloadable-personal-health-data

Chou, W. S., Hunt, Y. M., Beckjord, E. B., Moser, R. P., & Hesse, B. W. (2009). Social media use in the United States: Implications for health communication. *Journal of Medical Internet Research, 11*(4). Retrieved 30 December 2012 from http://www.jmir.org/2009/4/e48/

Cleverley, O. W., & Cameron, A. E. (2007). *Essentials of health care finance*. New York: Jones & Bartlett Learning Ed.

Danchev, S., Tsakanikas, A., & Ventouris, N. (2011). *Cloud computing: A driver for Greek economy*. Retrieved 14 September 2012 from http://www.iobe.gr/media/meletes/CloudComputing.pdf

Datta, G. (2010). HL7 international health level seven introduction. *HL7 Ambassador Presentation*. Retrieved 31 December 2012 from http://www.phdsc.org/standards/pdfs/naphit-Webinar-phdsc-business-case-gora-datta.pdf

DeVries, P. (2012). Electronic social media in the healthcare industry. *International Journal of Electronic Finance, 6*(1), 49–61. doi:10.1504/IJEF.2012.046593.

Donabedian, A. (1980). Explorations in quality assessment and monitoring: *Vol. I. The definition of quality approaches to its measurement*. Ann Arbor, MI: Health Administration Press.

Donabedian, A. (1982). Explorations in quality assessment and monitoring: *Vol. II. The criteria and standards of quality*. Ann Arbor, MI: Health Administration Press.

Donabedian, A. (1985). Explorations in quality assessment and monitoring: *Vol. III. The methods and findings of quality assessment and monitoring – An illustrated analysis*. Ann Arbor, MI: Health Administration Press.

Donabedian, A. (1993). Continuity and change in the quest for quality. *Clinical Performance and Quality Health Care, 1*, 9–16. PMID:10135611.

Donabedian, A., & Bashshur, R. (2003). *An introduction to quality assurance in health care*. Oxford, UK: Oxford University Press.

Doupi, P., et al. (2010). *eHealth strategies country brief: Iceland*. Retrieved 9 September 2012 from http://ehealth-strategies.eu/database/documents/Iceland_CountryBrief_eHStrategies.pdf

Ducrou, A. J. (2009). *Complete interoperability in healthcare: Technical, semantic and process interoperability through ontology mapping and distributed enterprise integration techniques*. (Doctor of Philosophy Thesis). University of Wollongong, Wollongong, Australia. Retrieved 31 December 2012 from http://ro.uow.edu.au/theses/3048

E-Health Governance Initiative. (2012). *Discussion paper on semantic and technical interoperability*. Retrieved 30 December 2012 from http://www.ehgi.eu/Download/eHealth%20Network%20-%20eHGI%20Discussion%20Paper%20Semantic%20and%20Technical%20Interoperability-2012-10-22.pdf

Eder, L. (2000). *Managing healthcare information systems with web enabled technologies*. Hershey, PA: Idea Group Publishing.

EIPA - European Institute of Public Administration. (2011). *European public sector award 2011, project catalogue, eprescribing in Estonia*. Retrieved 9 September 2012 from http://www.bka.gv.at/DocView.axd?CobId=45974

EpSOS. (2008). *epSOS home*. Retrieved from www.epsos.eu

EpSOS. (2009). *D2.1: Legal and regulatory constraints on epSOS, design- Participating member states T2.1.1: Analysis and comparison*. epSOS Project Deliverable. Retrieved September 14 2012 from http://www.epsos.eu/uploads/tx_epsosfileshare/D2.1.1_legal_requ_final_01.pdf

EpSOS. (2010). *D3.3.3 epSOS interoperability framework*. epSOS Project Deliverable. Retrieved September 14 2012 from http://www.epsos.eu/uploads/tx_epsosfileshare/D3.3.3_epSOS_Final_Interoperability_Framework_01.pdf

Ericsson. (2011). *More than 50 billion connected devices – Taking connected devices to mass market and profitability* (white paper). Retrieved September 14 2012 from http://www.ericsson.com/res/docs/whitepapers/wp-50-billions.pdf

European Commission. (2004). *Communication from the commission to the council: The European parliament, the European economic and social committee and the committee of the regions e-Health - Making healthcare better for European citizens: An action plan for a European e-Health area*. Retrieved 1 September 2012 from http://eur-lex.europa.eu/LexUriServ/LexUriServ.do?uri=COM:2004:0356:FIN:EN:PDF

European Commission. (2007). *eHealth priorities and strategies in European countries, eHealth ERA report, towards the establishment of a European eHealth research area*. Retrieved 8 September 2012 from http://www.ehealth-era.org/documents/2007ehealth-era-countries.pdf

European Commission. (2010a). *Communication from the commission Europe 2020: A strategy for smart, sustainable and inclusive growth*. Retrieved 1 September 2012 from http://ec.europa.eu/research/era/docs/en/investing-in-research-european-commission-europe-2020-2010.pdf

European Commission. (2010b). *Communication from the commission to the European parliament, the council, the European economic and social committee and the committee of the regions a digital agenda for Europe*. Retrieved 1 September 2012 from http://ec.europa.eu/information_society/digital-agenda/documents/digital-agenda-communication-en.pdf

European Commission. (2012c). *Communication from the commission to the European parliament, the council, the European economic and social committee and the committee of the regions, ehealth action plan 2012-2020 - Innovative healthcare for the 21st century*. Retrieved 30 December 2012 from https://ec.europa.eu/digital-agenda/en/news/ehealth-action-plan-2012-2020-innovative-healthcare-21st-century

Eysenbach, G. (2001). What is e-health? *Journal of Medical Internet Research, 3*(2), e20. doi:10.2196/jmir.3.2.e20 PMID:11720962.

Eysenbach, G. (2008). Medicine 2.0: Social networking, collaboration, participation, apomediation, and openness. *Journal of Medical Internet Research, 10*(3). Retrieved 30 December 2012 from http://www.ncbi.nlm.nih.gov/pmc/articles/PMC2626430/

Eysenbach, G., & Wyatt, J. (2002). Using the internet for surveys and health research. *Journal of Medical Internet Research, 4*(13). Retrieved 30 December 2012 from http://www.jmir.org/2002/2/e13/

Finkelstein, J., Knight, A., Marinopoulos, S., Gibbons, M. C., & Berger, Z. … Bass, E.B. (2012). Enabling patient-centered care through health information technology. Rockville, MD: Agency for Healthcare Research and Quality.

Flim, C., et al. (2010). *eHealth strategies country brief: The Netherlands*. Retrieved 9 September 2012 from http://www.ehealth-strategies.eu/database/documents/Netherlands_CountryBrief_eHStrategies.pdf

Forni, A., Chu, H. T., & Fanikos, J. (2010). Technology utilization to prevent medication errors. *Current Drug Safety*, *5*(1), 13–18. doi:10.2174/157488610789869193 PMID:20210714.

Fraunhofer, I. S. S. T. (2009). *Study on multilingualism*. Semantic Interoperability Centre Europe. Retrieved 14 September 2012 from https://www.opengroup.org/projects/si/uploads/40/19571/multilingualism-study.pdf

Gartner. (2009). *e-Health for a healthier Europe! Opportunities for a better use of healthcare resources*. Retrieved 20 September 2009 from http://www.se2009.eu/

Gibbons., et al. (2007). *Coming to terms: Scoping interoperability for health care*. Retrieved 31 December 2012 from http://www.hl7.org/documentcenter/public/wg/ehr/ComingtoTerms2007-03-22.zip

Glinos, I. (2012). Worrying about the wrong thing: Patient mobility versus mobility of health care professionals. *Journal of Health Services Research & Policy*, *17*, 254–256. doi:10.1258/jhsrp.2012.012018 PMID:22914545.

Grilo, A. (2010). *Interoperability frameworks, theories and models*. Retrieved 29 December from https://www.google.gr/url?sa=t&rct=j&q=&esrc=s&source=Web&cd=5&ved=0CEUQFjAE&url=http%3A%2F%2Fwww.fines-cluster.eu%2Ffines%2Fjm%2Fdocman%2FDownload-document%2F54-Interoperability-Frameworks-Theories-and-Models-Grilo.html&ei=nNDqUIfRB5T54QSoy4HYCg&usg=AFQjCNGUl_fR4QHqpkwH0n5p44nHBTBf_w&bvm=bv.1355534169,d.bGE

Gwee, S. (2011). 6 P's of social health. *Social Media Club Reporter*. Retrieved 14 September 2012 from http://socialmediaclub.org/blogs/from-the-clubhouse/6-ps-health

HL7. (2012a), *Press release: HL7 standards soon to be free of charge*. Retrieved 14 September 2012 from http://www.hl7.org/documentcenter/public_temp_BAC62A60-1C23-BA17-0C72E-CEC786D7A54/pressreleases/HL7_PRESS_20120904.pdf

HL7. (2012b). *Press release: First HL7 FHIR connectathon a success*. Retrieved 14 September 2012 from http://www.hl7.org/documentcenter/public_temp_BAC62A60-1C23-BA17-0C72E-CEC786D7A54/pressreleases/HL7_PRESS_20120912a.pdf

Hale, P. L. (2007). *Electronic prescribing for the medical practice: Everything you wanted to know but were afraid to ask*. Chicago: Healthcare Information Management Systems Society.

Hammar, T., Nyström, S., Petersson, G., Åstrand, B., & Rydberg, T. (2011). Patients satisfied with e-prescribing in Sweden: A survey of a nationwide implementation. *Journal of Pharmaceutical Health Services Research*, *2*, 97–105. doi:10.1111/j.1759-8893.2011.00040.x.

Harmoni, A. (2002). *Effective healthcare information systems*. Hershey, PA: IGI Global.

Hellström, L., Waern, K., Montelius, E., Åstrand, B., Rydberg, T., & Petersson, G. (2009). Physicians' attitudes towards eprescribing – Evaluation of a Swedish full-scale implementation. *BMC Medical Informatics and Decision Making*, *9*, 37. doi:10.1186/1472-6947-9-37 PMID:19664219.

Hider, P. (2002). *Electronic prescribing, a critical appraisal of the literature*. Retrieved 29 December 2012 from http://www.otago.ac.nz/christchurch/otago014044.pdf

Iakovidis, I. (1998). Towards personal health record: Current situation, obstacles and trends in implementation of electronic healthcare records in Europe. *International Journal of Medical Informatics*, *52*(123), 105–117. doi:10.1016/S1386-5056(98)00129-4 PMID:9848407.

Iakovidis, I. (2000). Towards a health telematics infrastructure in the European Union. In *Information technology strategies from US and the European Union: Transferring research to practice for healthcare improvement*. Amsterdam: IOS Press.

IDIKA. (2011). *Implementation and support of the national e-prescription system*. Retrieved 12 September 2012 from http://www.idika.gr/diabouleuseis/222-04-08-2011-26

IDIKA. (2012a). *The Greek e-prescription system is the larger online system in Greece*. Retrieved 14 September 2012 from http://www.idika.gr/files/deltiatypou/deltio_typoy__31.08.12.pdf

IDIKA. (2012b). *e-Prescription enterprise information bus presentation*. Retrieved 14 September 2012 from http://www.idika.gr/files/%20%CE%BC%CE%B7%CF%87%CE%B1%CE%BD%CE%B9%CF%83%CE%BC%CE%BF%CF%8D%20%CE%97%CE%9A%CE%95%CE%A3%2014-3-2012.pdf

IEEE-USA. (2009). *Interoperability for the national health information network*. Retrieved 30 December 2012 from http://www.ieeeusa.org/policy/positions/NHINInterooperability1109.pdf

Institute of Medicine. (2001). *Crossing the quality chasm: A new health system for the 21st century*. Retrieved 31 December 2012 from http://iom.edu/Reports/2001/Crossing-the-Quality-Chasm-A-New-Health-System-for-the-21st-Century.aspx

Interoperability Solutions for European Public Administrations – ISA. (2011). *European interoperability framework (EIF) towards interoperability for European public services*. Retrieved 10 September 2012 from http://ec.europa.eu/isa/documents/eif_brochure_2011.pdf

Kaiser, H. J. (2012). Family foundation. In *Health Care Costs: A Primer Key Information on Health Care Costs and their Impact*. The Henry J. Kaiser Family Foundation. Retrieved 31 December 2012 from http://www.kff.org/insurance/upload/7670-03.pdf

Kohn, L. T., Corrigan, J. M., & Donaldson, M. S. (2000). *To err is human, building a safer health system*. Washington, DC: National Academy Press.

Leon, D. A. (2011). Trends in European life expectancy: A salutary view. *International Journal of Epidemiology, 40*, 271–277. Retrieved 31 December 2012 from http://ije.oxfordjournals.org/content/early/2011/03/16/ije.dyr061.full

Lorenzo, V., Giesen, D., Jansen, P., & Klokgieters, K. (2010). *Business models for ehealth final report*. Retrieved 5 September 2012 from http://ec.europa.eu/information_society/activities/health/docs/studies/business_model/business_models_eHealth_report.pdf

MEDCOM. (2012). *eHealth in Denmark eHealth as a part of a coherent Danish health care system*. Retrieved 9 September 2012 from http://www.medcom.dk/dwn5350

Mirkin, B., & Weinberger, M. B. (2001). *The demography of population ageing, population ageing and living arrangements of, older persons: Critical issues and policy responses*. Retrieved 31 December 2012 from http://www.un.org/esa/population/publications/bulletin42_43/weinbergermirkin.pdf

Mitchell, R. (2010). *Patient-centred e-health: Helping to improve quality of care through e-health*. Retrieved 30 December 2012 from http://www.healthfirsteurope.org/uploads/Modules/Newsroom/HFE-EqualityInE-health_BROCH_LayA_V23_spreads-2.pdf

MoU. (2010). *Memorandum of understanding between the European Union and the United States related to information and communication technologies for health activities.* Retrieved 14 September 2012 from http://ec.europa.eu/information_society/newsroom/cf/document.cfm?action=display&doc_id=751

Mykkänen, J. A., & Tuomainen, M. P. (2006). An evaluation and selection framework for interoperability standards. *Information and Software Technology, 50*(3), 176–197. doi:10.1016/j.infsof.2006.12.001.

Neuhauser, L., & Kreps, G. L. (2003). Rethinking communication in the e-health era. *Journal of Health Psychology, 8*(1), 7–23. Retrieved 30 December 2012 from http://www.uk.sagepub.com/ciel/study/articles/Ch10_Article.pdf

NHMRC. (2010). *Australian guidelines for the prevention and control of infection in healthcare.* Commonwealth of Australia. Retrieved 30 December 2012 from http://www.nhmrc.gov.au/_files_nhmrc/publications/attachments/cd33_complete.pdf

OASIS. (2005a). *XACML - eXtensible access control markup language v2.0 normative XACML 2.0 documents.* Retrieved 30 December 2012 from http://docs.oasis-open.org/xacml/2.0/XACML-2.0-OS-NORMATIVE.zip

OASIS. (2005b). *SAML - Security assertion markup language v2.0, the complete SAML v2.0 OASIS standard set.* Organization for the Advancement of Structured Information Standards – OASIS.

OECD. (2010). *OECD health policy studies improving health sector efficiency: The role of information and communication technologies.* Paris: Organisation for Economic Co-operation and Development. Retrieved 1 September 2012 from http://www.oecd.org/els/healthpoliciesanddata/improvinghealthsectorefficiency.htm

OECD. (2011). *OECD-NSF workshop building a smarter health and wellness.* Retrieved 14 September from http://www.oecd.org/Internet/Interneteconomy/47039222.pdf

Official Journal of the European Union. (2006). *Directive 2006/123/EC of the European parliament and of the council of 12 December 2006 on services in the internal market* (L 376, 27/12/2006 P. 0036 - 0068). Retrieved 29 August 2012 from http://eur-lex.europa.eu/JOHtml.do?uri=OJ:L:2011:088:SOM:en:HTML

Official Journal of the European Union. (2011). *Directive 2011/24/EU of the European parliament and of the council of 9 March 2011 on the application of patients' rights in cross-border healthcare.* Retrieved 22 August 2012 from http://eur-lex.europa.eu/JOHtml.do?uri=OJ:L:2011:088:SOM:en:HTML

Purves, I., & Scholte, N. (2002). *The Danish ETP model.* Newcastle, UK: Sowerby Centre for Health Informatics at Newcastle, University of Newcastle.

Reuben, D. B., & Tinetti, M. E. (2012). Goal-oriented patient care — An alternative health outcomes paradigm. *The New England Journal of Medicine, 366,* 777–779. doi:10.1056/NEJMp1113631 PMID:22375966.

Rosenmöller, M., McKee, M., & Baeten, R. (2012). *Patient mobility in the European Union learning from experience.* Retrieved 31 December 2012 from http://www.euro.who.int/__data/assets/pdf_file/0005/98420/Patient_Mobility.pdf

Samb, B., Evans, T., & Dybul, M. (2009). An assessment of interactions between global health initiatives and country health systems. *Lancet, 373*(9681), 2137–2169. doi:10.1016/S0140-6736(09)60919-3 PMID:19541040.

Shortliffe, E. H., Perreault, L. E., Wiederhold, G., & Fagan, L. M. (2001). *Medical informatics, computer applications, healthcare and biomedicine* (2nd ed.). London: Springer Ed.

Stegwee, R., & Spil, T. (2001). *Strategies for healthcare information systems*. Hershey, PA: Idea Group Publishing.

Stroetmann, K. A., Artmann, J., & Stroetmann, V. N. (2011). *European countries on their journey towards national eHealth infrastructures final European progress report*. Retrieved 5 September 2012 from www.ehealth-strategies.eu/report/report.html

Stroetmann, V. N., Kalra, D., Lewalle, P., Rector, A., Rodrigues, J. M., & Stroetmann, K. A. … Zanstra, P. E. (2009). *Semantic interoperability for better health and safer healthcare research and deployment roadmap for Europe*. Retrieved 30 December 2012 from http://ec.europa.eu/information_society/activities/health/docs/publications/2009/2009semantic-health-report.pdf

Stuckler, D., Feigl, B. A., & Basu, S. (2010). *The political economy of universal health coverage*. Retrieved 30 December from http://www.hsr-symposium.org/images/stories/8political_economy.pdf

Surescripts. (2011). *The national progress report on e-prescribing and interoperable health care, year 2011*. Retrieved 6 September 2012 from http://www.surescripts.com/downloads/npr/National%20Progress%20Report%20on%20E%20Prescribing%20Year%202011.pdf

Teich, J., Bordenick, J., et al. (2004). *Electronic prescribing: Toward maximum value and rapid adoption recommendations for optimal design and implementation to improve care, increase efficiency and reduce costs in ambulatory care a report of the electronic prescribing initiative ehealth initiative*. Washington, DC: Foundation for eHealth Initiative. Retrieved 6 September 2012 from http://c.ymcdn.com/sites/www.azhec.org/resource/resmgr/files/erx_toward_maximum_value_and.pdf

Valeri, L., Giesen, D., Jansen, P., & Klokgieters, K. (2010). *Business models for ehealth, final report*. Retrieved 30 December 2012 from http://ec.europa.eu/information_society/activities/health/docs/studies/business_model/business_models_eHealth_report.pdf

Van Dijk, L. Villalba, De Vries, H., & Bell, D.S. (2011). Electronic prescribing in the United Kingdom and in The Netherlands. Rockville, MD: Agency for Healthcare Research and Quality.

Wald, J., & McCormack, L. (2012). *Patient empowerment and health information technology* (White Paper). Retrieved 30 December 2012 from http://www.himss.org/content/files/RTI_WhitePaper_patientEmpowerment.pdf

Warden, G., et al. (2012). *Health IT and patient safety: Building safer systems for better care*. Washington, DC: The National Academy Press. Retrieved 5 September 2012 from http://www.iom.edu/Reports/2011/Health-IT-and-Patient-Safety-Building-Safer-Systems-for-Better-Care.aspx

Wismar, M., Palm, W., Figueras, J., Ernst, K., & van Ginneken, E. (2011). *Cross-border health care in the European Union: Mapping and analysing practices and policies*. Retrieved 21 August 2012 from http://www.euro.who.int/__data/assets/pdf_file/0004/135994/e94875.pdf

World Health Organization. (2002a). *The world health report 2002, reducing risks, promoting healthy life*. Geneva, Switzerland: WHO. Retrieved 21 August 2012 from http://www.who.int/entity/whr/2002/en/index.html

World Health Organization. (2002b). *WHO global burden of disease (GBD) 2002 estimates (revised)*. Retrieved 30 December 2012 from http://www.who.int/healthinfo/bodestimates/en/

World Health Organization. (2005). *International health regulations (2005)* (2nd Ed.). Geneva, Switzerland: WHO. Retrieved 31 December 2012 from http://whqlibdoc.who.int/publications/2008/9789241580410_eng.pdf

World Health Organization. (2008a). *The world health report 2008 - Primary health care (now more than ever)*. Geneva, Switzerland: WHO. Retrieved 21 August 2012 from http://www.who.int/whr/2008/en/index.html

World Health Organization. (2008b). *Global burden of disease*. Retrieved 30 December 2012 from http://www.who.int/healthinfo/global_burden_disease/en/index.html

World Health Organization. (2010). *The world health report - Health systems financing: The path to universal coverage*. Geneva, Switzerland: WHO. Retrieved 21 August 2012 from http://www.who.int/whr/2010/en/index.html

WP 29. (2004). *Strategy document*. Retrieved 12 September 2012 from http://ec.europa.eu/justice/policies/privacy/docs/wpdocs/2004/wp98_en.pdf

Yasnoff, W. A., Humphreys, B. L., & Overhage, J. M. et al. (2004). A consensus action agenda for achieving the national health information infrastructure. *Journal of the American Medical Informatics Association, 11*(4), 332–338. doi:10.1197/jamia.M1616 PMID:15187075.

ADDITIONAL READING

American Medical Association. (2011). A clinician's guide to e-prescribing, 2011 update. Retrieved from http://www.ama-assn.org/resources/doc/hit/clinicians-guide-erx.pdf

Ash, J. S., Sittig, D. F., Poon, E. G., Guappone, K., Campbell, E., & Dykstra, R. H. (2007). The extent and importance of unintended consequences related to computerized provider order entry. *Journal of the American Medical Informatics Association, 14*, 415–423. doi:10.1197/jamia.M2373 PMID:17460127.

Åstrand, B. (1985). Doctor's use of VDUs for medical prescriptions. In Proceedings of the IFIP-IMIA Second Stockholm Conference on Communication in Health Care (pp. 267-269). Stockholm, Sweden: Elsevier Science Publishers B.V.

Åstrand, B. (2007). ePrescribing – Studies in pharmacoinformatics. Retrieved from http://urn.kb.se/resolve?urn=urn:nbn:se:hik:diva-32

Åstrand, B., Hovstadius, B., Antonov, K., & Petersson, G. (2007). The Swedish national pharmacy RegisterStud. *Health Technology and Informatics, 129*, 345–349. PMID:17911736.

Bates, D. W., Cohen, M., Leape, L. L., Overhage, J. M., Shabot, M. M., & Sheridan, T. (2001). Reducing the frequency of errors in medicine using information technology. *Journal of the American Medical Informatics Association, 8*, 299–308. doi:10.1136/jamia.2001.0080299 PMID:11418536.

Busse, R., Wörz, M., Foubister, T., Mossialos, E., & Berman, P. (2006). Mapping health services access: National and cross-border issues (HealthACCESS) final report, November 2006. Retrieved from http://ec.europa.eu/health/ph_projects/2003/action1/docs/2003_1_22_frep_en.pdf

Buurma, H., de Smet, P. A., Hoff, O. P., & Egberts, A. C. (2001). Nature, frequency and determinants of prescription modifications in Dutch community pharmacies. *British Journal of Clinical Pharmacology, 52*, 85–91. doi:10.1046/j.0306-5251.2001.01406.x PMID:11453894.

Campbell, E. M., Sittig, D. F., Ash, J. S., Guappone, K. P., & Dykstra, R. H. (2006). Types of unintended consequences related to computerized provider order entry. *Journal of the American Medical Informatics Association, 13*, 547–556. doi:10.1197/jamia.M2042 PMID:16799128.

Cap Gemini. (2004). Architecture for delivering pan-European e-government services version 1.0. Retrieved from http://europa.eu.int/Idabc

Carroll, N. V. (2003). Do community pharmacists influence prescribing? *Journal of the American Pharmaceutical Association, 43*, 612–621. doi:10.1331/154434503322452256 PMID:14626754.

Chrischilles, E. A., Fulda, T. R., Byrns, P. J., Winckler, S. C., Rupp, M. T., & Chui, M. A. (2002). The role of pharmacy computer systems in preventing medication errors. *Journal of the American Pharmaceutical Association, 42*, 439–448. doi:10.1331/108658002763316879 PMID:12030631.

Committee of the Regions. European Union. (2011). Dynamic health systems and new technologies: eHealth solutions at local and regional levels. Retrieved from http://80.92.67.120/en/documentation/studies/Documents/c24aa096-55a7-4e43-be10-d938dfad6251.pdf

Corley, S. T. (2003). Electronic prescribing: A review of costs and benefits. *Topics in Health Information Management, 24*, 29–38. PMID:12674393.

Cornell, S. (2001). Electronic prescribing: New technology can reduce errors and save time. *Advances in Nurse Practitioning, 9*, 107–108. PMID:12400283.

Dobrev, A., Jones, T., Stroetmann, V., Stroetmann, K., Vatter, Y., & Peng, K. (2010). Interoperable eHealth is worth it, securing benefits from electronic health records and ePrescribing, study report 2010. Luxembourg: Office for Official Publications of the European, Communities. Retrieved from http://ec.europa.eu/information_society/activities/health/docs/publications/201002ehrimpact_study-final.pdf

Dobrev, A., Jones, T., Stroetmann, V. N., Stroetmann, K. A., Artmann, J., & Kersting, A. … Lilischkis, S. (2008). Report on: Sources of financing and policy recommendations to member states and the European commission on boosting eHealth investment final study report version 1.0. Retrieved from http://ec.europa.eu/information_society/activities/health/docs/studies/boosting-ehealth-invest_report.pdf

Dovancescu, S., Meschede, J., Petre, C., Schleyer, M., & Mircea, V. F. (2010). The ePrescription system in Finland: A case study. University of Aachen. Retrieved from http://www.wi.rwth-aachen.de/Theses/Seminar/ePrescription.pdf

eHRQTN. (2009). CIP thematic network: eHRQTN: Thematic network on quality and certification of EHR systems. Retrieved from http://www.eurorec.org/RD/index.cfm

European Commission. (1995). 87/95/EC: Council decision of 22 December 1986 on standardization in the field of information technology and telecommunications. Retrieved from http://eur-lex.europa.eu/LexUriServ/LexUriServ.do?uri=CELEX:31987D0095:en:NOT

European Commission. (1998). Directive 98/34/Ec, of the European parliament and of the council of 22 June 1998: Laying down a procedure for the provision of information in the field of technical standards and regulations and of rules on information society services. Retrieved from http://ec.europa.eu/enterprise/tris/consolidated/index_en.pdf

European Commission. (2003). Communication from the commission concerning the introduction of a European health insurance card. Retrieved from http://eur-lex.europa.eu/LexUriServ/LexUriServ.do?uri=CELEX:52003DC0073:EN:HTML

European Commission. (2007a). Accelerating the development of the eHealth market in Europe. Luxembourg: Office for Official Publications of the European Communities. Retrieved from http://ec.europa.eu/information_society/activities/health/docs/publications/lmi-report-final-2007dec.pdf

European Commission. (2007b). SMART 2007/0059 study on the legal framework for interoperable eHealth in Europe final report. Retrieved from http://ec.europa.eu/information_society/activities/health/docs/studies/legal-fw-interop/ehealth-legal-fmwk-final-report.pdf

European Commission. (2008a). Communication 133 of 11.03.2008 towards an increased contribution from standardization to innovation in Europe. Retrieved from http://eur-lex.europa.eu/LexUriServ/LexUriServ.do?uri=COM:2008:0133:FIN:en:PDF

European Commission. (2008b). Commission recommendation of 2 July 2008 on cross-border interoperability of electronic health record systems. *Official Journal of the European Union, L, 190,* 37–43. Retrieved from http://eur-lex.europa.eu/LexUriServ/LexUriServ.do?uri=CELEX:32008H0594:EN:NOT.

European Commission. (2009a). White paper modernising ICT standardization in the EU – The way forward. Retrieved from http://eur-lex.europa.eu/LexUriServ/LexUriServ.do?uri=CELEX:52009DC0324:EN:NOT

European Commission. (2009b). (EC) mandate M/403 (eHealth-INTEROP) phase 1 report, 2009. Retrieved from http://eHealth-INTEROP.eu

European Commission. (2009c). Council conclusions of 1 December 2009 on a safe and efficient healthcare through eHealth. Official Journal of the European Union (2009/C 302/06), 2980th Employment, Social Policy, Health and Consumer Affairs Council meeting, Brussels, 1 December 2009

European Commission. (2009d). eHealth in action good practice in European countries good eHealth report January 2009. Office for Official Publications of the European Communities. Retrieved from http://ec.europa.eu/information_society/activities/health/docs/studies/good_ehealth/2009good_eHealth-report.pdf

European Commission. (2009e). Mandate M/403. Retrieved from http://ec.europa.eu/enterprise/standards_policy/action_plan/doc/mandate_m403en.pdf

European Commission. (2009f). Semantic interoperability for better health and safer healthcare, deployment and research roadmap for Europe. European Communities. Retrieved from http://ec.europa.eu/information_society/activities/health/docs/publications/2009/2009semantic-health-report.pdf

European Commission. (2010). Report of the expert panel for the review of the European standardization system: Standardization for a competitive and innovative Europe: A vision for 2020, February 2010. Retrieved from http://ec.europa.eu/enterprise/policies/european-standards/files/express/exp_384_express_report_final_distrib_en.pdf

European Communities. (2004). European interoperability framework for pan-European Egovernment services version 1.0. Luxembourg: Office for Official Publications of the European Communities. Retrieved from http://europa.eu.int/idabc

European Parliament. (2010). Report on the future of European standardisation, committee on internal market and consumer protection, European parliament, October 2010. Retrieved from http://www.europarl.europa.eu/sides/getDoc.do?pubRef=-//EP//NONSGML+REPORT+A7-2010-0276+0+DOC+PDF+V0//EN

Feifer, R. A., Nevins, L. M., McGuigan, K. A., Paul, L., & Lee, J. (2003). Mail-order prescriptions requiring clarification contact with the prescriber: Prevalence, reasons, and implications. *Journal of Managing Care and Pharmacology, 9*, 346–352. PMID:14613453.

Fulda, T. R., Lyles, A., Pugh, M. C., & Christensen, D. B. (2004). Current status of prospective drug utilization review. *Journal of Managing Care and Pharmacology, 10*, 433–441. PMID:15369426.

Gandhi, T. K., Weingart, S. N., Seger, A. C., Borus, J., Burdick, E., & Poon, E. G. et al. (2005). Outpatient prescribing errors and the impact of computerized prescribing. *Journal of General Internal Medicine, 20*, 837–841. doi:10.1111/j.1525-1497.2005.0194.x PMID:16117752.

Griffin, J. P. (2004). Venetian treacle and the foundation of medicines regulation. *British Journal of Clinical Pharmacology, 58*, 317–325. doi:10.1111/j.1365-2125.2004.02147.x PMID:15327592.

Halamka, J. (2006). Early experiences with e-prescribing. *Journal of Healthcare Information Management, 20*, 12–14. PMID:16669580.

Hawksworth, G. M., Corlett, A. J., Wright, D. J., & Chrystyn, H. (1999). Clinical pharmacy interventions by community pharmacists during the dispensing process. *British Journal of Clinical Pharmacology, 47*, 695–700. doi:10.1046/j.1365-2125.1999.00964.x PMID:10383549.

HITCH. (2010). HITCH: Interoperability testing and conformance harmonisation, SmartPersonalHealth: Interoperability of connected personal health systems (PHS) with the wider eHealth domain. Retrieved from http://www.hitch-project.eu/

Hyppönen, H., Salmivalli, L., & Suomi, R. (2005). Organizing for a national infrastructure project: The case of the Finnish electronic prescription. In Proceedings of 38th Hawaii International Conference on System Sciences (HICSS-38 2005). IEEE Computer Society.

ISA. (2009). Interoperability solutions for European public administrations (ISA) (OJ L 260, 3.10.2009, p. 20). Retrieved from http://ec.europa.eu/isa/documents/isa_lexuriserv_en.pdf

Johansen, I., Henriksen, G., Demkjaer, K., Jensen, H. B., & Jorgensen, L. (2003). Quality assurance and certification of health IT-systems communicating data in primary and secondary health sector. *Studies in Health Technology and Informatics, 95*, 601–605. PMID:14664053.

Kennedy, A. G., & Littenberg, B. (2004). A dictation system for reporting prescribing errors in community pharmacies. *International Journal of Pharmacy Practice, 12*, 13–19. doi:10.1211/096176704773048704.

Knapp, K. K., Katzman, H., Hambright, J. S., & Albrant, D. H. (1998). Community pharmacist interventions in a capitated pharmacy benefit contract. *American Journal of Health-System Pharmacy, 55*, 1141–1145. PMID:9626376.

Kohli, M., & Cook, B. G. (2005). Electronic prescribing at Johns Hopkins community physicians: A success story. *Maryland Medicine, 6*, 23–25. PMID:16454436.

Koppel, R., Metlay, J. P., Cohen, A., Abaluck, B., Localio, A. R., Kimmel, S. E., & Strom, B. L. (2005). Role of computerized physician order entry systems in facilitating medication errors. *Journal of the American Medical Association, 293*, 1197–1203. doi:10.1001/jama.293.10.1197 PMID:15755942.

Lapane, K. L., Dubé, C., Schneider, K. L., & Quilliam, B. J. (2007). Patient perceptions regarding electronic prescriptions: is the geriatric patient ready? *Journal of the American Geriatrics Society, 55*, 1254–1259. doi:10.1111/j.1532-5415.2007.01248.x PMID:17661966.

Lapane, K. L., Dubé, C. E., Schneider, K. L., & Quilliam, B. J. (2007). Misperceptions of patients vs providers regarding medication-related communication issues. *The American Journal of Managed Care, 13*, 613–618. PMID:17988186.

Lundkvist, J., & Jonsson, B. (2004). Pharmacoeconomics of adverse drug reactions. *Fundamental & Clinical Pharmacology*, 275–280. doi:10.1111/j.1472-8206.2004.00239.x PMID:15147278.

Mäkinen, M. (2007). Delivery of European cross-border healthcare and the relevance and effects of EU regulations and judicial processes with reference to delivery of drugs and blood donor information material. Retrieved from http://www.doria.fi/bitstream/handle/10024/33603/D790.pdf?sequence=1

Mjorndal, T., Boman, M. D., Hagg, S., Backstrom, M., Wiholm, B. E., Wahlin, A., & Dahlqvist, R. (2002). Adverse drug reactions as a cause for admissions to a department of internal medicine. *Pharmacoepidemiology and Drug Safety, 11*, 65–72. doi:10.1002/pds.667 PMID:11998554.

Montelius, E., Åstrand, B., Hovstadius, B., & Petersson, G. (2008). Individuals appreciate having their medication record on the web: A survey of attitudes to a national pharmacy register. *Journal of Medical Internet Research, 10*, e35. doi:10.2196/jmir.1022 PMID:19000978.

Nilsson, S., Ockander, L., Dolby, J., & Åstrand, B. (1983). A computer in the physician's consultancy. In Proceedings of the Fourth World Conference on Medical Informatics. Amsterdam: IFIP-IMIA.

Peterson, C. (1995). On-line prescribing: Keystrokes for quality. *HMO, 36*(5), 11–14. PMID:10153122.

Rupp, M. T. (1992). Value of community pharmacists' interventions to correct prescribing errors. *The Annals of Pharmacotherapy, 26*, 1580–1584. PMID:1482816.

Schiff, G. D., & Rucker, T. D. (1998). Computerized prescribing: Building the electronic infrastructure for better medication usage. *Journal of the American Medical Association, 279*, 1024–1029. doi:10.1001/jama.279.13.1024 PMID:9533503.

Schneck, L. H. (2006). E-prescribing can be new tool in quality-care arsenal. *MGMA Connexion, 6*, 32–37. PMID:16454076.

Tanne, J. H. (2004). Electronic prescribing could save at least 29bn dollars. *British Medical Journal, 328*, 1155. doi:10.1136/bmj.328.7449.1155 PMID:15142905.

Van Doosselaere, C., Herveg, J., Silber, D., & Wilson, P. (2008). Legally eHealth - Putting eHealth in its European legal context. Retrieved from http://ec.europa.eu/information_society/activities/health/docs/studies/legally_ehealth/legally-ehealth-report.pdf

Venot, A. (1999). Electronic prescribing for the elderly: Will it improve medication usage? *Drugs & Aging, 15*, 77–80. doi:10.2165/00002512-199915020-00001 PMID:10495067.

Von Laue, N. C., Schwappach, D. L., & Koeck, C. M. (2003). The epidemiology of medical errors: A review of the literature. *Wiener Klinische Wochenschrift, 115*, 318–325. doi:10.1007/BF03041483 PMID:12800445.

Westein, M. P., Herings, R. M., & Leufkens, H. G. (2001). Determinants of pharmacists' interventions linked to prescription processing. *Pharmacy World & Science*, *23*, 98–101. doi:10.1023/A:1011261930989 PMID:11468883.

Wettermark, B., Hammar, N., Fored, C. M., Leimanis, A., Otterblad Olausson, P., & Bergman, U. et al. (2007). The new Swedish prescribed drug register-Opportunities for pharmacoepidemiological research and experience from the first six months. *Pharmacoepidemiology and Drug Safety*, *16*, 726–735. doi:10.1002/pds.1294 PMID:16897791.

WHO. (2005). Connecting for health global vision, local insight report for the world summit on the information society. Retrieved from http://apps.who.int/iris/bitstream/10665/43385/1/9241593903_eng.pdf and country profiles at http://www.who.int/kms/resources/wsis_country_profiles.pdf

World Health Organization and International Telecommunication Union. (2012). National eHealth strategy toolkit. Retrieved from www.who.int

KEY TERMS AND DEFINITIONS

CDA: The HL7 Clinical Document Architecture (CDA) is an XML-based markup standard intended to specify the encoding, structure and semantics of clinical documents for exchange. CDA is part of the HL7 version 3 standard. Akin to other parts of the HL7 version 3 standard it was developed using the HL7 Development Framework (HDF) and it is based on the HL7 Reference Information Model (RIM) and the HL7 Version 3 Data Types. CDA documents are persistent in nature. The CDA specifies that the content of the document consists of a mandatory textual part (which ensures human interpretation of the document contents) and optional structured parts (for software processing). The structured part relies on coding systems (such as from SNOMED and LOINC) to represent concepts. CDA Release 2 has been adopted as an ISO standard, ISO/HL7 27932:2009.

Cloud Computing: Is the use of computing resources (hardware and software) that are delivered as a service over a network (typically the Internet). The name comes from the use of a cloud-shaped symbol as an abstraction for the complex infrastructure it contains in system diagrams. Cloud computing entrusts remote services with a user's data, software and computation.

Cross-Border Healthcare: Means healthcare provided or prescribed in a Member State other than the Member State of affiliation.

eHealth Interoperability: Is a characteristic of an ICT enabled system or service in the healthcare domain that allows its user to exchange, understand and act on citizens/patients and other health-related information and knowledge in a commonly interpreted way. In other words, it is a means of crossing linguistic, cultural, professional, jurisdictional and geographical border in eHealth.

Electronic Prescribing or E-Prescribing (e-Rx): Is the computer-based electronic generation, transmission and filling of a medical prescription, taking the place of paper and faxed prescriptions. E-prescribing allows a physician, nurse practitioner, or physician assistant to electronically transmit a new prescription or renewal authorization to a community or mail-order pharmacy. It outlines the ability to send error-free, accurate, and understandable prescriptions electronically from the healthcare provider to the pharmacy. E-prescribing is meant to reduce the risks associated with traditional prescription script writing. It is also one of the major reasons for the push for electronic medical records. By sharing medical prescription information, e-prescribing seeks to connect the patients team of healthcare providers to facilitate knowledgeable decision making.

E-Services: Are all electronic services together comprise integrated ICT supported health services to citizens. Examples of such services are electronic identification, authentication and authorisation services, telemonitoring, access to electronic health records, ePrescribing, e-dispensation, and e-reimbursement.

Health Level Seven (HL7): Is a non-profit organization involved in the development of international healthcare informatics interoperability standards."HL7" also refers to some of the specific standards created by the organization (e.g., HL7 v2.x, v3.0, HL7 RIM). HL7 and its members provide a framework (and related standards) for the exchange, integration, sharing, and retrieval of electronic health information. The 2.x versions of the standards, which support clinical practice and the management, delivery, and evaluation of health services, are the most commonly used in the world.

Healthcare: Means health services provided by health professionals to patients to assess, maintain or restore their state of health, including the prescription, dispensation and provision of medicinal products and medical devices.

Integrating the Healthcare Enterprise (IHE): Is an initiative by healthcare professionals and industry to improve the way computer systems in healthcare share information. IHE promotes the coordinated use of established standards such as DICOM and HL7 to address specific clinical need in support of optimal patient care. Systems developed in accordance with IHE communicate with one another better, are easier to implement, and enable care providers to use information more effectively.

Prescription: Means a prescription for a medicinal product or for a medical device issued by a member of a regulated health profession within the meaning of Article 3(1)(a) of Directive 2005/36/EC who is legally entitled to do so in the Member State in which the prescription is issued.

Representational State Transfer (REST): Is a style of software architecture for distributed systems such as the World Wide Web. REST has emerged as a predominant Web service design model. The term representational state transfer was introduced and defined in 2000 by Roy Fielding in his doctoral dissertation. Fielding is one of the principal authors of the Hypertext Transfer Protocol (HTTP) specification versions 1.0 and 1.1. Conforming to the REST constraints is generally referred to as being "RESTful."

Chapter 12
Incongruent Needs:
Why Differences in the Iron–Triangle of Priorities Make Health Information Technology Adoption and Use Difficult

Edward J. Cherian
George Washington University, USA

Tom W. Ryan
George Washington University, USA

ABSTRACT

Health Information Technology (HIT) has the potential to redefine the confines of traditional medicine. Yet, in over a decade, little has been shown in improvements from HIT investments. In order to understand the failures of health IT policy, this chapter examines the diverse priorities of stakeholders in the health system. Using kiviat diagrams as adaptations of the traditional iron-triangle of tradeoffs, the priorities of four stakeholder groups (patients, providers, pharmaceuticals, and payers) are mapped against the priorities of government and public health. The chapter finds that the priorities of these stakeholders within the United States healthcare system are incongruent and in conflict. To better understand the HIT needs of the future, policy makers and public health officials must understand these dichotomous priorities and work to bring them in line.

INTRODUCTION

Healthcare Information Technology (HIT) has been hailed by many to be the future of healthcare, a panacea that will lower costs, increase quality, and usher in a new age of personalized medicine.

However, the results of more than a decade of HIT research and development have been modest in the United States, at best (Lau, Kuziemsky, Price, & Gardner, 2010). HIT adoption has been slow, and as Vaitheeswaren (2011) notes, the "...zeal [for HIT innovations] has not extended to front-office transactions" (p. 133) in American doctors' offices. HIT has failed to make doctor's offices paper free and the risks of HIT adoption have

DOI: 10.4018/978-1-4666-4321-5.ch012

pushed many physicians away (Karsh, Weinger, Abbott, & Wears, 2010). Thus, the question remains, why haven't the vast investments in HIT yielded the promised improvements in patient and citizen health? Why, when HIT has the potential to advance America's health care system into a new era of care, have we seen the rise of ineffective products and incompatible systems? The recent spike in HIT federal funding through the HITECH Act has made understanding the failures thus far even more crucial.

In order to analyze the interactions and interdependencies of stakeholders in the healthcare system, and how HIT adoption in the United States has failed to facilitate these relationships, one must first understand the economics behind each stakeholder, the incentives that guide their practice, and thus the stakeholders' priorities related to cost, access, and quality. To aid in this understanding, this paper will use kiviat diagrams as adaptations of Kissick's (1994) iron triangle. Since each stakeholder has different priorities in the health field, each will have a different iron triangle of priorities. Our supposition is that Health Information Technology has failed to meet its expectations due to mismatched priorities of each of the HIT stakeholders. Hopefully, through studying these priorities and addressing the similarities and differences between the triangles, public health and public policy officials can work to better integrate the stakeholders and thus grow the iron-triangle.

THE IRON TRIANGLE AND HIT'S PROMISE

Within the public health field, policy analysts refer to an iron triangle of trade-offs that confines medicine's ability to provide the low cost, high quality treatment to a large number of patients. William Kissick's *Medicine's Dilemmas: Infinite Needs Versus Finite Resources* (1994) introduces this idea, noting that when a health care system is in equilibrium, better performance of the health care system within one of the three dimensions (cost-containment, quality, and accessibility of care) can cause decreased performance in one or both of the other dimensions. Cost-containment, quality, and access are in constant conflict, and an increase in one must be offset by the reduction of the other two. For example, increases in quality would be offset by either a decrease in accessibility or an increase in cost.

Kissick did, however, note in some instances, these tradeoffs between cost-containment, quality, and accessibility of care are not always required, and health information technology may be one such occasion. Donald Berwick, former Administrator of the Centers for Medicare and Medicaid Services, echoes these sentiments that the iron-triangle may be expanded, recently noting that at least twenty percent of United States healthcare spending is "waste" in that it provides no value to the patient or system (Birnbaum, 2012, p. 719). He lists five reasons for waste, three of which HIT can meet head on: "overtreatment of patients, the failure to coordinate care, [and] the administrative complexity of the health care system" (Pear, 2011). Berwick argues that this wasteful spending prevents investment in those areas that improve patients' health, decreasing the quality of healthcare all while keeping costs high (Birnbaum, 2012, pp. 719-720). Taken together, HIT has the potential to answer Berwick's call for improvements in patient care through reduction of waste, breaking from the confines of Kissick's iron-triangle by saving the United States billions in health care costs all while improving patient health and access to care.

Electronic Health Records (EHRs) provide an example of how health information technology may circumvent the traditional limits of the iron-triangle. EHRs offer physicians the ability, over time, to reduce administrative expenses through lessened paperwork and clerical necessities. In larger settings, this leads to clerks and administrative staff spending less time handling paper, reducing the administrative costs and increasing efficiency of staff remaining (Cusack, 2008). In smaller practice settings, lessened paperwork and reduced time spent on administrative efforts has the promise to free-up time for providers to see more patients, improving access—an important concern for public health as the United States is threatened with a physician shortage. Finally, quality of care is enhanced in two ways. On the macro-level, EHR use and interaction with Health Information Exchanges (HIEs) facilitate the work of public health entities, allowing for better public health investigation, emergency response, and overall quality of care (Shapiro, Mostashari, Hripcsak, Soulakis, & Kuperman, 2011). On a micro-level, EHRs can help make patient records more reliable and more accurate, helping to reduce medical errors and thus improving the quality of care. In a longitudinal study of physician perceptions around HIT and quality of care delivered, Fang et al.(2011) found that provider use of American physicians perceive HIT to increase the quality of care delivered. Patient perceptions also validate this, with a survey conducted by Gaylin et al.(2011) finding that 78 percent of American's surveyed believe that electronic medical records are "likely to improve medical care" (p. 925) and 59 percent believe that they are "likely to reduce the cost of medical care" (p.925). Thus, EHRs can potentially increase quality, increase accessibility, and decrease long-term cost, a seemingly impossible feat within the iron triangle framework.

Telehealth is another avenue by which HIT can circumvent the confines and traditional tradeoffs of Kissick's model. Telehealth has the promise of connecting providers, pharmacists, technicians, and patients in any locality, at any time, day or night. This has many potential benefits for patients and health care providers in the areas of quality, cost-containment, and access to care. Perhaps the most visible benefit is to access of care. With robust use, telehealth has the ability to provide patients with access to care any time they need it.

Chumbler et al. (2011) found that patient-centered Care Coordination/Home Telehealth (CCHT) implementation at the Veterans Health Administration helped patients self-manage chronic diseases from their home, decreasing their need to come into the office. Costs are another key driver of Telehealth use, as decreased costs can be realized by both the physician, with reduced need for office-related overhead expenses, and the patient, with reduced cost of time-lost and travel to receive care. In a sample of patients who enrolled in the Medicare Health Buddy telehealth program, Baker et al.(2011) found spending reductions between "7.7-13.3 percent per person, per quarter" (p. 1693). Perhaps the least discussed opportunity arising from telehealth is in the quality of care provided. Telehealth systems allow for real time access to specialists and expert opinions for both patients and their primary care physicians. The most poignant example of this comes with telepharmacy. In addition to electronic prescribing and drug-checking software that cross-references the EHR to identify potential adverse drug reactions for patient prescriptions (Cusack, 2008), telepharmacy technology can now provide for "round-the-clock medication review by pharmacists" (Wakefield, Ward, Loes, O'Brien, & Speery, 2010, p. 2052). This provides a crucial safety check for patients at risk for adverse drug reactions as a result of medical conditions or other medications they are receiving. In a computer simulation designed to show implementation of HIT designed to prevent adverse drug reaction, Anderson et al.(2002) found that such systems could prevent over 1000 days of unnecessary hospitalization and over $1 million annually in the United States (as cited in Hartzema, Winterstein, Johns, De Leon, Bailey, McDonald, & Pannell, 2007). Such opportunities for improved quality of care and cost reductions using telehealth can also be applied to tele-radiology, tele-cardiology, and other fields requiring expert analysis beyond the primary care setting.

STAKEHOLDERS AND THE IRON TRIANGLE

Despite HIT's opportunity to forever expand Kissick's iron-triangle and bring a new era of healthcare to America, widespread adoption and use of HIT has yet to come to fruition. We propose that the reason for this is the mismatched priorities of HIT stakeholders around cost, access and quality of care. To demonstrate this, we present an analysis of each stakeholder's priority and diagram the priorities accordingly. Whereas Kissick's model represents cost-containment, access, and quality priorities by the angles at each corner (the larger the angle, the more priority placed on it), the kiviat diagrams we employ will represent these priorities within the triangle as distances from the origin. The original diagram (Figure 1) represents government's and public health's priorities.

The economic models of each individual stakeholder shift the priorities in their own micro-level triangle. While we understand these groups are by no means homogenous, and that variances in circumstances will lead to individual members of the group to vary in their priorities, the analyses presented attempt to focus on typical member within the stakeholder group. Additionally, these analyses are merely notional representations of the priorities of stakeholder groups; future research will be helpful in identifying these priorities with greater precision. Each of these stakeholders will now be discussed in turn:

Patients

Any analysis of HIT stakeholders would be remiss not to start the discussion by focusing on patients, for they are the most critical stakeholder in a healthcare system ideally built around improving their health. Although patients, as a group, are extremely diverse, their priorities as group are perhaps easier to understand. Access is a must for patients of any geography, class, and income level. With regards to quality, Pauly (2011) suggests that "few people are willing to accept, or even discuss having, anything but the best in health care" (p. 576). However, quality of care is not easily discernible to the consumers of health care. Many consumers base their estimation of quality on how much they like their physician or how compassionate they are. In a recent survey by Lown et al. (2011), 85 percent of patients responded that compassionate care "is 'very important' to successful medical care" (p. 1774). As a result, much of patient search for healthcare is innately personalized, as Pauly and Satterthwaite (1981) argue, since health care is a reputation good. This implies both that health care providers are differentiated and that consumer search is a process of asking neighbors, friends, and families. While this understanding seemingly applies mainly to primary care, the underlying priorities are clear. Patients care about quality, or at least, as McPake et al. (2006) note, "easily observable aspects of quality" (p. 138). Cost-Containment for patients has two aspects: insurance costs and cost of care. Research tends to suggest that demand for healthcare is price-inelastic, meaning that the rise in healthcare cost only has minor effects on patient demand (p. 25). This has two causes. First, once consumers have insurance, the fees for care are usually minimal and thus unaffected by income

Figure 1. The iron triangle of priorities for public health and government

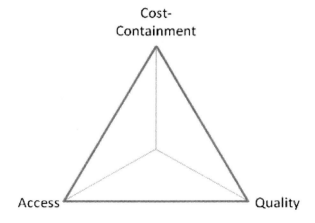

elasticity. Second, in many circumstances with expensive care, demand for such care is without choice, as it can determine the short-term health and life of the patient (Krugman, 2011). Insurance is much more price-elastic, but as Pauly et al. (2006) suggest, patient search tends to vary with premium; the more expensive the premium, for example those with preexisting conditions and the elderly, the more likely one is to engage in a deeper search process for insurance. Cost-containment is thus less important to the average patient than those in this higher extreme. Since this paper is examining patients as a group, the evidence suggests cost-containment is not as crucial a concern as quality and access. Figure 2 details these priorities.

Providers

Providers, as a group, exhibit great diversity, both in the patients they serve and the specialties in which they work. For the sake of clarity, we will examine the three most pervasive types of providers, small practice physicians (owners), large practice physicians (employees), and healthcare institutions.

Figure 2. The iron triangle of priorities for patients

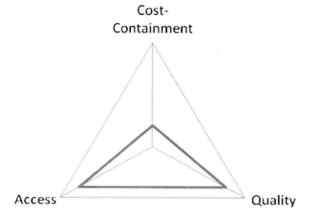

Small Practice Physicians (Owners)

The first group of providers are small practice physicians with ownership over their practice. Members of this group are dual-hatted in that they are both the physician and the business owner. While it may be difficult then to identify the typical physician/owner, it is not difficult to point to priorities across the group. Perhaps the most crucial need for these physicians is quality. The quality of care determines the word-of-mouth referrals, crucial to patients' searches, and especially important in small-group practices lacking robust advertising budgets. Due to demand being price-inelastic, competition in health care is based on quality. This suggests that as competition becomes fiercer for physicians in a geographic area (known as lower concentration), physicians react by increasing quality, not dropping price. As a result, increased competition leads to both increased cost and increased quality (McPake et al., 2006). However, in the past few decades, quality has become more important to basic survival of physicians due to medical malpractice. A United States Government Accountability Office Report (2003) noted that while malpractice insurance premiums vary both by specialty and location, the continual rise of these costs has greatly impacted the bottom line. Low quality care by physicians can hurt the practice not only by losing patients, but also by rising premiums and greater administrative and legal costs. This threat is evident in the current discussion of redundant tests. Redundant tests are beneficial to physicians' bottom lines, but more importantly, they protect them from malpractice suits (United States Executive Office of the President, 2010).

Access for patients is not of great importance to doctors past their ability to fill their patient rolls. Once physicians have a full load of patients, they must sacrifice quality or their time in order to grant access to others. Finally, cost-containment must be viewed through the lens of the owner in relation to these physicians. Physicians must worry more about margins than about cost-containment, but the underlying priority is similar. As we see with redundant tests, the increase in costs to patients actually increases the bottom line. While many physicians do not have the slim profit margins of other industries, they must still be concerned with costs that reduce their margins. Thus, overall cost-containment is not high a high priority of doctors; however, there are a few costs, such as administrative and overhead costs, that do make cost-containment important. To give an example, the administrative costs of interacting with insurance companies are unavoidable if doctors want to get paid. As the number of patients and physicians a practice holds increases, the overall administrative costs rise. However, the price per patient actually falls, and the cost is thus easier to disperse (Casalino, Nicholson, Gans, Hammons, Morra, Karrison, & Levinson, 2009). For small physician practices, these costs can be difficult to disperse among a small patient base. Financing costs on large purchases (such as an EHR) can also be much greater for the small physician practice due to limited access to capital and infrastructure (Gold, McLaughlin, Devers, Berenson, & Bovbjerg, 2012). Thus, small physician groups have priorities towards cost-containment, at least to an extent. Figure 3 demonstrates the priorities of these physician/owners.

Large Practice Physicians (Employees)

Large practice physicians, defined not by the size of their practice, but rather by their lack of ownership, exhibit many of the same priorities as the previous physician group, excluding those priorities most applicable to an owner. Quality of care still enhances word-of-mouth referrals, but this is less of a concern for the large practice

Figure 3. The iron triangle of priorities for small practice physicians (owners)

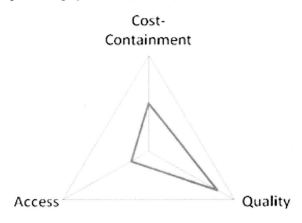

physician group as many are employed by health institutions with advertising budgets geared towards bringing in patients. Quality is, however, still crucial to avoiding medical malpractice suits and keeping malpractice insurance premiums low. Further, as with all physicians, definitive quality measurements related to a physician's work, whether it be the limited number of sentinel events a surgeon has under his watch or the cure rate of an oncologist, are important for the physician's reputation and longevity in the medical field. Access is not a high priority in the large practice physician group, and without the right incentive program from their institution, they may actually have the priority to avoid being overburdened by large patient rolls. Finally, cost-containment must be viewed through the lens of an employee in relation to these physicians. Again, without the right incentive and monitoring system, physicians have little reason to attempt to control costs above and beyond their normal routine. Figure 4 shows these priorities.

Health Care Institutions

Health Care institutions, such as hospitals, nursing homes, long term care, and hospice facilities exhibit many similarities to the physician groups.

Figure 4. The iron triangle of priorities for large practice physicians (employees)

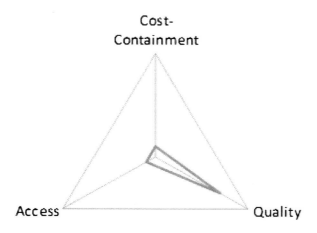

However, the salient differences between the groups deserve mention. Like physicians, health care institutions need to compete on quality, better understood as perceived quality, as a result of their position as provider. The need to provide quality is magnified by the larger number of patients. A major focus of health information technology has been to improve patient safety (indirectly quality of care) through better management of patient information and history (Parente & McCullough, 2009). The large number of patients increases the likelihood of mistakes through misidentification, allergens, and the like, increasing the priority placed on quality. Large overhead and administrative costs, in an absolute sense, and the ability to disperse these costs across a large customer base (Casalino et al, 2009) promotes cost-control measures and thus makes cost-containment a greater priority. Finally, access is a priority to health care institutions, to a degree. Facility location and capacity are important determinants both of access to health care for patients (Loh, Cobb, & Johnson, 2009) and of health institution business models. While rural hospitals may increase access most visibly (Ross, Normand, Wang, Nallamothu, & Lichtman, 2008), the inherent economics behind all health institutions, the need to fill beds and

make profit, aligns health institution priorities with access, at least up to a point. Figures 5 illustrates these priorities.

Pharmaceuticals

Pharmaceutical researchers and manufacturers have priorities that very much align with their economic needs. The pharmaceutical industry is built around innovation as the source of profit. A recent study on worldwide pharmaceutical innovation showed that the United States pharmaceutical industry accounts for over forty percent of new drugs among innovator countries worldwide (Keyhani, Wang, Herbert, Carpenter, & Anderson, 2010). The entrant of generic drug competition after the expiration of patents drives profit down, forcing brand name pharmaceuticals to lower their prices (Saha, Grabowski, Birnbaum, Greenberg, & Bizan, 2005) and resulting in lost revenue as consumers' business is spread among competitors.

Pharmaceutical priorities, thus, reflect these economic realities, as well as regulatory necessities under the Food and Drug Administration (FDA). Within the Iron-triangle framework, the pharmaceutical industry's greatest priority is quality. While the long and difficult drug approval process within the FDA does not ensure quality of drugs

Figure 5. The iron triangle of priorities for health care institutions

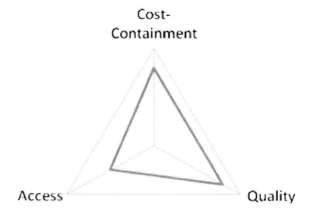

entering the market, as was seen with the Vioxx recall (Tong, Tong, & Tong, 2009), this gatekeeper approach does force pharmaceuticals to focus on quality. The drug approval process has three phases of trials, ranging from 18 months to 3.5 years to complete, while exposing more individuals to the drug at each phase (Beales, 2009). The length and liability of this drug approval process freezes capital and threatens profits, making quality of utmost concern. Tangential to quality is internal cost-containment within the drug manufacturing process. Like with any good, containing costs can yield greater profits at the same price. However, intense competition and the need to constantly innovate require intensive research and development expenditures, limiting the industry's ability to contain costs. Finally, while the industry is built on creating drugs for consumers, the inevitability of generic competition makes wide-spread consumer access to drugs possibly counterproductive to their economic model. Figure 6 illustrates the priorities of pharmaceuticals.

Payers

The two largest payers in the healthcare market are government (Medicaid, Medicare, VA, etc.) and health insurance companies. The economic

Figure 6. The iron triangle of priorities for pharmaceuticals

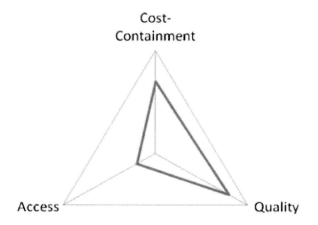

purpose of insurance in general, and health insurance specifically, is to spread the risk of large expenditures over a group of individuals. Health insurance companies and payers alike face two important, and perhaps contradictory, moral hazards that shape the overall economic priorities of the group. The first moral hazard is the perverse incentive to spend more when another is paying. Richard Zeckhauser (1970) explains it thusly:

Insurance provision will... introduce a perverse incentive toward over expenditure if, as usually is the case, the insured have substantial influence over the amount that is spent on their own behalf in any particular medical circumstance, and the level of reimbursement by the insurance plan is a positively associated function of the expenses incurred by its insured (p. 14).

This moral hazard, the rise of expenditures, is evident in the current health-spending environment in the United States. In order to make a profit in the case of insurance companies or make provision economically feasible in the case of government, payers must work to control these costs, prioritizing cost-containment.

The priority of quality is tangential to payers' cost structure, for quality and preventative care can reduce the likelihood of extremely costly procedures and long-term care. Here, ex ante moral hazard, or consumer reduction in healthy activities and prevention, conflicts with payer interest. Evidence of ex ante moral hazard shows that since insurance reduces the risk of large health expenditures for individuals, they reduce preventive and healthy activities (Dave and Kaestner, 2009; Stanicole, 2008). Since physician counseling can help promote healthy activities and prevention (Dave and Kaestner, 2009), quality care should be a priority for payers, if it is not already. Finally, access is a priority for only some payers, namely government payers. Medicare and Medicaid are built on access. However, government payers and insurance companies alike restrict access to consumers by controlling the network of providers one is able to access, gaining discounts and avoiding certain costly providers. Payers thus do not have the economic incentive to fully prioritize access to consumers. Figure 7 details these priorities.

EXAMPLES OF INCONGRUENCE

The differences between each stakeholder's iron-triangle demonstrate the difficulties in creating a health information technology framework that fulfills the needs and is cognizant of the priorities of each of these groups. While the complexity of digital record conversions, the lack of standards for record keeping and communications, and the natural reluctance to change all contribute to the enormity of the effort required, the overarching barrier standing in the way of a truly valuable HIT society is the incongruence of stakeholder priorities. Examples of this incongruence and its detrimental effects on HIT adoption and use are numerous in the HIT literature.

Perhaps the most poignant example of how incongruous priorities can lead to suboptimal results is electronic health record adoption and interoperability. As seen previously, EHR use has the immense potential to make healthcare cheaper, more effective, and more accessible for millions of

Figure 7. The iron triangle of priorities for payers

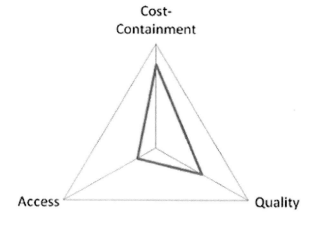

Americans, expanding the traditional iron-triangle and leading the way for a new health society. Yet, in order to maximize the benefits of EHRs, systems must be adopted and interoperable. Without these two facets: adoption and interoperability, EHRs function no different than electronic versions of their paper predecessors. However, with wide-spread adoption of EHRs and interoperable systems, the benefits of sharing information, of better quality prescriptions and diagnoses, and of operational efficiencies can be realized.

Unfortunately, the realities of adoption and interoperability are grim, and a result of the incongruous priorities of public health, physicians, and health institutions. Small-group and individual physician reservations regarding HIT have slowed EHR adoption, with an April 2010 study finding only "…18 percent reported having at least a basic electronic record system" (Hogan and Kissam, 2010, p. 601). The high costs of adoption are less able to be spread across a patient base and thus small-group physicians are less able to take on large purchases like electronic health records. While quality is a priority, the lack of observable improvements in EHR use assures small-group physicians remain late adopters. Since access is not a major priority, EHRs ability to allow patients to move between physicians does not drive physician adoption of electronic health records. Adoption is less problematic in health institutions, as the priority of cost-containment, the larger patient base over which to spread costs, and the immense operational efficiencies make EHR adoption and use a major opportunity. Quality improvements internally are more readily visible, as health institutions must be better able to track and understand the large number of patients that walk through their doors. Finally, the large network of patients and institutional facilities align access with EHR adoption in healthcare institutions.

While healthcare institutions may be leading the charge in EHR adoption, their size and priorities have many times come in the way of large-scale, societal interoperability. The "make or buy" decision for HIT investments has been a major consideration for healthcare institutions adopting EHRs in the past decade (National Institutes of Health, 2006). Many of the largest health institutions have chosen to make their own HIT systems that fit the idiosyncrasies of their own unique situations. Perhaps the most impressive example of this in the private sector has been Kaiser Permanente's KP Health Connect (Silvestre, Sue, & Allen, 2009). Unfortunately, as each health institution chooses to "make" a unique system rather than to "buy" one used by others, the interoperability decreases. However, even the pre-made EHRs that small physicians adopt and use are not always congruous. As Kleinke (2005) notes, "no single health care organization or HIT venture has attained anything close to the critical mass" (p. 1246). The mismatched priorities of physicians and health institutions have allowed a plethora of small HIT ventures to be created with none dominating the market. The result has been failed interoperability of HIT systems. While government and public health may value access and thus push for interoperability, the priorities of physicians and health institutions just do not align. The incentives to buy interoperable systems are not innate, the priorities are misaligned, and the failure of interoperability thus far is the result.

FUTURE RESEARCH DIRECTIONS

We have presented an analysis of the classic conundrum in healthcare; the iron-triangle. By representing the issues of cost-containment, quality, and access by stakeholder group, this work adds insight into the dilemma faced by healthcare professionals and government officials. Although useful, our analysis suffers for lack of quantitative data to assure readers and researchers of the validity and specificity of these assertions. Future research should focus on the gathering of data to populate the dimensions of the stakeholder triangles with greater precision.

CONCLUSION

The failure of health information technology to provide America with a new health society, one more accessible, less costly, and of greater quality, must be overcome. While many have looked for solutions to the issues of complexity, technological standardization, and change management, the most crucial barrier to HIT's promise is being ignored. The basic economic priorities of stakeholders in the HIT field are incongruent and working against each other. Incentives are misaligned, and the health field is suffering as a result. The disappointments of health information technology are thus an example of market failure, one in which government can step in to correct. With the HITECH Act, the Federal government has headed this call, and has started setting standards for meaningful use and creating incentives for HIT adoption, Health information exchange use, and other HIT endeavors (Williams, Mostashari, Mertz, Hogin, & Atwal, 2012). While these are important steps towards realizing the benefits of health information technology in America, it must go further to address the true problem. Once government and public health realize that the issue is incongruity in stakeholder priorities, they can begin to work to realign these priorities. Only then will HIT prove Kissick's words prophetic and expand the iron-triangle, making healthcare less expensive, of better quality, and more accessible for all Americans.

REFERENCES

Baker, L., Johnson, S., Macaulay, D., & Birnbaum, H. (2011). Integrated telehealth and care management program for medicare beneficiaries with chronis disease linked to savings. *Health Affairs*, *30*(9), 1689–1697. doi:10.1377/hlthaff.2011.0216 PMID:21900660.

Beales, H. (2009). Prescription drug regulation. In *Business and Governmental Relations: An Economic Perspective*. Dubuque, IA: Kendall Hunt.

Birnbaum, M. (2012). A conversation with donald berwick on implementing national health reform. *Journal of Health Politics, Policy and Law*, *37*(4), 709–727. doi:10.1215/03616878-1597511 PMID:22466046.

Casalino, L., Nicholson, S., Gans, D., Hammons, T., Morra, D., Karrison, T., & Levinson, W. (2009). What does it cost physician practices to interact with health insurance plans? *Health Affairs*, *28*(4), w533–w543. doi:10.1377/hlthaff.28.4.w533 PMID:19443477.

Chumbler, N., Haggstrom, D., & Saleem, J. (2011). Implementation of health information technology in veterans health administration to support transformational change: Telehealth and personal health records. *Medical Care*, *49*(12), S36–S42. doi:10.1097/MLR.0b013e3181d558f9 PMID:20421829.

Cusack, C. (2008). Electronic health records and electronic prescribing: Promise and pitfalls. *Obstetrics and Gynological Clinics of North America*, *35*, 63–79. doi:10.1016/j.ogc.2007.12.010 PMID:18319129.

Dave, D., & Kaestner, R. (2009). Health insurance and ex ante moral hazard: Evidence from Medicare. *International Journal of Health Care Finance and Economics*, *9*(4), 367–390. doi:10.1007/s10754-009-9056-4 PMID:19277859.

Fang, H., Peifer, K., Chan, J., & Rizzo, J. (2011). Health information technology and physicians' perceptions of healthcare quality. *The American Journal of Managed Care*, *17*(3), e66–e70. PMID:21504261.

Gaylin, D., Moiduddin, A., Mohamoud, S., Lundeen, K., & Kelly, J. (2011). Public attitudes about health information technology, and its relationship to health care quality, costs, and privacy. *Health Services Research*, *46*(3), 920–934. doi:10.1111/j.1475-6773.2010.01233.x PMID:21275986.

Gold, M., McLaughlin, C., Devers, K., Berenson, R., & Bovbjerg, R. (2012). Obtaining providers' 'buy-in' and establishing effective means of information exchange will be critical to HITECH's success. *Health Affairs*, *31*(3), 514–526. doi:10.1377/hlthaff.2011.0753 PMID:22392662.

Hartzema, A., Winterstein, A., Johns, T., De Leon, J., Bailey, W., McDonald, K., & Pannell, R. (2007). Planning for pharmacy health information technology in critical access hospitals. *American Journal of Health-System Pharmacists*, *64*, 315–321. doi:10.2146/ajhp060134 PMID:17244881.

Hogan, S., & Kissam, S. (2010). Measuring meaningful use. *Health Affairs*, *29*(4), 601–606. doi:10.1377/hlthaff.2009.1023 PMID:20368588.

Karsh, B., Weinger, M., Abbott, P., & Wears, R. (2010). Health information technology: Fallacies and sober realities. *Journal of the American Medical Informatics Association*, *17*, 617–623. doi:10.1136/jamia.2010.005637 PMID:20962121.

Keyhani, S., Wang, S., Hebert, P., Carpenter, D., & Anderson, G. (2010). US pharmaceutical innovation in an international context. *American Journal of Public Health*, *100*(6), 1075–1080. doi:10.2105/AJPH.2009.178491 PMID:20403883.

Kissick, W. L. (1994). *Medicine's dilemmas: Infinite needs versus finite resources*. New Haven, CT: Yale University Press.

Kleinke, J. (2005). Dot-gov: Market failure and the creation of a national health information technology system. *Health Affairs*, *24*(5), 1246–1262. doi:10.1377/hlthaff.24.5.1246 PMID:16162569.

Krugman, P. (2011, April 22). Patients are not consumers. *New York Times*, p. A23.

Lau, F., Kuziemsky, C., Price, M., & Gardner, J. (2010). A review on systematic reviews of health information system studies. *Journal of the American Medical Informatics Association*, *17*, 637–645. doi:10.1136/jamia.2010.004838 PMID:20962125.

Loh, C., Cobb, S., & Johnson, C. (2009). Potential and actual accessibility to hospital and hospital services in northeast Florida. *Southeastern Geographer*, *49*(2), 171–184. doi:10.1353/sgo.0.0043.

Lown, B., Rosen, J., & Marttila, J. (2011). An agenda for improving compassionate care: A survey shows about half of patients say such care is missing. *Health Affairs*, *30*(9), 1772–1778. doi:10.1377/hlthaff.2011.0539 PMID:21900669.

McPake, B., Kumaranayake, L., & Normand, C. (2006). *Health economics: An international perspective*. New York, NY: Routledge Publishing.

National Institutes of Health National Center for Research Resources. (2006). *Electronic health records overview*. Retrieved April 10, 2010, from http://www.ncrr.nih.gov/publications/informatics/ehr.pdf

Parente, S., & McCullough, J. (2009). Health information technology and patient safety: Evidence from panel data. *Health Affairs*, *28*(2), 357–360. doi:10.1377/hlthaff.28.2.357 PMID:19275990.

Pauly, M. (2011). The trade-off among quality, quantity, and cost: How to make it-if we must. *Health Affairs*, *30*(4), 574–580. doi:10.1377/hlthaff.2011.0081 PMID:21471475.

Pauly, M., Herring, B., & Song, D. (2006). Information technology and consumer search for health insurance. *International Journal of the Economics of Business*, *13*(1), 45–63. doi:10.1080/13571510500519970.

Pauly, M., & Satterthwaite, M. (1981). The pricing of primary care physicians services: A test of the role of consumer information. *The Bell Journal of Economics*, *12*(2), 488–506. doi:10.2307/3003568.

Pear, R. (2011, December 3). Health official takes parting shot at 'waste'. *New York Times*, p. A23.

Ross, J., Normand, S., Wang, Y., Nallamothu, B., & Lichtman, J. (2008). Hospital remoteness and thirty-day mortality from three serious conditions. *Health Affairs*, *27*(6), 1707–1717. doi:10.1377/hlthaff.27.6.1707 PMID:18997230.

Saha, A., Grabowski, H., Birnbaum, H., Greenberg, P., & Bizan, O. (2005). Generic competition in the US pharmaceutical industry. *International Journal of the Economics of Business*, *13*(1), 15–38. doi:10.1080/13571510500519905.

Shapiro, J., Mostashari, F., Hripcsak, G., Soulakis, N., & Kuperman, G. (2011). Using health information exchange to improve public health. *American Journal of Public Health*, *101*(4), 616–623. doi:10.2105/AJPH.2008.158980 PMID:21330598.

Silvestre, A., Sue, V., & Allen, J. (2009). If you build it, will they come? The Kaiser Permanente model of online health care. *Health Affairs*, *28*(2), 334–344. doi:10.1377/hlthaff.28.2.334 PMID:19275988.

Stanciole, A. (2008). Health insurance and lifestyle choices: Identifying ex ante moral hazard in the US market. *The Geneva Papers on Risk and Insurance*, *33*, 627–644. doi:10.1057/gpp.2008.27.

Tong, H., Tong, L., & Tong, J. (2009). The Vioxx recall case and comments. *International Business Journal*, *29*(2), 114–118.

United States Executive Office of the President. President's Council of Advisors on Science and Technology. (2010). *Report to the President realizing the full potential of health information technology to improve healthcare for Americans: The path forward*. Retrieved August 20, 2012, from http://www.whitehouse.gov/sites/default/files/microsites/ostp/pcast-health-it-report.pdf

United States Government Accountability Office. (2003). *Medical malpractice insurance: Multiple factors have contributed to increased premium rates* (GAO Publication No. GAO-03-702). Retrieved August 20, 2012, from http://www.gao.gov/new.items/d03702.pdf

Vaitheeswaran, V. (2011, March 31). A very big HIT. *The Economist: The World in 2011, 133.*

Wakefield, D., Ward, M., Loes, J., O'Brien, J., & Speery, L. (2010). Implementation of a telepharmacy service to provide round-the-clock medication order review by pharmacists. *American Journal of Health-System Pharmacists, 67*, 2052–2057. doi:10.2146/ajhp090643 PMID:21098378.

Williams, C., Mostashari, F., Mertz, K., Hogin, E., & Atwal, P. (2012). From the office of the national coordinator: The strategy for advancing the exchange of health information. *Health Affairs, 31*(3), 527–536. doi:10.1377/hlthaff.2011.1314 PMID:22392663.

Zeckhauser, R. (1970). Medical insurance: A case study of the tradeoff between risk spreading and appropriate incentives. *Journal of Economic Theory, 2*(1), 10–26. doi:10.1016/0022-0531(70)90010-4.

KEY TERMS AND DEFINITIONS

Accessibility of Care: One of the three pillars of the Iron-triangle, Accessibility describes the priority to ensure all patients are able to receive health services when needed or requested.

Cost-Containment: One of the three pillars of the Iron-triangle, Cost-containment describes the priority to deliver healthcare for the lowest cost.

EHR: Electronic Health Records (EHR) are electronic versions of the patient records health care providers use to identify and treat patients. The complexity of the EHR and the integration within clinical practice varies by institution and provider.

HIE: Health Information Exchanges (HIE) organize and mobilize public health and healthcare information across geographies and health service organizations. They often link the health information systems of disparate entities within specified geographic region, but can be organized in various other ways to accomplish the goals of the specific HIE.

HIT: Health Information Technology (HIT) is a discipline focused on the integration of technological tools and processes within the delivery and study of health care. It draws on various disciplines including computer science, information technology, operations research, management, public health, and health sciences to develop methods and solutions that optimize the use of information in the healthcare.

Iron-Triangle: First developed by Kissick, the Iron-Triangle of trade-offs within healthcare describes that in equilibrium, improved performance in one of three pillars (cost-containment, quality, and access to care) can cause decreased performance in one or both of the other pillars.

Quality of Care: One of the three pillars of the Iron-triangle, Quality of care describes the priority to deliver healthcare that will provide to the greatest benefit to the patient's health.

Chapter 13
Home Telecare, Medical Implant, and Mobile Technology:
Evolutions in Geriatric Care

Vishaya Naidoo
York University, Canada

Yedishtra Naidoo
Wayne State University, USA

ABSTRACT

With a rapidly expanding global aging population, alternatives must be developed to minimize the inevitable increase in acute and long-term care admissions to the health care system. This chapter explores the use of home telecare as an alternative medical approach to managing this growing trend, while also providing superior care to geriatric patients. To address some of the emergent disadvantages of home telecare concerning usability, self-management, and confinement to the home, the use of a cardiac implant in conjunction with a mobile device—to assist in the management of chronic heart failure in seniors—is proposed as a promising technological solution to overcoming these limitations. Ultimately, it seems that the growth of home telecare, as well as the great potential to enhance its services with the use of mobile wireless technology, stands to drastically improve clinical decision-making and management of health services in the future.

INTRODUCTION

We are living in an era when the world's aging population is rapidly expanding. In the year 2000, 600 million people were aged 60 and over, with this number projected to increase to 1.2 billion in

2025 and 2 billion by the year 2050 (WHO, 2006). At this rate of growth, the inevitable increase in acute and long-term care admissions is a significant concern for policymakers, managers and providers of health care. Concerns arise from the increased economic cost, as well as the potentially lower standard of care that is likely to result from a higher volume of patients seeking treatment in

DOI: 10.4018/978-1-4666-4321-5.ch013

an over-burdened system. Currently, international trends indicate that health care needs increase as people become older, and that the number of people requiring *daily* health care over the age of 85 is now four times more than those aged 65 to 75 (Botsis et al., 2008). One proposed solution to managing this problem is home telecare – a sub-specialty within the larger field of telemedicine. This involves a shift in care with the use of new and emergent information technology in the home, utilizing an array of hardware, software and network services (Roback & Herzog, 2003). With this system, patients can be monitored, consult with their physicians, and receive care without physically leaving their private homes; thereby allowing them to maintain their independence, more conveniently and efficiently manage chronic conditions, and ultimately reduce health care costs to the system (Hébert et al., 2006; Koch, 2006).

In this chapter, we examine the growing arena of home telecare and assess its potential to enhance treatment and clinical decision-making in geriatric medicine. Following a review of important facets of home telecare, as well as a discussion of the advantages of this medical technology for policymakers and patients, we then outline the challenges that arise with this system, proposing the use of an implantable device—under the skin—as a means through which to increase convenience and overcome user-related challenges for seniors with chronic Heart Failure (HF). The use of a cardiac implant in conjunction with mobile wireless technology is a potentially promising solution that addresses some of the emergent challenges of home telecare concerning usability, self-management, and confinement to the home. This proposed technology would allow seniors in chronic HF, and under the monitoring of a home telecare system, to leave their home while maintaining a similarly comprehensive level of medical monitoring and management for their condition. Ultimately, it seems that the growth of home telecare, as well as the great potential to enhance its services with

the use of mobile wireless technology, stands to drastically improve clinical decision-making and management of health services in the future.

BACKGROUND

Telemedicine refers to the delivery of medical care—and the sharing of health knowledge—from a distance with the use of telecommunication devices, the Internet, and various monitoring technologies (Allen & March, 2002; Hersh et al., 2002). Home telecare operates on the same premise, allowing health care practitioners to manage and treat patients in their homes from a remote location (Celler et al., 2003; Coughlin et al., 2006). Services encompass a wide array of technologies, including "virtual visiting, reminder systems, home security, and social alarm systems," all of which support the larger goal of home telecare: to manage the care of geriatric patients where they live, and avoid lengthy stays in hospitals or nursing homes (Magnusson, 2004, pp. 224-225). It is a method of health care delivery that addresses many of the existing gaps and weaknesses in the current primary health care system, by providing a higher level of monitoring and medical consultation for patients in their everyday lives. The services provided by this branch of telemedicine are meant to increase convenience for patients, their families, and practitioners, where a higher level of patient autonomy and independence is supported, while also enhancing clinical management and decision-making.

Much of the strength in this system lies in the ability to extensively record and monitor patient data electronically. Clayton and Hripcsak (1995) suggest that the availability of patient information in an electronic format has been one of the most valuable and widely used Decision Support Systems (DSS) in health care. With patient information stored and tracked through home-based DSS, clinicians can potentially make more informed decisions with convenient access to entire patient histories and vital statistics (Cardozo & Steinberg, 2010). Clinicians rely upon timely access to test results and patient records in order to manage care and make efficient treatment decisions. The rapid or real-time transmission of accurate and organized data provided by the monitoring tools of home telecare technologies serve to facilitate this process (Klonoff & True, 2009). Devices are currently in existence to track a number of patient vitals and biostatistics over a period of time, including basic clinical measurements such as temperature, weight, blood pressure, and lung function (Magrabi et al., 2001; Rahimpour et al., 2008). Falas et al. (2003) suggest that providing real-time access to this information allows physicians to rank cases in terms of medical priority, as well as electronically manage how they are handled. This level of monitoring is of particular value to older adults with chronic conditions, who may otherwise find it difficult to physically visit their general practitioner for consultation and treatment of minor symptoms. With this technology, the physical barriers to accessing care are eliminated because minor concerns or changes in vital signs can be dealt with quickly and remotely.

Thornett (2001) indicates that computer-based access to individual patient data can also assist with diagnosis and enhance clinical decision-making through the vast amounts of information that modern practice databases can potentially hold. This allows aging patients to receive more carefully monitored care than if they were to rely upon less-frequent in-person physician visits. Home telecare technologies are used to manage such symptoms as "chronic heart failure, asthma, diabetes, and hypertension" (Celler et al., 2003, p. 242). One of the technological applications used with this form of case management is the videophone system, allowing nurses and physicians the opportunity to speak directly with and see patients via video monitoring technology, while also wirelessly gathering and assessing data on their vital signs from health monitoring equipment (p. 242).

With this more accessible format to gather and display patient information, a clinician may then also more easily consult electronic decision support materials and evidence – using the Internet or some other form of health information database – to assist in treatment plans and diagnosis.

In addition to videophone technology, and the increased level of decision support that comes with real-time access to patient history and information, another prominent facet of home telecare is teleconsulting. Here, general practitioners can remotely consult with specialists when managing a particular case, thereby interacting with a panel of "experts" when treating a patient (Vitacca et al., 2006). Given that distance is not a barrier with telemedical technology, the geographic location of the consulting panel can potentially include a wide array of international experts. This aspect of telemedicine enables the globalization of medical practice and group decision-making – an important transition in an era when information sharing is becoming increasingly ubiquitous. Here, patients may be treated from a far larger pool of knowledge than they would otherwise receive from traditional care in a physician's office. Instead of one clinician assessing and making decisions about a complex case, there is now the potential to rely upon multiple experts in the delivery of care.

BENEFITS AND CHALLENGES OF HOME TELECARE

Strengths of Home Telecare for Policymakers and Patients

With new home telecare technologies—and access to a more extensive pool of medical expertise—there are several noteworthy aspects of home telecare that are superior to methods of traditional medicine for both policymakers and patients. The first is the reduced economic cost to the health care system itself. This can be seen with less outpatient visits, as well as a reduction in hospital inpatient stays and fewer admissions to nursing homes (Magnusson et al., 2004). Though the initial implementation costs associated with home telecare equipment may be high, it is likely to become lower with the widespread adoption and greater prevalence of such technologies – particularly with the resultant competitive pricing and lowered cost of goods that comes in any rapidly growing market of this nature (Dansky et al., 2001). The benefit of a lesser financial burden to the health care system is particularly important in a time when the scarcity of health care resources is becoming an increasing concern as society's largest age cohort enters the later stages of life. Health care provision has transformed through free market enterprise, to become an increasingly commodified entity, where resources are scarce and care may be compromised (Bambra, et al., 2005; Kearns & Barnett, 1999). As a result, the system is faced with the prospect of being unable to accommodate the needs of all patients equally. The increased use of new information technologies to minimize costs by providing care in the home therefore offers an economic benefit that will enable a greater number of older adults in the growing senior population to efficiently receive treatment and care.

The use of in-home technologies that monitor vital signs and symptoms also benefit patients by allowing individuals to maintain their independence and remain active members of their community. The movement of forcing seniors into a nursing home or other form of long term care facility can be a difficult experience, sometimes fostering a degree of physical, emotional, and/or intellectual decline. When older adults remain in their homes, rather than moving to an institutional environment, they are able to enjoy an overall better quality of life and continue to benefit from enriched social networks (Hébert et al., 2001).

Another important benefit of home telecare technologies is the ability of policymakers to better support patients in rural and other underserved regions (Magnusson et al., 2004). For example,

with the use of home telecare technologies, older adults in northern Aboriginal communities of Canada – where the shortage of physicians is a significant concern – may benefit from the medical expertise of physicians that are remotely located in more populated urban centers. Due to a significant shortage of physicians and specialists in rural areas of Canada, for example, many do not receive medical attention (Dove, 2009). Members of vulnerable groups who require specialized services—particularly women, older adults, and racialized individuals—are at an even greater risk of experiencing compromised care. The use of home telecare technologies has the potential to allow governments to cater to the health care needs of even their most geographically underserved populations.

Finally, home telecare—as with many other branches of telemedicine—allows for greater opportunity to facilitate group clinical decision-making and the sharing of knowledge between clinicians. Quintero et al. (2001) refer to this as "collaborative medical reasoning," where physicians can draw upon knowledge produced in group meetings comprised of both experts and novices (p. 4). This exchange of information ultimately allows for more informed decisions that draw upon a large knowledge base to aid in making treatment and care decisions. With the expertise of more health care professionals, a reduction in medical errors is likely to be realized in treatment and diagnosis. From an international perspective, there is also the added benefit of forging strong partnerships and connections amongst those in the global medical community, while also providing the best possible care from an expansive medical pool of expertise.

Challenges of Home Telecare

Despite the aforementioned benefits of home telecare technologies, prominent research questions, perspectives, as well as concerns emerge with regards to self-management, the changing role of the health care professional, and usability for patients – particularly older adults. The new role of both the patient and the clinician in managing and making decisions about care is an important perspective for consideration. With the growth of home telecare mechanisms and technologies comes a greater emphasis on self-management by the patient and a potentially lesser role for health care professionals. Celler et al. (2003) explore this shift, describing a patient-managed system:

A patient-managed Home Telecare System with integrated clinical signs monitoring, automated scheduling and medication reminders, as well as access to health education and daily logs, is presented as an example of information and communication technology use for chronic disease self-management (p. 242).

This trend is motivated by the economic goals of the home telecare effort, where an important aim is to alleviate cost to the health care system by shifting the responsibility away from the hospital or primary care facility, toward technological solutions to assist in clinical decisions. The de-personalization of medical care, and potential reduction of human contact in clinical care, is one prominent dilemma that has yet to be reconciled (Percival & Hanson, 2006). One aspect of home telecare, for example, is that of "self-assessed patient health status," which essentially monitors and assesses one's health status through electronic questionnaires and provides health information to the patient electronically (Magrabi et al., 2001). A central question that emerges with this increased role of the patient in managing his or her own health is how this will impact both patient care and clinical decision-making at large.

Questions around usability also emerge as a related challenge in discussions about home telecare. Botsis et al. (2008) write of the importance of usability, given that patients and their families are likely to be directly utilizing these technologies in their homes and the design of the information system must be such that it is useable for clinicians *and* their patients. This may be

particularly difficult given that geriatric patients are less likely to be technologically inclined and are also more likely to be distrustful of newer methods of care than their younger counterparts (Rahimpour et al., 2008). This concern will only grow as information technology and the field of telemedicine continues to advance. Adaptability, usability, and accessibility are therefore important perspectives of consideration with home telecare for older adults.

Older adults also express reservations about the loss of autonomy and privacy that arises with the self-management and monitoring tools utilized by home telecare systems (Percival & Hanson, 2006). Given that many of these patients are older in age, some prefer human interaction with their health care providers and might be hesitant toward the shifting reliance on technology to assist clinicians with making decisions concerning their care and treatment. Use of computers and the Internet tend to be under-utilized amongst seniors (Kaufman et al., 2003; Magnusson et al., 2004). Given that home telecare is geared mainly toward the aged, accessibility and the use of adaptive technology to make these mechanisms as user-friendly as possible are crucial to the full implementation of the system.

There is also concern with home telecare and the scope of medical conditions that can be effectively managed and monitored with its services. While home telecare efforts have been found to be feasible and effective for monitoring and treating chronic conditions, it is difficult to sustain with more life-threatening and serious conditions given the physical distance between the physician and the patient (Botsis et al., 2008). Such cases potentially require immediate in-person response and action from a treating physician.

Furthermore, technological difficulties from misuse or mis-handling of equipment, faulty devices, or other malfunctioning errors can be frustrating for both providers and patients, making the monitoring process more complex (Roback & Herzog, 2003). Examples include devices that may require manual data entry—such as one's blood pressure level—allowing for the input of potentially incorrect or missing information, depending on who is operating the device and how well-trained or skilled they are in such mechanisms. In the event of technical or human error, there are a number of problems that can result, not the least of which is compromised care or increased risk that can be fatal for the patient.

Finally, given that home telecare is a fairly new field involving a number of technological advancements that could completely alter the way we interact with health care providers, a number of change management challenges are also involved in its implementation and in how the scheme would "operate, define, deliver, and manage care at home and throughout the health care system" (Coughlin et al., 2006, p. 206). With the increased number of actors involved in this transition, for example, significant integration efforts make it difficult to co-ordinate and operationalize a system that is completely aligned with a telemedical effort. This creates not only a potentially difficult transition for those working within the system, but also for patients themselves. In the subsequent section, we propose the use of a medical implant device to address some of these challenges involved with geriatric home telecare for health policymakers, clinical decision-makers and patients.

Mergence of Medical Implant and Mobile Wireless Technology

As has emerged throughout this discussion, usability, accessibility and efficiency are significant areas of concern for home telecare technology in geriatric medicine. One technology that has the potential to address these challenges, and assist physician decision-making in remote patient care, is the implantation of a device—under the skin—that can be used as a tool to monitor physiological statistics and wirelessly transmit real-time patient data. Such technologies currently exist in some forms to assist physicians in monitoring, treating,

and diagnosing conditions related to "heart disease, gastrointestinal tract, neurological disorders, cancer detection, handicap rehabilitation, and general health monitor[ing]" (Zhen et al., 2009, p. 23). Yet, one aspect of this technology that does not emerge in the literature is the potential use of such implants for older patients with chronic Heart Failure (HF).

Chronic HF is a condition that affects an increasing number of older adults each year, impacting more than 350,000 Canadians (Godfrey et al., 2007; Liu et al., 2001). With the rapidly growing aging population, the number of cases is projected to increase in the coming years. Currently, in order to properly manage a chronic condition like HF frequent hospitalization or cardiac monitoring is required (Abraham et al., 2011). Hospitalization rates for this particular condition are therefore high and on the rise, posing some concern over the increased cost of caring for this influx of patients. In treating this condition, the Canadian health care system must sustain a cost of over $1 billion per year for inpatient hospital care (Godfrey et al., 2007). A mechanism for constant monitoring of this condition outside of a health care facility therefore stands to dramatically decrease cost to the primary health care system.

While a home telecare system provides one such solution, it is likely to involve confinement to the home, making it difficult for patients to sustain a high level of social activity and engagement in the community – an integral part of life for older adults who are particularly vulnerable to social isolation. Therefore, the use of an implantable monitoring device for chronic HF would allow those in the vulnerable senior population to more easily leave the home telecare environment, knowing that their condition is still being closely monitored. This also eases the concerns of caregivers who may otherwise have reservations about accompanying these individuals outside of the home and away from monitoring equipment.

To address this need, we propose the merging of two existing technologies with seemingly compatible properties. This proposed amalgamation would allow patient data collected through a specific type of body implant—known as Micro Electro-Mechanical Systems (MEMS)—to be transmitted to a mobile device that the patient carries on their person, allowing for clinical management and decision-making by the patient or caregiver in addition to the remotely located physician. Currently, MEMS transmit detailed health information to the remote physician via the Internet, but not to the patient. Before discussing the proposed use of these technologies together, it is important to first establish how they each separately operate.

First, MEMS are miniature electronic implantable devices that monitor and transmit hemodynamic information directly from a body implant to a secure Website (Botsis et al., 2008). With regards to chronic HF, data recorded by these implants currently include pulmonary artery pressures, systolic and diastolic pressures, heart rate and cardiac output. The purpose of such monitoring is to reduce the number of hospitalizations due to the worsening of chronic HF in patients. Heart failure is broadly defined as the inability of the heart to output sufficient blood to meet the metabolic demands of the body (Borlaug et al., 2006). While it may have numerous causes, it is most commonly due to coronary artery disease and hypertension. Clinical signs and symptoms of the condition include shortness of breath, fatigue, dizziness, and cough. Patients experiencing these symptoms commonly present to emergency departments to alleviate their clinical symptoms. The worsening of chronic HF leads to increased emergency department visits and higher instances of inpatient hospitalization. If a treating physician could monitor blood pressure levels remotely and adjust medications as necessary, however, hospitalization could be prevented, improving the lifestyle of patients and ultimately reducing health-care costs to the system.

CardioMEMS—the company that produces this particular implant—utilizes this technology to monitor symptoms of HF in patients by inserting the implant directly into one of the ventricles of the heart (Raskovic et al., 2004). Transmission occurs when the patient is lying down on a pillow with a built-in antenna. From here, the device records the hemodynamic data previously mentioned, and transmits it via a telephone line to a private Internet database system, allowing remote and real-time access to the information through a secure Web-based server (Abraham et al., 2011). At present, the MEMS device data transmits exclusively to a private Website which can only be accessed by healthcare professionals. Through access to the database, physicians can adjust blood pressure medication dosage or recommend hospitalization, if necessary. After a pressure reading is taken, the patient may then be advised to adjust their medication dosage fairly quickly if a change in levels is detected.

The secure online medical database available to the physician while tracking vital signs in this way greatly assists clinicians in the clinical decision-making process by allowing easy and electronic access to patient histories, teleconsultation with other physicians, as well as access to various health databases and resources to assist in diagnosis. The capability of remote real-time monitoring is a potentially more efficient and direct method that is comparable to patients with diabetes who are similarly given blood glucose monitoring and subsequent prescription medication adjustments. The benefit of this technology for patients is that it allows physicians to frequently monitor cardiac data in a way that many other current non-invasive methods of management for chronic HF cannot (Abraham, et al., 2011). Implant technology is effective for management of this particular condition because if caught early, HF can be efficiently observed before clinical signs and systems manifest themselves, requiring the patient to be hospitalized. This is where mobile device transfer to a portable unit on the patient's person would be the next logical step in utilization of the MEMS device.

The second existing technology that we are suggesting should be adapted for more efficient results with MEMS in the treatment of HF is a mobile device that wirelessly records and processes information directly from the body implant. This device does so in close proximity to the patient – as they would be expected to carry this on their person. Milenković et al. (2006) describe such a system where a personal server application is run on a mobile device and wirelessly linked to medical body sensors, providing feedback through a "user friendly and intuitive graphical or audio user interface," thereby providing an interface custom to the user as well as an interface distinct to the medical server (p. 2523).

The combined use of both of these technologies, as illustrated in Figure 1, involves the short distance transmission of data from the implant to a mobile device, as well as the long distance transmission of patient data to a remotely located physician. In essence, the patient or caregiver is alerted to real time changes in their condition—

Figure 1. Flow of data in telecare system utilizing a body implant in conjunction with a mobile device

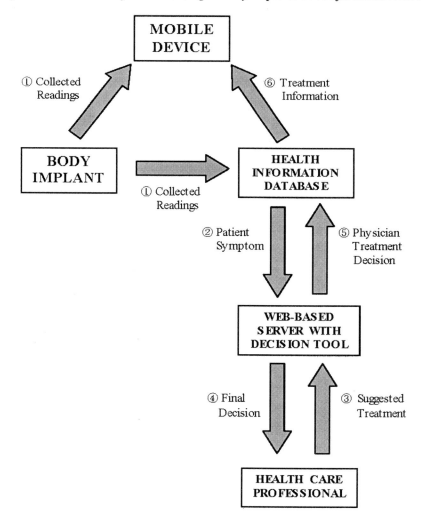

through the mobile device—and provided with appropriate health information and feedback in instances where symptoms do not necessarily require emergency treatment and can be self-managed. Hospitalization rates can in turn also be reduced by optimization of blood pressure symptoms that may lead to the exacerbation of chronic HF (Abraham et al., 2011).

The value of the combined use of these technologies is that the patient can more easily move to a different location or travel without the fear of losing data, and the physician can better assess their condition by monitoring cardiac output during normal daily activities – as opposed to doing so when the patient is bed-ridden or immobile (Tan et al., 2009). Efficiency of monitoring also increases with the use of a mobile device in conjunction with a body monitoring implant such as MEMS by "increasing the amount of data obtained, and streamlining its storage and processing" for faster results (p. 260). Using the example of blood pressure levels, Figure 2 illustrates the efficient use of a Web-based decision support tool in providing accurate diagnosis and treatment. With the combined use of these technologies, and the element of self-care management that it allows, the

task of clinical decision-making now has the potential to extend beyond the sole practitioner, to encompass a medical community of both physicians and patients.

Benefits of an Implant

There are several practical applications for this proposed use of MEMS with a mobile device in the monitoring of HF. Firstly, disease management and care are not compromised for aging patients if they leave the confines of their home. Therefore, they are not restricted to one location and can enjoy a more enhanced social life with family and friends – something that is of particular importance to older adults who are already at greater risk of isolation.

Second, the regular and consistent monitoring of HF symptoms provided by the technology allows patients or caregivers the opportunity to more efficiently manage treatment regimes. Users can be trained to use the health tools provided by the mobile device application that would be designed with a simple and highly usable interface. Of course—as established earlier—usability is always a concern when dealing with technology

Figure 2. Web-based server with decision support system for monitoring blood pressure

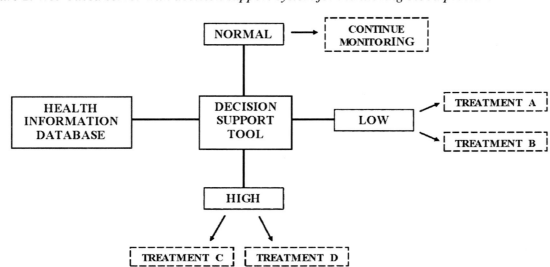

and older adults, but the advent of touch screen devices and large icons with minimalist displays could minimize these limitations. For example, including warning mechanisms for symptoms associated with chronic HF could alert healthcare professionals and patients to the need for more urgent intervention via the emergency department. In less serious instances, patients with blood pressure readings that are either too high or low may also benefit from real-time or immediate adjustment of medication dosages via the mobile device. These elements serve the important goal of alleviating the burden on the health care system by shifting care toward self-management whenever possible.

Another important benefit with this proposed technology concerns medication compliance. One major cause for the worsening of chronic HF in older adults is failing to adhere to medication regimens assigned by a physician. Much of this is due to poor follow up with primary care practitioners, which can result in the worsening of this condition (Schiff et al., 2003). Convenient access to care, self-monitoring and reinforcement are all factors, which have been shown to improve compliance with medication regimes because patients are not required to make multiple visits to their physician for treatment (Haynes et al., 2008). Although further research is needed to explore the extent to which the use of a body implant device with mobile wireless technology would achieve this, it is likely to result in better compliance and in turn, reduced hospitalizations.

Finally, the mobile device also has the potential to facilitate communication with a physician via instant messaging, or make use of videophone technologies that would allow live consultation with a health care professional directly on the screen of the device. Of course, one potential limitation of this is the availability of health care professionals, which may become problematic if the widespread use of this technology involves

long wait times for consultation. Ultimately, the goal is a shift towards self-management, where the physician is not over-burdened with treatment decisions if a case can be efficiently managed remotely by a patient or caregiver using assistive tools and devices.

FUTURE RESEARCH DIRECTIONS

There is little doubt that as the aging population continues to grow, policymakers, managers and patients must adapt to the changing landscape of health care delivery. As has been discussed throughout this chapter, the increased use of information technologies and home telecare services are an important avenue through which to meet the needs of aging patients; while also lessening the reliance on what are becoming more limited resources of the primary health care system. With this drastic transition, there are a number of important considerations and difficulties that will require extensive research and effort going forward. As home telecare efforts expand, policymakers will be faced with the ethical questions that will inevitably arise as medicine is delivered at a distance (Botsis & Hartvigsen, 2008). The line between patient- and physician- managed care becomes blurred as the two can now function in entirely different geographic locations during consultation and treatment. The legal aspects of telemedicine also emerge as an immense concern in the future, particularly where medical malpractice policies and technological malfunction and errors are concerned. Additionally, Botsis and Hartvigsen (2008) discuss that while cost savings to the system may be high with these new technologies, a number of countries are not equipped to provide reliable and consistent methods of reimbursement to patients for the purchase of home telecare equipment. Given that older adults are likely to experience greater levels of poverty than their younger counterparts; proper government assistance programs must also be explored and implemented by policymakers.

In addition to these policy considerations, managers of care must also be mindful of the complexities involved in the testing, research and development of new telecare technologies, each of which is likely to involve a number of different dimensions. In order to properly test and determine the efficacy of adapting a technology such as the MEMS cardiac implant for use with a mobile device, for example, a number of actors would need to be involved. First, as a primary corporate actor, the CardioMEMS company would need to invest in research and development to adapt the MEMS implant for use with a mobile device. Once a prototype version of the device is developed and ready for testing, a willing health care facility or hospital must be selected to test the product, in conjunction with a leading academic research team to conduct the study. Here, a lead physician is needed to manage a clinical trial involving an appropriately selected group of geriatric participants with chronic HF. In the trial phase of the study, a team of experts in information technology would also be required to facilitate and guide the creation, implementation and maintenance of the software tools and health information database to be accessed by patients on the mobile device, as well as by physicians at a distance. Such a process is likely to take time and involve a number of patient safety considerations from both managers and health care providers.

Finally, future research and effort must also be concentrated on the increasing trend of self-care amongst patients and caregivers who are required to take a more prominent role in the delivery of telecare – alongside physicians. User-friendly technology is critical in this endeavour. Patients, along with policymakers and managers will need to adapt to constant changes in the rapidly changing and evolving sphere of information technology and health. In this effort, more comprehensive studies and literature on the efficacy and efficiency of home telecare will be needed as new avenues—including the adaptation of mobile wireless technology in this field—emerge.

CONCLUSION

In this chapter, we have explored the use of home telecare technology as a promising application for enhanced clinical decision-making in geriatric medicine. With the growing aging population, telemedicine is likely to become a very attractive option to increase efficiency in health care management. Throughout this analysis, several challenges arise in the areas of usability, privacy, patient autonomy, self-management and group clinical decision-making. To address some of these concerns, particularly with self-management and usability, we suggest the use of the MEMS cardiac implant in conjunction with a mobile device to assist in more efficient clinical decision-making for physicians, as well as an improved standard of care for patients and caregivers. Ultimately, it seems certain that home telecare is an expanding field that is sure to be met with significant innovation in the coming years. Going forward, despite the immense promise for clinical management that stands to result from the use of these new methods, the inevitable dramatic shift in the way that medicine is delivered must be handled carefully so that patient care remains as a fundamental priority.

REFERENCES

Abraham, W. T., Adamson, P. B., Bourge, R. C., Aaron, M. F., Costanzo, M. R., & Stevenson, L. W. et al. (2011). Wireless pulmonary artery haemodynamic monitoring in chronic heart failure: A randomised control trial. *Lancet, 377*(9766), 658–666. doi:10.1016/S0140-6736(11)60101-3 PMID:21315441.

Abraham, W. T., Adamson, P. B., Hasan, A., Bourge, R. C., Pamboukian, S. V., Aaron, M. F., & Raval, N. Y. (2011). Safety and accuracy of a wireless pulmonary artery pressure monitoring system in patients with heart failure. *American Heart Journal*, *161*(3), 558–566. doi:10.1016/j.ahj.2010.10.041 PMID:21392612.

Allen, A., & March, A. (2002). Telemedicine at the community cancer center. *Oncology Issues*, *17*(1), 18–24.

Bambra, C., Fox, D., & Scott-Samuel, A. (2005). Towards a politics of health. *Health Promotion International*, *20*(2), 187–193. doi:10.1093/heapro/dah608 PMID:15722364.

Borlaug, B. A., Melenovsky, V., Russell, S. D., Kessler, K., Pacak, K., Becker, L. C., & Kass, D. A. (2006). Impaired chronotropic and vasodilator reserves limit exercise capacity in patients with heart failure and a preserved ejection fraction. *Circulation*, *114*(20), 2138–2147. doi:10.1161/CIRCULATIONAHA.106.632745 PMID:17088459.

Botsis, T., Demiris, G., Pedersen, S., & Hartvigsen, G. (2008). Home telecare technologies for the elderly. *Journal of Telemedicine and Telecare*, *14*, 333–337. doi:10.1258/jtt.2008.007002 PMID:18852311.

Botsis, T., & Hartvigsen, G. (2008). Current status and future perspectives in telecare for elderly people suffering from chronic diseases. *Journal of Telemedicine and Telecare*, *14*, 195–203. doi:10.1258/jtt.2008.070905 PMID:18534954.

Cardozo, L., & Steinberg, J. (2010). Telemedicine for recently discharged older patients. *Telemedicine and e-Health*, *16*(1), 49-55.

Celler, B. G., Lovell, N. H., & Basilakis, J. (2003). Using information technology to improve the management of chronic disease. *The Medical Journal of Australia*, *179*(5), 242–246. PMID:12924970.

Clayton, P. D., & Hripcsak, G. (1995). Decision support in healthcare. *International Journal of Bio-Medical Computing*, *39*(1), 59–66. doi:10.1016/0020-7101(94)01080-K PMID:7601543.

Coughlin, J. F., Pope, J. E., & Leedle, B. R. (2006). Old age, new technology, and future innovations in disease management and home health care. *Home Health Care Management & Practice*, *18*(3), 196–207. doi:10.1177/1084822305281955.

Dansky, K. H., Palmer, L., Shea, D., & Bowles, K. H. (2001). Cost analysis of telehomecare. *Telemedicine Journal and e-Health*, *7*(3), 225–232. doi:10.1089/153056201316970920 PMID:11564358.

Dove, N. (2009). Can international medical graduates help solve Canada's shortage of rural physicians? *Canadian Journal of Rural Medicine*, *14*(3), 120–123. PMID:19594998.

Falas, T., Papadopoulos, G., & Stafylopatis, A. (2003). A review of decision support systems in telecare. *Journal of Medical Systems*, *27*(4), 347–356. doi:10.1023/A:1023705320471 PMID:12846466.

Godfrey, C. M., Harrison, M. B., Friedberg, E., Medves, J. M., & Tranmer, J. E. (2007). The symptom of pain in individuals recently hospitalized for heart failure. *The Journal of Cardiovascular Nursing*, *22*(5), 368–374. PMID:17724418.

Haynes, R. B., Ackloo, E., Sahota, N., McDonald, H. P., & Yao, X. (2008). Interventions for enhancing medication adherence [review]. *Cochrane Database of Systematic Reviews*, 2(2), 1–127.

Hébert, M. A., Korabek, B., & Scott, R. E. (2006). Moving research into practice: A decision framework for integrating home telehealth into chronic illness care. *International Journal of Medical Informatics*, 75, 786–794. doi:10.1016/j.ijmedinf.2006.05.041 PMID:16872892.

Hébert, R., Dubios, M., Wolfson, C., Chambers, L., & Cohen, C. (2001). Factors associated with long-term institutionalization of older people with dementia: Data from the Canadian study of health and aging. *Journal of Gerontology*, 56(11), 693–699.

Hersh, W., Helfand, M., Wallace, J., Kraemer, D., Patterson, P., Shapiro, S., & Greenlick, M. (2002). A systematic review of the efficacy of telemedicine for making diagnostic and management decisions. *Journal of Telemedicine and Telecare*, 8, 197–209. doi:10.1258/135763302320272167 PMID:12217102.

Kaufman, D. R., Patel, V. L., Hilliman, C., Morin, P. C., Pevzner, J., Weinstock, R. S., & Starren, J. (2003). Usability in the real world: Assessing medical information technologies in patients' homes. *Journal of Biomedical Informatics*, 36(1-2), 45–60. doi:10.1016/S1532-0464(03)00056-X PMID:14552846.

Kearns, R. A., & Barnett, J. R. (1999). Auckland's starship enterprise: Placing metaphor in a children's hospital. In Williams, A. (Ed.), *Therapeutic landscapes: The dynamic between place and wellness* (pp. 169–200). Lanham, MD: University Press of America Inc..

Klonoff, D. C., & True, M. W. (2009). The missing element of telemedicine for diabetes: Decision support software. *Journal of Diabetes Science and Technology*, 3(5), 996–1001. PMID:20144411.

Koch, S. (2006). Home telehealth–Current state and future trends. *International Journal of Medical Informatics*, 75(8), 565–576. doi:10.1016/j.ijmedinf.2005.09.002 PMID:16298545.

Liu, P., Arnold, M., Belenkie, I., Howlett, J., Huckell, V., & Ignazewski, A. et al. (2001). The 2001 Canadian cardiovascular society consensus guideline update for the management and prevention of heart failure. *The Canadian Journal of Cardiology*, 17(Suppl E), 5E–25E. PMID:11773943.

Magnusson, L., Hanson, E., & Borg, M. (2004). A literature review study of information and communication technology as a support for frail older people living at home and their family carers. *Technology and Disability*, 16(4), 223–235.

Magrabi, F., Lovell, N. H., Huynh, K., & Celler, B. G. (2001). *Home telecare: System architecture to support chronic disease management*. Paper presented at the 23rd Annual International Conference of the IEEE Engineering in Medicine and Biology Society. Istanbul, Turkey.

Milenković, A., Otto, C., & Jovanov, E. (2006). Wireless sensor network for personal health monitoring: Issues and implementation. *Computer Communications*, 29, 2521–2533. doi:10.1016/j.comcom.2006.02.011.

Percival, J., & Hanson, J. (2006). Big brother or brave new world? Telecare and its implications for older people's independence and social inclusion. *Critical Social Policy*, 26(4), 888–909. doi:10.1177/0261018306068480.

Quintero, J., Abraham, M., Aguilera, A., Villegas, H., Montilla, G., & Solaiman, B. (2001, October). *Collaborative medical reasoning in telemedicine.* Paper presented at the 23rd Annual International Conference of the IEEE Engineering in Medicine and Biology Society. Istanbul, Turkey.

Rahimpour, M., Lovell, N. H., Celler, B. G., & McCormick, J. (2008). Patients' perceptions of a home telecare system. *International Journal of Medical Informatics, 77,* 486–498. doi:10.1016/j.ijmedinf.2007.10.006 PMID:18023610.

Raskovic, D., Martin, T., & Jovanov, E. (2004). Medical monitoring applications for wearable computing. *The Computer Journal, 47*(4), 495–504. doi:10.1093/comjnl/47.4.495.

Roback, K., & Herzog, A. (2003). Home informatics in healthcare: Assessment guidelines to keep up quality of care and avoid adverse effects. *Technology and Health Care, 11,* 195–206. PMID:12775936.

Schiff, G. D., Fung, S., Speroff, T., & McNutt, R. A. (2003). Decompensated heart failure: Symptoms, patterns of onset, and contributing factors. *The American Journal of Medicine, 114*(8), 625–630. doi:10.1016/S0002-9343(03)00132-3 PMID:12798449.

Tan, R., McClure, T., Lin, C. K., Jea, D., Dabiri, F., & Massey, T. et al. (2009). Development of a fully implantable wireless pressure monitoring system. *Biomedical Microdevices, 11,* 259–264. doi:10.1007/s10544-008-9232-1 PMID:18836836.

Thornett, A. M. (2001). Computer decision support systems in general practice. *International Journal of Information Management, 21,* 39–47. doi:10.1016/S0268-4012(00)00049-9.

Vitacca, M., Assoni, G., Pizzocaro, P., Guerra, A., Marchina, L., & Scalvini, S. et al. (2006). A pilot study of nurse-led, home monitoring for patients with chronic respiratory failure and with mechanical ventilation assistance. *Journal of Telemedicine and Telecare, 12*(7), 337–342. doi:10.1258/135763306778682404 PMID:17059649.

World Health Organization. (2006). *Active aging – A policy framework.* Retrieved September 3, 2012, from http://whqlibdoc.who.int/hq/2002/who_nmh_nph_02.8.pdf

Zhen, B., Li, H., & Kohno, R. (2009). Networking issues in medical implant communications. *International Journal of Multimedia and Ubiquitous Engineering, 4*(1), 23–37.

ADDITIONAL READING

Amala, L., Turner, T., Gretton, M., Baksh, A., & Cleland, J. (2003). A systemic review of telemonitoring for the management of heart failure. *European Journal of Heart Failure, 5*(5), 583–590. doi:10.1016/S1388-9842(03)00160-0 PMID:14607195.

Audebert, H. J., Boy, S., Jankovits, R., Pilz, P., Klucken, J., Fehm, N. P., & Schenkel, J. (2008). Is mobile teleconsulting equivalent to hospital-based telestroke services? *Stroke, 39*(12), 3427–3430. doi:10.1161/STROKEAHA.108.520478 PMID:18787198.

Barlow, J., Bayer, S., Curry, R., Hendy, J., & McMahon, L. (2010). From care closer to home to care in the home: The potential impact of telecare on the healthcare built environment. In Kagioglou, M., & Tzortzopoulos, P. (Eds.), *Improving healthcare through built environment infrastructure* (pp. 131–150). Malden, MA: Blackwell Publishing Ltd. doi:10.1002/9781444319675.ch9.

Barlow, J., Singh, D., Bayer, S., & Curry, R. (2007). A systemic review of the benefits of home telecare for frail elderly people and those with long-term conditions. *Journal of Telemedicine and Telecare, 13*(4), 172–179. doi:10.1258/135763307780908058 PMID:17565772.

Bates, D. W., & Bitton, A. (2010). The future of health information technology in the patient-centered medical home. *Health Affairs, 29*(4), 614–621. doi:10.1377/hlthaff.2010.0007 PMID:20368590.

Bellazzi, R., Montani, S., Riva, A., & Stefanelli, M. (2001). Web-based telemedicine systems for home-care: Technical issues and experiences. *Computer Methods and Programs in Biomedicine, 64*(3), 175–187. doi:10.1016/S0169-2607(00)00137-1 PMID:11226615.

Bertera, E. M., Tran, B. Q., Wuertz, E. M., & Bonner, A. (2007). A study of the receptivity to telecare technology in a community-based elderly minority population. *Journal of Telemedicine and Telecare, 13*(7), 327–332. doi:10.1258/135763307782215325 PMID:17958932.

Cartwright, L. (2000). Reach out and heal someone: Telemedicine and the globalization of health care. *Health, 4*(3), 347–377.

Coleman, E. A. (2003). Falling through the cracks: Challenges and opportunities for improving transitional care for persons with continuous complex care needs. *Journal of the American Geriatrics Society, 51*(4), 549–555. doi:10.1046/j.1532-5415.2003.51185.x PMID:12657078.

Freedman, V. A., & Martin, L. G. (1998). Understanding trends in function among older Americans. *American Journal of Public Health, 88*(10), 1457–1462. doi:10.2105/AJPH.88.10.1457 PMID:9772844.

Hersh, W. R., Hickam, D. H., Severance, S. M., Dana, T. L., Krages, K. P., & Helfand, M. (2006). Diagnosis, access and outcomes: Update of a systematic review of telemedicine services. *Journal of Telemedicine and Telecare, 12*(Suppl. 2), 3–31. doi:10.1258/135763306778393117 PMID:16884561.

Jerant, A. F., Azari, R., & Nesbitt, T. S. (2001). Reducing the costs of frequent hospital admissions for congestive heart failure: A randomized trial of a home telecare intervention. *Medical Care, 39*(11), 1234–1245. doi:10.1097/00005650-200111000-00010 PMID:11606877.

Koch, S. (2006). Meeting the challenges – The role of medical informatics in an ageing society. *Studies in Health Technology and Informatics, 124*, 25–31. PMID:17108500.

Koch, S., & Hägglund, M. (2009). Health informatics and the delivery of care to older people. *Maturitas, 63*(3), 195–199. doi:10.1016/j.maturitas.2009.03.023 PMID:19487092.

Lehoux, P., Sicotte, C., Denis, J., Berg, M., & Lacroix, A. (2002). The theory of use behind telemedicine: How compatible with physicians' clinical routines? *Social Science & Medicine, 54*(6), 889–904. doi:10.1016/S0277-9536(01)00063-6 PMID:11996023.

Liddy, C., Dusseault, J. J., Dahrouge, S., Hogg, W., Lemelin, J., & Humber, J. (2008). Telehomecare for patients with multiple chronic illnesses. *Canadian Family Physician Medecin de Famille Canadien, 54*(1), 58–65. PMID:18208957.

Mann, W. C., Marchant, T., Tomita, M., Fraas, L., & Stanton, K. (2002). Elder acceptance of health monitoring devices in the home. *Care Management Journals, 3*(2), 91–98. PMID:12455220.

McColl, M. A., Jarzynowska, A., & Shortt, S. E. D. (2010). Unmet health care needs of people with disabilities: Population level evidence. *Disability & Society, 25*(2), 205–218. doi:10.1080/09687590903537406.

Meredith, S., Feldman, P. H., Frey, D., Hall, K., Arnold, K., Brown, N. J., & Ray, W. A. (2001). Possible medication errors in home healthcare patients. *Journal of the American Geriatrics Society, 49*(6), 719–724. doi:10.1046/j.1532-5415.2001.49147.x PMID:11454109.

Nebeker, J. R., Hurdle, J. F., & Bair, B. D. (2003). Future history: Medical informatics in geriatrics. *Journal of Gerontology, 58*(9), 820–825.

Rialle, V., Duchêne, F., Noury, N., Bajolle, L., Demongeot, J. Health 'smart' home: Information technology for patients at home. *Telemedicine and e-Health, 8*(4), 395-409.

Rialle, V., Lamy, J., Noury, N., & Bajolle, L. (2003). Telemonitoring of patients at home: A software agent approach. *Computer Methods and Programs in Biomedicine, 72*(3), 257–268. doi:10.1016/S0169-2607(02)00161-X PMID:14554139.

Vitacca, M., Scalvini, S., Spanevello, A., & Balbi, B. (2006). Telemedicine and home care: Controversies and opportunities. *Breathe, 3*(2), 149–158.

Wyatt, S., Henwood, F., Hart, A., & Platzer, H. (2004). Extending patient's world: The internet, health information and everyday life. *Sciences Sociales et Sante, 22*(1), 45–68. doi:10.3406/sosan.2004.1608.

Xiao, Y., & Chen, H. (2008). *Mobile telemedicine: A computing and networking perspective.* Boca Raton, FL: Auerbach Publications.

KEY TERMS AND DEFINITIONS

Decision Support System: An electronic system that stores data and assists in decision making. In a clinical context, it can be used to store detailed patient data and vital statistics that can then be accessed and used by clinicians to assist in treatment decisions.

Home Telecare: A subspecialty within the larger field of telemedicine that involves clinical monitoring and the collection of patient data—with the use of information technologies—in a private home.

Medical Implant Device: A device placed under the skin that both records and transmits data to a sensor or other device located outside of the body.

Mobile Device: A handheld device with a display screen that can be used as a communicative tool to convey information to a user.

Self-Management: In clinical practice, a process by which a patient takes responsibility in managing their own care.

Telemedicine: Medicine performed at a distance using telecommunications technology. This branch of medicine allows for the exchange of clinical information and provision of care by physicians and other medical professionals from a remote location.

Usability: The extent to which a technology is user friendly and accessible to a patient who may lack technological expertise.

Chapter 14
How Web 2.0 Shapes Patient Knowledge Sharing:
The Case of Diabetes in Italy

Chiara Libreri
Università Cattolica del Sacro Cuore, Italy

Guendalina Graffigna
Università Cattolica del Sacro Cuore, Italy

ABSTRACT

Web 2.0 has totally changed the health communication world. In particular, it has reconfigured peer exchanges about health. These exchanges are important because they allow knowledge sharing and construction between patients, in particular chronic patients. Although their importance is well established, this field of study brings together a variety of theories not uniformly shared or understood. It is not clear how patients use Web for knowledge processes: what kind of knowledge processes happen in Web 2.0 between patients? How does Web 2.0 sustain or impede these processes? The aim of this research is to map virtual exchanges about diabetes in Italy by developing a systematic exploration of Web using the main search engines (Google, Yahoo) and analyzing the site that hosts posts and exchanges about diabetes. According to a psychosocial perspective, findings highlight the main features of online knowledge processes among patients.

INTRODUCTION

The Internet, and in particular Web 2.0, has totally changed the healthcare prevention and communication world. According to Turner et al. (2011), the Web 2.0 is "the transition of use of the Internet from primarily information receiving to information generating [...] Web 2.0 tools are seen

by some as a revolutionary leap in the ability to manage, remix, and transform health information" (p. 103). Indeed, the advent of Web 2.0 has offered even more potential than the Internet alone by particularly encouraging participation. Using Web 2.0, we consider all the sites that allow people to interact with each other to the Website's content, in contrast to Websites where people are limited to just read the information that is provided to them. Tim O'Reily defines Web 2.0 activities, such

DOI: 10.4018/978-1-4666-4321-5.ch014

as based on "participation architecture" (Grivet Foiaia, 2007). This means that Web 2.0 and its applications structure is constructed to promote cooperation and sharing between participants (Norris, Mason, & Lefrere, 2003).

In practice, the use of Web 2.0 dramatically increased in the last ten year in the Western society (the 78,6% of the USA population and the 61.3% of the European one use the Internet[1]). More than the half of the Internet users[2] has employed this technology to search for health information. Moreover, people who suffer from chronic conditions use the Internet significantly more than healthy people (Siliquini et al., 2011).

As a matter of fact, patients are becoming increasingly independent in the process of information-seeking and decision-making about their self-care (de Boer, Versteegen, & van Wijhe, 2007). So, thanks to Web 2.0, not only searching for information but also participation in online peer exchanges is more and more a growing phenomenon, also for topic that concerns to health and in particular chronic disease issues (Nambisan, & Nambisan, 2009).

In literature, it is well established the role that offline peer exchanges and peer support groups have on the management of chronic diseases, such as diabetes, cancer or cardiac diseases (McPherson, Jospeh, & Sullivan, 2004); scholars more and more agree on the importance of online peer exchanges between patients (Ancker et al., 2009) who face with a daily and active care&cure management, and/or between family caregivers (such as parents or children): they use the online exchanges to get informed about their condition (Nettleton, Burrows, & O'Malley, 2005), to seek support from other patients (Bar-Lev, 2008) and to share experiences, opinions and knowledge about care management (Graffigna, Libreri, & Bosio, 2012).

This is even more evident as far as chronic conditions are concerned: in this case the engagement of patients (Barello, Graffigna, & Vegni, 2012) in

their daily management of care and cure, as well as their psychological endurance and ability to cope with the disease may benefit from support received in the online exchange with peers (Mo, & Coulson, 2010).

Even if the importance of this phenomenon and the great interest toward it in literature:

- It's not clear how chronic patients share and construct their knowledge online (O'Grady, Witteman, & Wathen, 2008); in particular, which conditions favor or hinder the activation of "good" processes of knowledge sharing and construction among patients are still a matter for debate.
- Even more confuse is the role of the medium (and its different formats) in shaping the processes of peer exchanges and the kind of achieved knowledge outputs.

On the basis of these premises, in this chapter, starting from the discussion of pragmatic and psychological relevance of patients knowledge sharing and moving through the theoretical positions toward the knowledge sharing and construction processes in the online context, we will outline the role of Web 2.0 and of its different formats (i.e. blogs, forum, social networks...) in shaping the processes and their outcomes. In order to empirically support our arguments, we will discuss the results achieved by an exploratory study of the online exchanges which take place among diabetic patients in Italy.

BACKGROUND

To examine online exchanges and knowledge processes requires the use of different theoretical points of view (often external to the health field) within a quickly expanding literature and within the increasingly complex and continuous evolvement of the Web.

A Taxonomy of Online Knowledge Processes

As already said, there is a lack of literature regarding online knowledge sharing processes between patients.

Concepts like "knowledge sharing" and "knowledge construction" do not have a shared definition and they are labeled in several different ways. The overlapping among the definitions (e.g., knowledge dissemination, knowledge translation, knowledge sharing, knowledge building, knowledge creation, knowledge mobilization) is not clear and the specific role of Web 2.0 (and its formats) in shaping these processes is even less define (see Table 1).

The following taxonomy (Table 1) clarifies the panorama of the online knowledge processes (because of the variety of definition in considering knowledge sharing and construction processes, from now we refer to them using the term knowledge processes); starting from a literature review of contributes regarding knowledge processes in the online context, the Table 1 shows the main labels attributed to the online knowledge processes, giving a definition and stating the reference field and the main actors of each process.

The definitions proposed are examples that maximize the differences between processes. In fact, shared definitions do not exist and the different labels are often used as synonymous.

The variety of definitions reported in Table 1 claims for some reflections.

Firstly, even if all the labels and definitions derive from contributes referring to online group or peer conditions, some of them refers to processes and activities that happen neither in the online context nor in a peer group, but they consider individual processes of elaboration of knowledge (such as knowledge absorption).

Moreover, the presented concepts refer to three disciplinary areas: health, Internet and communication, learning processes (in education and in organization). The traditional interest of health field to knowledge processes is focused on the comprehension and improvement of the passage of knowledge from the scientific and medical world to the lay world. Health research always tries to find solutions to improve people's health and life but often the research results don't reach interested people and health decision makers. Web is a way to connect health world with lay people, showing them what they can do in order to solve their problem (Curran-Smith, Abidi, & Forgeron, 2005). Instead, the Internet and communication studies' approach refers to peer exchanges. In this perspective it is really important to underline how, thanks to Web 2.0, the knowledge is more and more constructed and owned by lay or common people (Baez et al, 2010). According to this perspective there is not interest about how the knowledge is constructed and produced; the focus is the possibility to disseminate knowledge to the larger number of people as possible in order to give more power to more people (Wei & Yan, 2010). Finally, the learning studies focus on how people acquire and construct knowledge. Considering the taxonomy above, we are interested in those approaches who consider learning as a processes happening in a group of peers and aimed to give to them useful knowledge. In this way the concepts knowledge building, knowledge construction, knowledge creation and knowledge sharing can be considered as appropriate to label the processes we are interested in.

Moreover, even if it was possible to define the processes we are interested into, some points need to be deepen:

- Firstly, this variety of labels and concepts is symptom of a major focus on the outcomes of these knowledge processes and not on their process of development.
- Secondly, dimensions that configure, support or impede or shape the knowledge processes are unclear.
- Finally, even if all these definitions refer to the online context, this dimension is not re-

Table 1. Knowledge processes taxonomy

Label	Main Field of Study	Actors and Relations	Definition
Knowledge absorption	Learning	Individual	"Mechanisms used by scholars to absorb and apply knowledge such as pursuing an academic degree, attending online courses, doing tests in labs, applying knowledge in new settings, and so forth. Absorption refers to using the knowledge acquired; it does not mean to create new." (Echeverri, & Abels, 2008, p. 149)
Knowledge acquisition	Learning	Individual	"Brings to mind the activity of accumulating material goods. The language of 'knowledge acquisition' and 'concept development' makes us think about the human mind as a container to be filled with certain materials and about the learner as becoming an owner of these materials. (Hamilton et al., 2004, p. 848)
Knowledge building	Learning	Peers (mainly students) with a moderator or a facilitator	"Collaborative knowledge building defines a useful paradigm for conceptualizing learning as social practice in which shared knowledge is constructed [...] as the result of inter- related group and personal perspectives." (Ang et al., 2011, p. 539)
Knowledge collaboration	Internet studies	Peer	"Knowledge collaboration is defined as the sharing, transfer, recombination, and reuse of knowledge among parties. Collaboration is a process that allows parties to leverage their differences in interests, concerns, and knowledge. Knowledge collaboration online refers to the use of the Internet (or Intranet) to facilitate the collaboration." (Jarvenpaa & Majchrzak, 2010, p. 774)
Knowledge construction	Learning	Peers (mainly students) (with a moderator or a facilitator)	"Knowledge construction [...] is based on the assumption that individuals engage in specific discourse activities and that these discourse activities are related to the sharing and negotiation of knowledge" (Hew & Cheung, 2010, p. 304)
Knowledge creation	Learning, organization and management	Peer, mainly: work groups, companies, organizations, (van Aalst, 2009)	"Knowledge creation refers to developing new content or replacing existing content; the above activities are performed through the conversion between two types of knowledge – tacit and explicit knowledge [...] knowledge creation involves the conversion from existing knowledge to new knowledge" (Chou et al., 2010, p. 557)
Information/ Knowledge diffusion	Internet studies	Peer	"When information diffusion in the blog world is analyzed, the information diffusion paths can be found. In social network theory, information diffusion in the social network is said to occur through the established relations between members" (Kwon, Kim, & Park, 2009, p. 28)
Knowledge dissemination	Internet studies	Peer	"Mechanisms used by scholars, libraries, and publishers to communicate the new knowledge created such as posting documents on the Web, publishing articles in a journal, publishing new books, and so forth. Dissemination implies to make new knowledge accessible to other people so they can acquire it to begin again the cycle and doing that, to move forward the topic under consideration." (Echeverri, & Abels, 2008, p. 149)
Knowledge mobilization	Health and political communication	Expert and lay people	"Mobilization theories highlight how the Internet can facilitate activities with a political purpose, or how the Internet forms a 'political playground' where people can exercise civic skills and obtain the knowledge deemed important for political participation" (Hirzalla, van Zoonen, & de Ridder, 2011, p. 2)
Knowledge production	Communication and political studies	Peer	"The production of knowledge is no longer controlled by social elites thanks to the diffusion of the Internet. Web 2.0 applications, which not only allow but encourage individuals' production and sharing of their own information, break the bureaucratic monopoly of knowledge." (Wei & Yan, 2010, p. 239)

continued on following page

Table 1. Continued

Label	Main Field of Study	Actors and Relations	Definition
Knowledge sharing	Learning and organizational	Peers that usually share the same role (all students, all colleagues…)	"Knowledge sharing refers to the transmission of knowledge between people" (Van Aalst, 2009, p. 260) "Knowledge sharing is the process where individuals mutually exchange their (implicit and explicit) knowledge and jointly create new knowledge" (van den Hoof et al., 2003, p. 121)
Knowledge transfer	Health (mainly health communication and promotion)	Expert to lay people and decision makers	"Knowledge transfer can be defined as the activity of transforming knowledge into a format which can be used to improve clinical practice and service delivery" (Wilkinson et al., 2009, p. 118)
Knowledge translation	Health (mainly health communication and promotion)	Expert and lay people	"Knowledge translation is the synthesis, exchange, and application of knowledge by relevant stakeholders to accelerate the benefits of global and local innovation in strengthening health systems and improving people's health" (Arnold et al., 2007, p. 1047)

ally considered: A better consideration on the role played by Internet (in its different format and applications) in shaping knowledge processes is needed.

According to this perspective, it will be necessary to understand the conditions (subjective, interactive and contextual) which may foster or hinder the different knowledge processes. In particular is unclear the role of the medium in shaping these processes.

Web 2.0 in the Health Field

As we already said, Web 2.0 helps patients to become really protagonists of their care management throughout the possibility to participate in sharing and construction of knowledge about their illness, their care (Nambisan & Nambisan, 2009) and their identity (Miles, 2009).

The shared aim of Web 2.0 is to favor participation and collaboration between users, facilitating production of culture and knowledge (Bakardjieva, 2003). However, Web 2.0 is very heterogenic in terms of different applications, such as blogs, forums, wikis, podcast, social networks and all the emergent social medias that have both technical and social aspects (others define them hard and soft features) (Grivet Foiaia, 2007). The features

and specificities of each Web 2.0 application are very well defined (Korica, Maurer, & Schinagl, 2006) and are consistently updated (Holt, 2011).

Table 2 defines main types of Web 2.0 applications.

As mentioned above, the role that these different applications may have in configuring patients online exchanges and knowledge processes hasn't been deepened.

Indeed, literature regarding online patient exchanges and knowledge processes substantially considers exchanges happening on different platforms as the same phenomenon: "online environments in which users interact with one another around a set of common interests or shared purpose related to health using a variety of tools including discussion boards, chat, virtual environments, and direct messaging" (Newman et al., 2011, p. 342); focuses of interest of literature about this topic are: contents of the online patients exchanges (e.g., Greene et al., 2010), motivation to participate into them (e.g., Blank & Adam-Blodnieks, 2007), perceived benefits and outcomes of the participation (e.g., Mo, & Coulson, 2010). Less attention is given to the exchange processes themselves and to the role of the Web into define these processes.

The situation in the knowledge processes field is almost the same. Practically, in this field there is more interested into the comprehension of the

Table 2. Main web 2.0 applications

Label	Definition	Types
Blog	"The term Web-log, or blog, refers to a simple Webpage consisting of brief paragraphs of opinion, information, personal diary entries, or links, called posts, arranged chronologically with the most recent first" (Anderson; 2007 p. 7)	• Personal blog (one authors) • Collaborative blog (many authors)
Forum	"Online forums provide a virtual environment to conduct discussion between a defined group" (Burr, & Dawson, 2003)	• Forum • Bullettin boards
Wiki	"Wikis in general are self-organising Web-sites, where anyone on the Internet can edit existing pages and add new documents any time they wish. This means that every reader can instantly become an author." (Kolbisch & Maurer,2006, p. 191)	
Social networking	"We define social network sites as Web-based services that allow individuals to (1) construct a public or semi-public profile within a bounded system, (2) articulate a list of other users with whom they share a connection, and (3) view and traverse their list of connections and those made by others within the system" (boyd & Ellison; 2008 p. 211)	• Social network sites • File sharing sites

functioning of knowledge processes - such as knowledge sharing and construction (e.g., Zenios, 2011) – than in the health field, but these processes are studied especially by using forums and discussion boards (e.g., Nor, Razak, & Aziz, 2010) (considering them as representative for all the Web applications) and no attention is given to the medium of exchange.

The Literature Gap

Because of this, it is fundamental to study how Web 2.0 applications and their usage affect the construction of different knowledge processes. Practically, it is not clear:

- If and how Web 2.0 activate knowledge processes and what are the basic conditions for the development of knowledge sharing processes.
- If and how different Web 2.0 applications support different type of knowledge processes.

In the following section, we will present a research work aimed to clear this question.

THE RESEARCH

The Case

According to these assumptions, we present a research case focused on the online peer exchanges between diabetic patients in Italy.

As we said in the "Introduction," online peer exchanges may be really relevant in the care and management of chronic conditions. In this frame, across chronic disease, diabetes appears a paradigmatic in case. Diabetes involves everyday behavior and daily management of care (Kneck, Klang, & Fagerberg, 2011). This means that diabetic patients have to be active and attentive in their daily care (MacPherson, Joseph, & Sullivan, 2004), and knowledge and experiences sharing taking place offline (Joseph, Griffin, Hall, & Sullivan, 2001) and more and more online are a crucial source of pragmatic and psychological support for their illness management (Greene et al., 2010).

Moreover, the research was developed in the Italian context. According to the number of Internet users, Italy is ranked 32nd in Europe. Despite that, the number of Internet users in the last ten years is more than duplicated (from 22.8% of the total population in 2000 to 51.7% in the 2010)[3]. For these characteristics, it seems a good context in which to understand the online peer exchanges in health: it's a really relevant phenomenon, but there is enough possibility to address these exchanges to make them more supportive of good knowledge sharing processes for patients.

Aims

The main aim of this research is to provide an overview of the online exchanges between diabetic patients, understanding what kind of knowledge processes they activate and defining what are the basic conditions for the development of knowledge sharing processes.

Practically, since a shared definition of online knowledge processes, their features and their boundaries do not exist in the literature, this research will propose a map of online exchange contexts, considering how and if different online contexts may shape different knowledge processes.

In practice this inquiry wants to comprehend how different Web 2.0 applications shape knowledge processes, considering:

1. What are the conditions of Web 2.0 contexts that define different online peer exchanges and knowledge processes (focus on different Web tools and their features)?
2. Who are the different actors involved in them?
3. What the contents dealt in the exchanges?

Method

The presented work is an exploratory research to empirically study online exchanges and online knowledge processes. An ethnographic perspective (Mayan, 2009) is the best method to reach our aim as it allows us to explore the online world by assuming the Internet users' perspective.

The first step was the search and the identification of the Web contexts in which sharing,

participation and discussion about diabetes were possible. A sample of Web 2.0 sites (defining them as sites where people could interact about something), were found using the Google, Yahoo, Google discussions, Google Blog, and Facebook search engines, with the key word: "Diabetes." We chose Google and Yahoo because they are the most used search engines in Italy. Google Blog and Google discussions were added to pay as much as possible attention on Web 2.0 sites. Additionally, we included Facebook as it is the main social network in Italy.

Our search included only Italian sites: keyword is the Italian word for Diabetes [diabete] and we used Italian version of the search engines (e.g., Google.it).

The search was performed from February to September 2011.

Then the first 100 references for each search engine (excluding Facebook search that had less references) were analyzed to yield 344 references (in some cases, we found the same references in more than one search engine).

Then, according to the aims of this work, we developed three main steps of analysis:

1. The first step of analysis regarded the features of the online exchange context. To analyze the data we developed a grid, in part developed by theory (e.g. trust toward the site derived from Orizio et al., 2010) and in part, inductively developed from the initial analysis. The grid had the following sections:
   a. Web 2.0 applications and their features description (e.g., exchange activities allowed, site topic/s, number of visiting people).
   b. Trust indexes towards the site (e.g., affiliation, logo and copyright presence, contacts availability).
   c. Information toward other participants (e.g., enrollment, profile, shared interests).

The analysis was organized using ATLAS. Ti software.

2. Secondly, we analyzed the exchanges. Also for this step we developed a grid focused on:

    a. Exchange descriptions (e.g., lasting how long, number of posts, number of participants, exchange mean).
    b. Participants in the exchanges (e.g., patients, caregivers, experts, admin or moderator);
    c. Exchange aims (e.g., information, support, sharing).

As for the first step, the analysis was organized using ATLAS.Ti software

This analysis helped us in drafting a conceptual map for summarizing and visualizing the main characteristics and differences of each context.

3. Finally, content textual analysis was provided using T-Lab software. Contents of post and discussion were analyzed, according to the main following variables:

    a. Web applications in which the contents were written.
    b. Actors who wrote the contents[4].

Results

Of the 344 references found, we considered 156 Web 2.0 sites about diabetes.

We chose to exclude 84 sites that did not allow any type of exchanges (e.g. to post a comment, to share posts or discussions, to link content to/ from other sites); 79 sites where exchanges about diabetes happened before the chosen period; 20 sites that were off topic (e.g. animal diabetes,) and 5 sites that were not in Italian. Table 3 shows the typology of Web 2.0 applications found.

Table 3. Types of web 2.0 applications (frequencies and percentage)

	N	%
Blogs	77	51
Personal blogs	14	9
Forums	40	25
Chats	1	0,5
Social networks: pages	12	8
Social Networks: groups	8	4
Q&A sites	4	2,5
TOTAL	**156**	**100**

Blogs, forums and social networks seem to be the most used contexts to post something about diabetes; anyway, many different Web applications deal with diabetes.

These data make evident the consistent presence of online peer exchanges about diabetes and the variety of online supports which make them possible. However, at a closer analysis it appears clear that these different channels influence in a specific way not only the contents of online peer exchanges, but also their goals of knowledge and the activated processes.

The qualitative analysis, supported by ATLAS. ti, of the Web sites permitted to define a conceptual descriptive map of the online peer exchanges (see Figure 1).

This map is based on two main axes:

1. **Legitimation of Knowledge:** This axis describes the "model" of knowledge legitimization (i.e. the reliability and credibility of the posts and exchanges contents) in the online exchange. On the negative pole are described the exchanges where there is a "top down" legitimization of the exchange contents and directions, throughout the role of an institutional expert (for example: a health professional, the blog manager...) perceived

Figure 1. Web 2.0 exchanges map

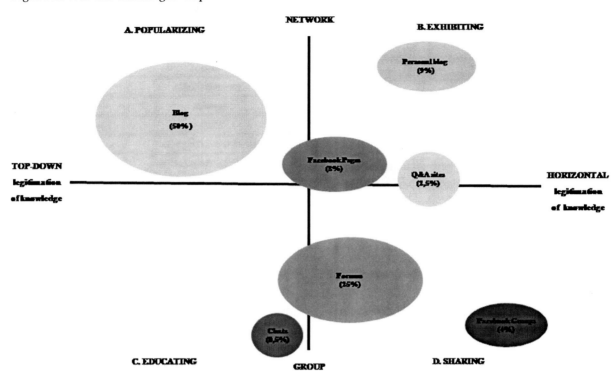

as a grantor. On the other side, the credibility and usefulness of information shared are guaranteed in a "horizontal" way, by people who participate in the online exchanges themselves. In this "model of legitimization", thus, there is no an institutional expert who can guarantee for the contents produced, but contents are legitimated because people who produce them experienced the problem and its solutions.

2. **Relational Aim:** The vertical axis describes the type of linkage sought by patients taking part in the exchange. On the positive pole are positioned all the Websites where patients aim is spreading information within the biggest network of people as possible. In practice, the kind of exchange achieved in these Websites is limited to the posting of news/information and to their forwarding within their reference networks, without adding other comments or knowledge. The other

pole is characterized by Website frequented by patients who seek affiliation and feeling of group belonging. In this case the exchange is animated by, people asking for and sharing opinion, information experiences, within that particular group.

According to the presented map, it is possible to define four main clusters that characterize different type of exchanges and knowledge processes that those exchanges support. The Web applications easily fit into these clusters:

1. **Popularizing:** The aim of exchanges in these sites is to spread information toward the Web, reaching the main number of interested people. The blogs are the main characters of this area. Indeed, blogs are used to share and disseminate information and in particular, news. People do not use blogs to discuss (only 8 blogs presented dis-

cussions after the first post). It makes sense then, that in some blogs (17) people cannot discuss about the news or the topic posted, but they can only share with their reference network. Practically, in this area exchanges are mainly based on RSS and social bookmarking, namely the possibility to share what the person is reading with his/her reference networks (Facebook friends, Google or email contacts, readers of his/her own blog). The aim of participants to these contexts is to spread a content they found interesting, without add anything more. The few discussions retrievable in these Websites are limited to the publication of links to other Websites. For example, it is interesting to note that exactly the same news/information (using exactly the same wording) is posted on many different blogs since those who post do not share personal ideas, but just something they think is interesting or may be useful for their networks. People trust into the expertise and credibility of the ones that manage the blog. Blogs are furnished by many classic trust indexes like logos, copyrights, and contact information. They are mainly managed by Web communication agencies or by experts (e.g., physicians, nurses, nutritionists) that likely need to build trust with people. Many blogs don't require enrollment to post; you can just put your name and e-mail address in order to comment. Only 10 blogs required enrollment to post. Just one blog (autoblog) presented how many people are enrolled and some blogs (19 sites) show how many people have visited the site (this kind of indexes is important for the group construction).

2. **Exhibiting:** In this area someone or some groups (such as an association) are interested into show information about themselves. This area is mainly covered by social network pages and personal blogs. They are really similar to blogs; one person or group or organization post something about diabetes but there are few interactions. The difference is in the topic. The news doesn't deal some aspects of the disease, but they refer to: a person (personal blog) or news about projects, associations or organizations to inform/update people that are interested/involved in this project. Substantially they seem display windows: people and organizations use them to show their activities and their interest to the world. For example: the BCD (Buon Compenso Diabete) Facebook page is about a temporary project for diabetes care. The Fondazione Italian Diabete Facebook page is mainly a place where people (e.g., administration, other associations, patients) share information about for example books, conferences, and scientific papers.

3. **Educating:** This is the "realm" of health experts. This area is covered by few forums and less blogs in which recognized expert (such as practitioners, nutritionists, psychologists) discuss with people, addressing them towards diagnosis and cure. It's important to underline that when the expert participates in the discussion, the exchange become dyadic and polarized (i.e. expert – patient) and the peer exchange tends to be inhibited.

4. **Sharing:** In this area, the aim is to discuss and to share opinions, experiences, emotions and knowledge with other people recognized as qualified (for example for their experience as patients) to say something about the topic. This area is mainly covered by forums and Facebook groups. Here it is possible to track a greater variety of exchange activities: not only related to posting experiences and comments, but also to the possibility to express appreciation for other participants' messages (many forums have tools to express that people like others' comments or to thank or to quote other people's words). Exchanges are not only a series of comments but often a person posts something, a second person responds (quoting the first person's words),

and the first person provides yet another answer. In fact, in blog discussions the number of posts and the number of participants are the same. In forums, there are almost always less participants than posts. This means that participants are involved into the exchange and in the output that this exchange will eventually provide and not only into state their opinion. Moreover, in the forums, people trust toward other participants; there are a lot of indicators that give people information about other participants from which they can evaluate their trustworthiness. For example, in all forums, enrollment is mandatory for participation and in 7 forums, we found enrollment was required to even read the discussion. Other common indicators of trust toward other participants in forum are: the possibility to see each other's profiles (26 sites), a sharing of similar interests (e.g., swimming) (33 sites) and recalling prior conversations/discussions where the person participated (6 sites). Facebook groups are really similar to the forums. People share information and experiences and try to support others. A great example is "Mamme e diabete" where caregivers (mothers) participate in the discussion in order to improve their children care and to support each others. The legitimation of knowledge works similar to forums. People have to be enrolled in Facebook and also in all the specific pages or groups. Further, people have to be accepted to post on these pages or groups. Some groups are closed, so people have to send a request in order to read the posts. As a matter of fact, Facebook groups present more discussions than forums. A first impressive explanation may be based on the fact that Facebook groups exist in a big social network where participants are not connected only to the group on diabetes

but to people who are part of their offline life and to other group they are involved in. Participants do not have to "go" on the diabetes group, but the group is "where they live."

After, the qualitative analysis of sites and their features, we analyzed the content dealt in the posts and discussion on diabetes by using T-lab software. According to this analysis is possible to show the main relevant—in terms of frequency—contents (see Figure 2) and to articulate them according to the Web 2.0 application engaged in the discussion style described in Figure 1.

It seems possible to articulate the contents about diabetes covered by online exchanges on a continuum that opposites a "private" to a "public" sphere of meanings and experiences.

The public sphere (especially linked to blogs) is mainly linked to: 1) scientific contents, such as new research or innovation in diabetes care (e.g., "Association between diabetes type 1 and enterovirus") and 2) general posts referring: facts, connected to diabetes, happened in the real world (e.g., "The spot above, commissioned by FID, Italian Diabetes Foundation, and realized by Armando Testa advertising agency, opens a big discussions between diabetes associations"[5]); exchanges to giving/receiving information about diabetes in general, mainly in Q&A sites ("What is the difference between diabetes 1 and diabetes 2?"); and the diabetes association and group activities, mainly in social networks pages ("This is a picture of some of our friends who joint us this week end in Garibaldi square").

There is instead a private sphere of diabetes concerning mainly: the daily management of diabetes and all the topic related (devices, food…) ("try to control in the wizard bolus settings what values the device has and maybe you can high them up, or check how much activity time you set for your insulin… now I don't have any other

Figure 2. Content maps (from T-lab output)

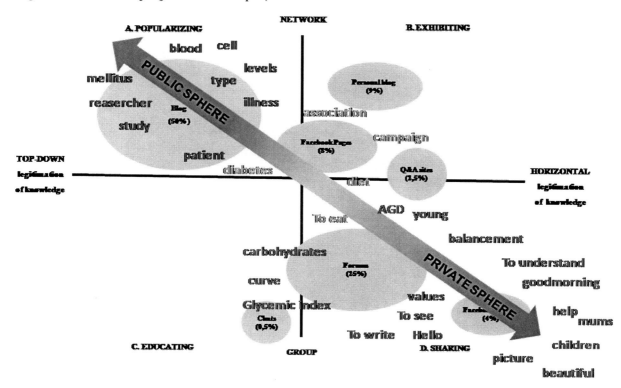

idea....") and the emotional and social support ("To talk here is different.... We totally understand each other . . . without seeing us . . . . . !! ! ! ! ;)").

Finally, it is possible to show on our map the types of participants (see Figure 3). In practice, different actors activate and participate to different type of exchanges and they focus on different types of content.

Both exchanges and contents[6] analysis (see "Method") shows four main clusters of participants:

- **Cluster 1 (Others and Experts):** The content of the exchanges between these actors is mainly medical and scientific. They deal more with a public sphere of the disease (the left side of the map). As we already said, when some kind of expert (e.g. practitioner, psychologist) participates in the

discussion, the exchange is only between a single person and the expert (not between a group). So no knowledge sharing happen, but this kind of process is more similar to a transfer of knowledge in its classical conception: from expert to lay.

- **Cluster 2 (Mixed):** When exchanges happen between mixed actors the focus of the exchanges is informative; we can find two kind of discussion: a. sharing opinion about a relevant topic ([talking about a TV adv] "In my opinion if you don't shock people, in terms of pictures and contents, no one cares about your spot"); b. asking/ receiving general information about diabetes ("What is diabetic foot syndrome?"). These exchanges are positioned between public and private contents (in the center of the map).

Figure 3. Types of participants clusters

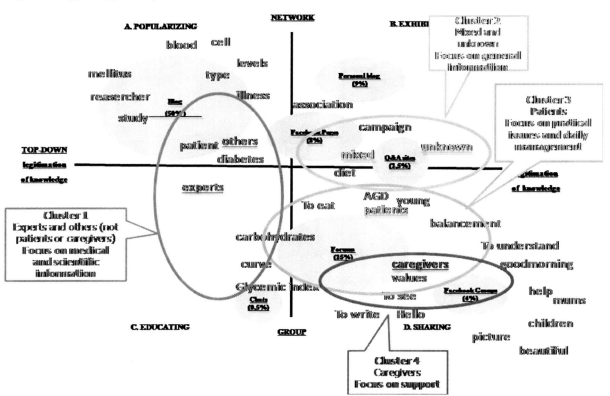

- **Cluster 3 (Patients):** Exchanges and posts in this cluster are mainly focused on practical issues and daily management of diabetes. The discussion deals with private contents and it is mainly developed in a problem solving logic. In practice, the discussion is activated by a request to help in solving practical problem ("there is someone of you that is living with diabetes and can give me some suggestions? They give me all the furniture to check my blood glycemic index..."). They share experiences and knowledge in order to solve a problem.

- **Cluster 4 (Caregivers):** Caregivers mainly exchange support ("To talk here is different. . . . We totally understand each other . . . without seeing us . . . . . !! ! ! ! ;))"). Their discussions can be considered as another type of problem-solving exchanges.

Discussion and Recommendations

The study allowed the generation of a descriptive framework of online exchanges about diabetes. We shall briefly discuss why these results can be important into literature debate.

Firstly, different Web contexts make possible different type of knowledge processes. The variety of labels and definitions in literature correspond to different processes and it's fundamental understanding which conditions brings out different knowledge processes.

According to our analysis, two main axes articulated typologies of processes.

The first axis ("knowledge legitimation") describes the "model" of knowledge legitimation: vertical is the classical model of knowledge legitimation where an expert proposes, diffuses and discusses his/her knowledge, throughout

Web based "knowledge transfer" activities (Ekberg et al., 2008). As opposite, it's possible an horizontal way of knowledge legitimation, in which lay actors are perceived as "experts" (namely trustable and knowledgeable) since they "experienced the disease". The interest toward the patient "expertise" topic is gaining growing relevance in the health studies (Civan & Pratt, 2007; Civan et al., 2009).

The second axis refers to the "relational aim" that users want to reach: network or group oriented. In a network perspective, the aim is really similar to the knowledge dissemination (Meyer, & Schroeder, 2009) or information and knowledge diffusion (Kwon, Kim, & Park, 2009) processes. According to this view we are "in the age of the Web called liquid. [....] The goal of the model is to disseminate knowledge in the best possible way" (Baez et al., 2010, p. 395).

On the other side online peer exchanges are conceived as a way to share and participate in a discussion to construct new knowledge. This perspective directly answers to the idea of O'Reily that considers Web 2.0 participation architecture (Grivet Foiaia, 2007); in these exchanges actors participate in the discussion and they really contribute to construct new knowledge.

This structure makes clear that online exchanges about diabetes may be divide into four main type: popularizing: diffusion and dissemination of knowledge (mainly scientific) produced by someone else; exhibiting: diffusion and spreading of knowledge toward the activities of single individuals or specific group; educating: discussion with experts of relevant topic; sharing: participation into the construction of knowledge useful for pragmatic aims.

According to our results, the type of Web 2.0 context has an important role into shape the knowledge processes; both its technical and social features affect the type of exchanges and knowledge processes developed between patients. In particular the different types of knowledge processes are characterized by:

- **Different Type of Web Tools:** Blogs are used mainly for knowledge spread, instead forums support knowledge construction processes within a group. Social networks have different type of applications that can support different type of processes. This topic need to be deepen; in particular if we found that different Web tools support different knowledge processes, it will be central to understand what role the Web and its tools play into the development of the different knowledge processes.
- **Different Type of Contents:** It is clear that a double set of contents discussed toward diabetes does exist. A public sphere of diabetes, regarding scientific advances and general information on diabetes is spread mainly throughout blogs. On the other side, it's possible to find a variety of contexts in which a private dimension of diabetes is discussed in a protect group of peers, such as in a dedicated forums.
- **Different Type of Actors:** Different actors have different aims and they use the Web tools to reach their aim and to find useful knowledge. Our data confirm literature on the topic: patients and caregivers look for sharing knowledge (useful and practice) and support (Ancker et al., 2009). It's a new and relevant result to understand that diabetic patients look more for practical knowledge; instead their caregivers are more interested in emotional support. This result will help professional to better understand the different needs of all the actors involved in the care process.

This conceptual map allow us to move a step forward in the plethora of peer exchanges and knowledge processes toward the diabetes; in our opinion similar processes may happen toward other chronic conditions, even if it will be really important to verify the role of the disease in shaping knowledge processes.

Moreover, these first explorative results need to be deepened by more dept study on the functioning of the different knowledge processes supported by different Web tools.

Finally, we want to propose some reflections specifically referring to those contexts able to support knowledge sharing between patients and caregivers; as we said at the beginning of this chapter, these types of exchanges can be really relevant for the management of chronic disease. Knowledge sharing processes are supported mainly by group oriented contexts in which the model of "legitimation of knowledge" is horizontal (such as forums of Facebook groups), where the actors of exchanges are patients and their caregivers and the exchange is focused on private and practical aspects of diabetes management.

Starting from these results, we propose some theoretical interpretations acted to guide future research on this topic.

Firstly, online contexts that show more information about participants will be the most supportive for the knowledge construction. In our opinion, Websites that want to sustain exchanges has to join the media richness approach: "the media richness of various technologies is defined by its capacity for immediate feedback, its ability to support natural language, the number of cues (non-verbal) it provides, and the extent to which the channel creates social presence for the receiver [xxx]. The researchers found that people prefer to use richer channels to be able to more efficiently and more effectively understand one another "(Dalkir, 2008, p. 93). Social networks, due to their technical features, seem to be a good online tool to develop good context for online patient exchanges.

Secondly, to sustain building processes, trust and credibility toward other participants is mandatory. This aspect is strongly linked to a classic concept of psychosocial studies on the computer-mediated interactions that is the "social presence", "the feeling to be with others selves in a real or virtual environment, as the result of the ability to

intuitively recognize others intentions in the environment" (Riva, Milani, & Gaggioli, 2010). Our analysis shows the importance of this concept in the Web world. Now it will be necessary to deepen the role of this concept in knowledge processes.

FUTURE RESEARCH DIRECTIONS

This research is an explorative work providing interesting results and insights for further intervention and research.

In our opinion, the main interesting research lines for the future should be:

- To operationalize the research insight: this is an explorative work; a great effort needs to be done in order to categorize and measure these explorative results.
- To deepen the study of the functioning of knowledge processes: if we have studied the main conditions that can support online knowledge sharing processes between diabetic patients, it will be fundamental deepen the study of the ways (e.g., discursive and rhetoric acts) in which the knowledge processes happen in these contexts.
- To generalize the results of this work into other chronic conditions.

CONCLUSION

These results give us interesting suggestions for further research and practical outcomes.

It will be fundamental for researchers interested in online communications, but also for health care practitioners, to understand how these knowledge processes work and how we can support good knowledge building processes.

Our results showed that different Web 2.0 contexts support different knowledge processes. In particular, we were able to define 4 types of online contexts supporting different knowledge processes and characterized by different Web 2.0 applications, contents, and actors. To conclude the chapter we want to present practical outcomes that each online context can have in the health communication world.

1. Popularizing for prevention: throughout the use of blogs, it is possible to make general public aware of the diabetes world. In particular, blogs are able to transfer knowledge to an indefinable number of people. That make evident the relevance these type of Web 2.0 tools may have in the prevention world.
2. Exhibiting for fund and resources raising: here it's possible to make the general public aware of the practical efforts of associations and organizations towards diabetes. These types of contents may help these organization in fund and resources raising.
3. Educating for clinical relations: throughout synchronous and asynchronous tools, the Web 2.0 is able to practically sustain relation between practitioners and patients. This area is not really used for now in Italy, but it has a big practical potential into facilitate the clinical relation.
4. Sharing for patient empowerment: this area spontaneously born by the need of patients and their caregivers to find help and support. The world of association and organization haven't so far totally understand the potential of this area in order to orientate good care&cure practices. Moreover it's evident that patients and caregivers needs are not the same and they need adequate tool to find the adequate type of support for them.

The opportunity to orientate online contexts on the basis of the aims we want to reach is fundamental for health communication success.

REFERENCES

Ancker, J. S., Carpenter, K. M., Greene, P., Kukafka, R., Marlow, L. A., & Prigerson, H. G. (2009). Peer-to-peer communication, cancer prevention, and the internet. *Journal of Health Communication, 14*, 38–46. doi:10.1080/10810730902806760 PMID:19449267.

Anderson, P. (2007). What is web 2.0? Ideas, technologies and implications for education. *JISC Technology and Standards Watch*. Retrieved from http://www.jisc.ac.uk/media/documents/techwatch/tsw0701b.pdf

Ang, C. S., Zaphiris, P., & Wilson, S. (2011). A case study analysis of a constructionist knowledge building community with activity theory. *Behaviour & Information Technology, 30*(5), 537–554. doi:10.1080/0144929X.2010.490921.

Arnold, L. K., Alomran, H., Anantharaman, V., Halpern, P., Hauswald, M., & Malmquist, P. et al. (2007). Knowledge translation in international emergency medical care. *Academic Emergency Medicine: Official Journal of the Society for Academic Emergency Medicine, 14*(11), 1047–1051. PMID:17967967.

Baez, M., Mussi, A., Casati, F., Birukou, A., & Marchese, M. (2010). Liquid journals: Scientific journals in the web 2.0 era. In J., Hunter (Ed.), *Proceedings of the 10th Annual Joint Conference on Digital Libraries* (pp. 395-396). New York: ACM.

Bakardjieva, M. (2003). Virtual togetherness: An everyday-life perspective. *Media Culture & Society, 25*(3), 291–313.

Bar-Lev, S. (2008). We are here to give you emotional support: Performing emotions in an online HIV/AIDS support group. *Qualitative Health Research, 18*(4), 509–521. doi:10.1177/1049732307311680 PMID:18192435.

Barello, S., Graffigna, G., & Vegni, E. (2013). Patient engagement as an emerging challenge for health-care services: Mapping the literature. *Nursing Research and Practice.*

Blank, T. O., & Adam-Blodnieks, M. (2007). The who and the what of usage of two cancer online communities. *Computers in Human Behavior, 23,* 1249–1257. doi:10.1016/j.chb.2004.12.003.

boyd, D.M., & Ellison, N.B. (2007). Social network sites: Definition, history, and scholarship. *Journal of Computer-Mediated Communication, 13,* 210-230.

Burr, L., & Dawson, S. (2003). Codification of interaction within a large scale online forum environment. In *Proceedings of Educause.* EDUCAUSE.

Chou, S.-W., Min, H.-T., Chang, Y.-C., & Lin, C.-T. (2010). Understanding continuance intention of knowledge creation using extended expectation–confirmation theory: An empirical study of Taiwan and China online communities. *Behaviour & Information Technology, 29*(6), 557–570. doi:10.1080/01449290903401986.

Civan, A., McDonald, D. W., Unruh, K. T., & Pratt, W. (2009). Locating patient expertise in everyday life. In *Proceedings of the International ACM SIGCHI Conference on Supporting Group Work* (pp. 291-300). ACM.

Civan, A., & Pratt, W. (2007). Threading together patient expertise. In *Proceedings of the AMIA Annual Symposium* (pp. 140-144). AMIA.

Curran-Smith, J., Abidi, S. S. R., & Forgeron, P. (2005). Towards a collaborative learning environment for children's pain management: Leveraging an online discussion forum. *Health Informatics Journal, 11*(1), 19–31. doi:10.1177/1460458205050682.

Dalkir, K. (2008). Computer-mediated knowledge sharing. In Bolisani, E. (Ed.), *Building the Knowledge Society on the Internet: Sharing and Exchanging Knowledge in Networked Environments* (pp. 89–109). New York: Information Science Reference. doi:10.4018/978-1-59904-816-1.ch005.

de Boer, M. J., Versteegen, G. J., & van Wijhe, M. (2007). Patients' use of the internet for pain-related medical information. *Patient Education and Counseling, 68*(1), 86–97. doi:10.1016/j.pec.2007.05.012 PMID:17590563.

Echeverri, M., & Abels, E. G. (2008). Opportunities and obstacles to narrow the digital divide: Sharing scientific knowledge on the internet. In Bolisani, E. (Ed.), *Building the Knowledge Society on the Internet: Sharing and Exchanging Knowledge in Networked Environments* (pp. 146–171). Hershey, PA: Information Science Publishing. doi:10.4018/978-1-59904-816-1.ch008.

Ekberg, J., Ericson, L., Timpka, T., Eriksson, H., Nordfeldt, S., Hanberger, L., & Ludvigsson, J. (2008). Web 2.0 systems supporting childhood chronic disease management: Design guidelines based on information behaviour and social learning theories. *Journal of Medical Systems, 34*(2), 107–117. doi:10.1007/s10916-008-9222-0 PMID:20433049.

Graffigna, G., Libreri, C., & Bosio, A. C. (2012). Online exchanges among cancer patients and caregivers: Constructing and sharing health knowledge about time. *Qualitative Research in Organizations and Management: An International Journal, 7*(3). Retrieved September 10, 2012 from http://www.emeraldinsight.com/journals.htm?articleid=17053129

Greene, J. A., Choudhry, N. K., Kilabuk, E., & Shrank, W. H. (2010). Online social networking by patients with diabetes: A qualitative evaluation of communication with facebook. *Journal of General Internal Medicine*. doi: doi:10.1007/s11606-010-1526-3 PMID:20945113.

Grivet Foiaia, L. (2007). *Web 2.0: Guida al nuovo fenomeno della rete*. Milano, Italy: Ulrico Hoepli Editore.

Hamilton, D., Dahlgren, E., Hult, A., Roos, B., & Söderström, T. (2004). When performance is the product: Problems in the analysis of online distance education. *British Educational Research Journal, 30*(6), 841–854. doi:10.1080/0141192042000279530.

Hew, K. F., & Cheung, W. S. (2010). Higher-level knowledge construction in asynchronous online discussions: An analysis of group size, duration of online discussion, and student facilitation techniques. *Instructional Science, 39*(3), 303–319. doi:10.1007/s11251-010-9129-2.

Hirzalla, F., van Zoonen, L., & de Ridder, J. (2011). Internet use and political participation: Reflections on the mobilization/normalization controversy. *The Information Society, 27*, 1–15. doi:10.1080/01972243.2011.534360.

Holt, C. (2011). Emerging technologies: Web 2.0. *Health Information Management Journal, 40*(1), 33–35.

Jarvenpaa, S. L., & Majchrzak, A. (2010). Vigilant interaction in knowledge collaboration: Challenges of online user participation under ambivalence. *Information Systems Research, 21*(4), 773–784. doi:10.1287/isre.1100.0320.

Joseph, D., Griffin, M., Hall, R., & Sullivan, E. (2001). Peer coaching: An intervention for individuals struggling with diabetes. *The Diabetes Educator, 27*, 703–710. doi:10.1177/014572170102700511 PMID:12212020.

Kneck, A., Klang, B., & Fagerberg, I. (2011). Learning to live with illness: experiences of persons with recent diagnoses of diabetes mellitus. *Scandinavian Journal of Caring Sciences, 12*. doi: doi:10.1111/j.1471-6712.2010.00864.x PMID:21244458.

Kolbitsch, J., & Maurer, H. (2006). The transformation of the web: How emerging communities shape the information we consume. *Journal of Universal Computer Science, 12*(2), 187–213.

Korica, P., Maurer, H., & Schinagl, W. (2006). *The growing importance of e-communities on the web*. Paper presented at IADIS International Conference on Web Based Communities. San Sebastian, Spain.

Kwon, Y.-S., Kim, S.-W., & Park, S. (2009). An analysis of information diffusion in the blogworld. In J. Wang & S. Zhou (Eds.), *CNIKM '09 Proceedings of the 1st ACM International Workshop on Complex Networks meet Information and Knowledge Management* (pp. 27-30). New York: ACM.

MacPherson, S. L., Joseph, D., & Sullivan, E. (2004). The benefits of peer support with diabetes. *Nursing Forum, 39*(4), 5-12. Retrieved September 10, 2012, from http://www.ncbi.nlm.nih.gov/pubmed/15700481

Mayan, M. (2009). *Essential of qualitative inquiry*. Walnut Creek, CA: Left Coast Press.

Meyer, E. T., & Schroeder, R. (2009). The world wide web of research and access to knowledge. *Knowledge Management Research & Practice, 7*(3), 218–233. doi:10.1057/kmrp.2009.13.

Miles, A. (2009). Of butterflies and wolves: enacting lupus transformations on the internet. *Anthropology & Medicine, 16*(1), 1–12. doi:10.1080/13648470802425906.

Mo, P. K. H., & Coulson, N. S. (2010). Empowering processes in online support groups among people living with HIV/AIDS: A comparative analysis of 'lurkers' and 'posters'. *Computers in Human Behavior, 26,* 1183–1193. doi:10.1016/j.chb.2010.03.028.

Nambisan, P., & Nambisan, S. (2009). Models of consumer value cocreation in health care. *Health Care Management Review, 34*(4), 344–354. doi:10.1097/HMR.0b013e3181abd528 PMID:19858919.

Nettleton, S., Burrows, R., & O'Malley, L. (2005). The mundane realities of the everyday lay use of the Internet for health, and their consequences for media convergence. *Sociology of Health & Illness, 27*(7), 972–992. doi:10.1111/j.1467-9566.2005.00466.x PMID:16313525.

Newman, M. W., Lauterbach, D., Munson, S. A., Resnick, P., & Morris, M. E. (2011). It's not that I don't have problems, I'm just not putting them on Facebook: Challenges and opportunities in using online social networks for health. In *Proceedings of the ACM 2011 Conference on Computer Supported Cooperative Work* (pp. 341-350). Hangzhou, China: ACM.

Nor, F. M., Razak, N. A., & Aziz, J. (2010). E-learning: Analysis of online discussion forums in promoting knowledge construction through collaborative learning. *WSEAS Transactions on Communications, 9*(1), 53–62.

Norris, D., Mason, J., & Lefrere, P. (2003). *Transforming e-knowledge: A revolution in the sharing of knowledge.* Ann Arbor, MI: Society for College and University Planning.

O'Grady, L. A., Witteman, H., & Wathen, C. N. (2008). The experiential health information processing model: Supporting collaborative web-based patient education. *BMC Medical Informatics and Decision Making, 8,* 58. doi:10.1186/1472-6947-8-58 PMID:19087353.

Orizio, G., Schulz, P., Gasparotti, C., Caimi, L., & Gelatti, U. (2010). The world of e-patients: A content analysis of online social networks focusing on diseases. *Telemedicine and e-Health, 16*(10), 1060-1066.

Riva, G., Milani, L., & Gaggioli, A. (2010). Networked flow. In *Comprendere e sviluppare la creatività in rete.* Milan, Italy: LED.

Siliquini, R., Ceruti, M., Lovato, E., Bert, F., Bruno, S., & De Vito, E. … La Torre, G. (2011). Surfing the Internet for health information: An Italian survey on use and population choices. *BMC Medical Informatics and Decision Making, 11*(21). Retrieved September 10, 2012, from http://www.biomedcentral.com/1472-6947/11/21

Turner, A., Kabashi, A., Guthrie, H., Burket, R., & Turner, P. (2011). Use and value of information sources by parents of child psychiatric patients. *Health Information and Libraries Journal, 28*(2), 101–109. doi:10.1111/j.1471-1842.2011.00935.x PMID:21564493.

van Aalst, J. (2009). Distinguishing knowledge-sharing, knowledge- construction, and knowledge-creation discourses. *Computer-Supported Collaborative Learning, 4,* 259–287. doi:10.1007/s11412-009-9069-5.

van den Hooff, B., Elving, W., Meeuwsen, J. M., & Dumoulin, C. (2003). Knowledge sharing in knowledge communities. In Huysman, M., Wenger, E., & Wulf, V. (Eds.), *Communities and Technologies* (pp. 119–141). Dordrecht, The Netherlands: Kluwer Academic Publishers. doi:10.1007/978-94-017-0115-0_7.

Wei, L., & Yan, Y. (2010). Knowledge production and political participation: Reconsidering the knowledge gap theory in the web 2.0 environment. In D. Wen & J. Zhu (Eds.), *The 2nd IEEE International Conference on Information Management and Engineering (ICIME)* (pp. 239-243). Los Alamitos, CA: IEEE Computer Society.

Wenger, E. (1998). *Communities of practice, learning, meaning and identity.* Cambridge, UK: Cambridge University Press.

Wenger, E., McDermott, R., & Snyder, W. R. (2002). *Cultivating communities of practice.* Boston: Harvard Business School Press.

Wenger, E., White, N., & Smith, J. D. (2009). Digital habitats stewarding technology for communities. Portland, OR: CPsquare.

Wilkinson, A., Papaioannou, D., Keen, C., & Booth, A. (2009). The role of the information specialist in supporting knowledge transfer: A public health information case study. *Health Information and Libraries Journal, 26*(2), 118–125. doi:10.1111/j.1471-1842.2008.00790.x PMID:19490150.

Yan, P., & Yang, X. (2009). To trade or to teach: Modeling tacit knowledge diffusion in complex social networks. In Q. Luo & J. Zhu (Eds.), *Second International Conference on Future Information Technology and Management Engineering* (pp. 151-154). Los Alamitos, CA: IEEE Computer Society.

Zenios, M. (2011). Epistemic activities and collaborative learning: Towards an analytical model for studying knowledge construction in networked learning settings. *Journal of Computer Assisted Learning, 27*(3), 259–268. doi:10.1111/j.1365-2729.2010.00394.x.

ADDITIONAL READING

Arduser, L. (2011). Warp and weft: Weaving the discussion threads of an online community. *Journal of Technical Writing and Communication, 41*(1), 5–31. doi:10.2190/TW.41.1.b.

Boulos, M. N. K., & Wheeler, S. (2007). The emerging web 2.0 social software: an enabling suite of sociable technologies in health and health care education. *Health Information and Libraries Journal, 24*, 2–23. doi:10.1111/j.1471-1842.2007.00701.x PMID:17331140.

Buraphadeja, V., & Dawsona, K. (2008). Content analysis in computer-mediated communication: Analyzing models for assessing critical thinking through the lens of social constructivism. *American Journal of Distance Education, 22*(3), 130–145. doi:10.1080/08923640802224568.

Consalvo, M., & Ess, C. (Eds.). (2011). *The handbook of internet studies.* Chichester, UK: Blackwell Publishing. doi:10.1002/9781444314861.

Dasgupta, S. (Ed.). (2006). *Encyclopedia of virtual communities and technologies.* Hershey, PA: Idea Group Reference.

El Morr, C. (2010). Health care virtual communities: Challenges and opportunities. In Cruz-Cunha, M., Tavares, A., & Simoes, R. (Eds.), *Handbook of Research on Developments in E-Health and Telemedicine: Technological and Social Perspectives* (pp. 278–298). Hershey, PA: IGI Global.

Eysenbach, G. (2008). Medicine 2.0: Social networking, collaboration, participation, apomediation, and openness. *Journal of Medical Internet Research*, *10*(3), e22. doi:10.2196/jmir.1030 PMID:18725354.

Falcone, P. (2010). Online communication and healthcare: The diffusion of health-related virtual communities. In Cruz-Cunha, M. M., Tavares, A. J., & Simoes, R. (Eds.), *Handbook of Research on Developments in E-Health and Telemedicine: Technological and Social Perspectives* (pp. 336–356). Hershey, PA: IGI Global.

Gavin, J., Rodham, K., & Poyer, H. (2008). The presentation of pro-anorexia in online group interactions. *Qualitative Health Research*, *18*(3), 325–333. doi:10.1177/1049732307311640 PMID:18235156.

Graffigna, G. (2009). *Interpersonal exchanges about HIV-AIDS through different media*. Saarbucken, Germany: VDM Verlag Dr. Muller.

Hara, N., & Hew, K. F. (2007). Knowledge-sharing in an online community of health-care professionals. *Information Technology & People*, *20*(3), 235–261. doi:10.1108/09593840710822859.

Hara, N., Shachaf, P., Haigh, T., Mackey, T. P., Sandusky, R. J., & Davenport, E. (2007). Knowledge sharing in online communities of practice: Digital trends. *Proceedings of the American Society for Information Science and Technology*, *43*(1), 1–10. doi:10.1002/meet.14504301141.

Joinson, A., McKenna, K. Y. A., Postmes, T., & Reips, U. (2007). *The Oxford handbook of internet psychology*. Oxford, UK: Oxford University Press.

Josefsson, U. (2003). Patients' online communities experiences of emergent Swedish self-help on the internet. In M. Huysman, E. Wenger, & Wulf (Eds.), Communities and Technologies (pp. 369-389). Dordrecht, The Netherlands: Kluwer Academic Publishers.

Ke, F., Chavez, A. F., Causarano, P. L., & Causarano, A. (2011). Identity presence and knowledge building: Joint emergence in online learning environments? *Computer-Supported Collaborative Learning*, *6*, 349–370. doi:10.1007/s11412-011-9114-z.

Kolbitsch, J., & Maurer, H. (2006). The transformation of the web: How emerging communities shape the information we consume. *Journal of Universal Computer Science*, *12*(2), 187–213.

Kvasny, L., & Igwe, C. F. (2008). An African American weblog community's reading of AIDS in Black America. *Journal of Computer-Mediated Communication*, *13*(3), 569–592. doi:10.1111/j.1083-6101.2008.00411.x.

Leimeister, J. M., Schweizer, K., Leimeister, S., & Krcmar, H. (2008). Do virtual communities matter for the social support of patients? Antecedents and effects of virtual relationships in online communities. *Information Technology & People*, *21*(4), 350–374. doi:10.1108/09593840810919671.

Leung, Z. C. S. (2009). Knowledge management in social work: Types and processes of knowledge sharing in social service organizations. *British Journal of Social Work*, *39*, 693–709. doi:10.1093/bjsw/bcp034.

Lewis, D., Eysenbach, G., Kukafka, R., Stavri, P. Z., & Jimison, H. B. (Eds.). (2005). Consumer health informatics. In Informing Consumers and Improving Health Care. New York: Springer Science+Business Media.

Markauskaite, L., & Sutherland, L. (2008). Exploring individual and collaborative dimensions of knowledge building in an online learning community of practice. *Informatics in Education*, *7*(1), 105–126.

Nambisan, P. (2011). Evaluating patient experience in online health communities: Implications for health care organizations. *Health Care Management Review*, *36*(2), 124–133. doi:10.1097/HMR.0b013e3182099f82 PMID:21317657.

Pachler, N., & Daly, C. (2009). Narrative and learning with web 2.0 technologies: towards a research agenda. *Journal of Computer Assisted Learning*, *25*(1), 6–18. doi:10.1111/j.1365-2729.2008.00303.x.

Roos, I. A. G. (2003). Reacting to the diagnosis of prostate cancer: Patient learning in a community of practice. *Patient Education and Counseling*, *49*, 219–224. doi:10.1016/S0738-3991(02)00184-2 PMID:12642193.

Sharratt, M., & Usoro, A. (2003). Understanding knowledge-sharing in online communities of practice. *Electronic Journal of Knowledge Management*, *1*(2), 187–196.

Slaughter, L. T., & Sandaunet, A. (2010). Technology-enhanced health communities. In Zaphiris, P., & Siang Ang, C. (Eds.), *Social Computing and Virtual Communities* (pp. 91–120). Boca Raton, FL: Chapman & Hall/CRC, Taylor & Francis Group.

Winkelman, W. J., & Choo, C. W. (2003). Provider-sponsored virtual communities for chronic patients: Improving health outcomes through organizational patient centered knowledge management. *Health Expectations*, *6*, 352–358. doi:10.1046/j.1369-7625.2003.00237.x PMID:15040797.

KEY TERMS AND DEFINITIONS

Chronic Patient: Someone who suffer from a chronic condition, namely a disease that persists over a long period. Chronic patients have to cope with physical, emotional and pragmatic dimensions connected to the last of the disease.

Ethnographic Perspective: A qualitative research approach that studies behaviors, practices, patterns, perspectives and mainly culture of people in their natural setting.

Online Knowledge Processes: All the possible ways throughout knowledge is spread, shared, negotiated, built, and produced in the online environments.

Online Knowledge Sharing: Construction of new knowledge, based on a shared and negotiated set of knowledge and happening within an online group.

Online Peer Exchanges: Online contexts in which people interact and exchange information and knowledge with others perceived as peers (not experts, but people who share the same experience).

Self-Care Management: Strategies used by people affected by chronic conditions comprehending individual ability to manage t symptoms, cures, physical and psychosocial consequences and life style changes inherent in living with a chronic condition.

Web 2.0: It does not refer to a specific version of the Web, but to a set of technological improvements. Practically, Web 2.0 provides a level users interaction that was not available before, sustaining the sharing and the production of knowledge and culture.

ENDNOTES

[1] Source: www.Internetworldstats.com.

[2] It depends on the single country. For example in USA the 80% of Internet users look for health information (Turner et al., 2011); in Italy, the 45.1% of the Internet users search for health information. Source: Italian National Statistics Institute (http://www.istat.it/it/archivio/48388).

[3] Source: www.Internetworldstats.com.

[4] Between the technical options offered by T-lab, we used specificities analysis: it defines which lexical units (words or lemmas) are the most typical lemmas (over-used lemmas) and those which are typically absent (under-used lemmas) in a text subset (defined by a variable) (Graffigna, 2009). This analysis allows determining lexical specificities of specific subsets, comparing it to the entire data corpus or to another subset. Outcomes significance is based on chi-square test. Practically, we used it to compare contents produced: 1) in different Web 2.0 application; 2) by different actors.

[5] To better explain the meaning of our speech, we add some quotations from the posts analyzed.

Compilation of References

Abraham, W. T., Adamson, P. B., Bourge, R. C., Aaron, M. F., Costanzo, M. R., & Stevenson, L. W. et al. (2011). Wireless pulmonary artery haemodynamic monitoring in chronic heart failure: A randomised control trial. *Lancet, 377*(9766), 658–666. doi:10.1016/S0140-6736(11)60101-3 PMID:21315441.

Abraham, W. T., Adamson, P. B., Hasan, A., Bourge, R. C., Pamboukian, S. V., Aaron, M. F., & Raval, N. Y. (2011). Safety and accuracy of a wireless pulmonary artery pressure monitoring system in patients with heart failure. *American Heart Journal, 161*(3), 558–566. doi:10.1016/j.ahj.2010.10.041 PMID:21392612.

Abujudeh, H. H., Kaewlai, R., Asfaw, B. A., & Thrall, J. H. (2010). Quality initiatives: Key performance indicators for measuring and improving radiology department performance. *Radiographics, 30*(3), 571–580. doi:10.1148/rg.303095761 PMID:20219841.

Accreditations Canada. (2012). *Leading practice: Recognizing innovation and creativity in Canadian health care delivery*. Retrieved 12 16, 2012, from http://www.accreditation.ca/news-and-publications/publications/leading-practices/

ACEP. (n.d.). Quality of care and the outcomes management movement. *American College of Emergency Physicians*. Retrieved 30 December 2012 from http://www.acep.org/content.aspx?id=30166

Agrawal, A. (2009). Medication errors: Prevention using information technology systems. *British Journal of Clinical Pharmacology, 67*(6), 681–686. doi:10.1111/j.1365-2125.2009.03427.x PMID:19594538.

AHRQ. (2003). *AHRQ's patient safety initiative, building foundations, reducing risk*. Interim Report to the Senate Committee on Appropriations. Retrieved 28 December from http://www.ahrq.gov/qual/pscongrpt/

Ajayi, J., Denson, C., Health, B., & Wilmot, K. (2010). *2010 Toronto food sector update*. Toronto, Canada: City of Toronto Economic Development & Culture.

Alberta Centre for Child, Family and Community Research. (2012). *Child and youth data laboratory so innovative, it's the first of its kind in the world*. Retrieved September 13, 2012, from http://www.research4children.com/admin/contentx/default.cfm?h=9999996&grp=1&PageId=9999996

Allen, A., & March, A. (2002). Telemedicine at the community cancer center. *Oncology Issues, 17*(1), 18–24.

Althaus, C., Bridgman, P., & Davis, G. (2007). *The Australian policy handbook* (4th ed.). Sydney, Australia: Allen & Unwin.

American Planning Association. (2007). *Policy guide on community and regional food planning*. Retrieved June 25, 2011, from http://www.planning.org/policy/guides/pdf/foodplanning.pdf

Ancker, J. S., Carpenter, K. M., Greene, P., Kukafka, R., Marlow, L. A., & Prigerson, H. G. (2009). Peer-to-peer communication, cancer prevention, and the internet. *Journal of Health Communication, 14*, 38–46. doi:10.1080/10810730902806760 PMID:19449267.

Anderson, P. (2007). What is web 2.0? Ideas, technologies and implications for education. *JISC Technology and Standards Watch*. Retrieved from http://www.jisc.ac.uk/media/documents/techwatch/tsw0701b.pdf

Andru, P., & Botchkarev, A. (2008). *Using financial modelling for integrated health care databases.* Retrieved December 18, 2012 from http://www.gsrc.ca/1569094939.pdf

Ang, C. S., Zaphiris, P., & Wilson, S. (2011). A case study analysis of a constructionist knowledge building community with activity theory. *Behaviour & Information Technology, 30*(5), 537–554. doi:10.1080/014492 9X.2010.490921.

Apostolakis, I., Koulierakis, G., Berler, A., Chryssanthou, A., & Varlamis, I. (2012). Use of social media by healthcare professionals in Greece: An exploratory study. *International Journal of Electronic Healthcare, 7*(2). doi:10.1504/IJEH.2012.049873 PMID:23079026.

Archer, N., & Fevrier-Thomas, U. (2010). An empirical study of Canadian consumer and physician perceptions of electronic personal health records. In *Proceedings of the Annual Conference, Administrative Sciences Association of Canada* (pp. 512-522). Regina, Canada: ASAC.

Archer, N., Fevrier, U., Lokker, C., McKibbon, K., & Straus, S. (2011). Personal health records: A scoping review. *Journal of the American Medical Informatics Association, 18*, 515–522. doi:10.1136/amiajnl-2011-000105 PMID:21672914.

Arman, R., Dellve, L., Wikström, E., & Törnström, L. (2009). What health care managers do: Applying Mintzberg's structured observation method. *Journal of Nursing Management, 17*(6), 718–729. doi:10.1111/j.1365-2834.2009.01016.x PMID:19694915.

Arnold, L. K., Alomran, H., Anantharaman, V., Halpern, P., Hauswald, M., & Malmquist, P. et al. (2007). Knowledge translation in international emergency medical care. *Academic Emergency Medicine: Official Journal of the Society for Academic Emergency Medicine, 14*(11), 1047–1051. PMID:17967967.

Asada, Y., & Kephart, G. (2007). Equity in health services use and intensity of use in Canada. *BMC Health Services Research.* doi:10.1186/1472-6963-7-41 PMID:17349059.

Ash, J. S., Gorman, P. N., Seshadri, V., & Hersh, W. R. (2004). Computerized physician order entry in U.S. hospitals: Results of a 2002 survey. *Journal of the American Medical Informatics Association, 11*(2), 95–99. doi:10.1197/jamia.M1427 PMID:14633935.

Åstrand, B., Montelius, E., Petersson, G., & Ekedahl, A. (2009). Assessment of e-prescription quality: An observational study at three mail-order pharmacies. *BMC Medical Informatics and Decision Making, 9*(8). doi: doi:10.1186/1472-6947-9-8 PMID:19171038.

Baez, M., Mussi, A., Casati, F., Birukou, A., & Marchese, M. (2010). Liquid journals: Scientific journals in the web 2.0 era. In J., Hunter (Ed.), *Proceedings of the 10th Annual Joint Conference on Digital Libraries* (pp. 395-396). New York: ACM.

Baghbanian, A., Hughes, I., Kebriaei, A., & Khavarpour, F. A. (2012). Adaptive decision-making: How Australian healthcare managers decide. *Australian Health Review, 36*(1), 49–56. doi:10.1071/AH10971 PMID:22513020.

Bakardjieva, M. (2003). Virtual togetherness: An everyday-life perspective. *Media Culture & Society, 25*(3), 291–313.

Baker, G. R., Norton, P. G., Flintoft, V., Blais, R., Brown, A., & Cox, J. et al. (2004). The Canadian adverse event study: The incidence of adverse events among hospital patients in Canada. *Canadian Medical Association Journal, 170*(11), 1678–1686. doi:10.1503/cmaj.1040498 PMID:15159366.

Baker, L., Johnson, S., Macaulay, D., & Birnbaum, H. (2011). Integrated telehealth and care management program for medicare beneficiaries with chronis disease linked to savings. *Health Affairs, 30*(9), 1689–1697. doi:10.1377/hlthaff.2011.0216 PMID:21900660.

Ballas, D., Clarke, G., Dorling, D., Rigby, J., & Wheeler, B. (2006). Using geographical information systems and spatial microsimulation for the analysis of health inequalities. *Health Informatics Journal, 12*(1), 65–79. doi:10.1177/1460458206061217 PMID:17023399.

Bambra, C., Fox, D., & Scott-Samuel, A. (2005). Towards a politics of health. *Health Promotion International, 20*(2), 187–193. doi:10.1093/heapro/dah608 PMID:15722364.

Barello, S., Graffigna, G., & Vegni, E. (2013). Patient engagement as an emerging challenge for health-care services: Mapping the literature. *Nursing Research and Practice.*

Bar-Lev, S. (2008). We are here to give you emotional support: Performing emotions in an online HIV/AIDS support group. *Qualitative Health Research, 18*(4), 509–521. doi:10.1177/1049732307311680 PMID:18192435.

Bates, D., Kuperman, G., Wang, S., Gandhi, T., Kittler, A., & Volk, L. et al. (2003). Ten commandments for effective clinical decision support: Making the practice of evidence-based medicine a reality. *Journal of the American Medical Informatics Association, 10*(6), 523–530. doi:10.1197/jamia.M1370 PMID:12925543.

Beacom, A. M. (2010). Communicating health information to disadvantaged populations. *Family & Community Health, 33*(2), 152–162. doi:10.1097/FCH.0b013e3181d59344 PMID:20216358.

Beales, H. (2009). Prescription drug regulation. In *Business and Governmental Relations: An Economic Perspective.* Dubuque, IA: Kendall Hunt.

Bédard, Y., Gosselin, P., Rivest, S., Proulx, M.-J., Nadeau, M., & Lebel, G. et al. (2003). Integrating GIS components with knowledge discovery technology for environmental health decision support. *International Journal of Medical Informatics, 70*, 79–94. doi:10.1016/S1386-5056(02)00126-0 PMID:12706184.

Bédard, Y., Rivest, S., & Proulx, M.-J. (2007). *Spatial on-line analytical processing (SOLAP): Concepts, architectures and solutions from a geomatics engineering perspective.* Quebec City, Canada: Centre for Research in Geomatics.

Begoyan, A. (2007). An Overview of interoperability standards for electronic health records. *Integrated Design and Process Technology,* 1-8.

Begun, J. W., Zimmerman, B., & Dooley, K. (2003). Health care organizations as complex adaptive systems. In Mick, S. M., & Wyttenbach, M. (Eds.), *Advances in health care organization theory* (pp. 253–288). San Francisco, CA: Jossey-Bass.

Bell, E. (2010). *Research for health policy.* Oxford, UK: Oxford University Press.

Berk, M., & Monkeit, A. (2001). The concentration of health care expenditures, revisited. *Health Affairs, 20*(2), 9–18. doi:10.1377/hlthaff.20.2.9 PMID:11260963.

Berler, A. (2009). *Service oriented information management model in a citizen centred regional healthcare network.* (Doctoral dissertation). National Technical University of Athens and the Medical School of the University of Patras, Patras, Greece. Retrieved 30 August 2012 from http://nemertes.lis.upatras.gr/dspace/handle/123456789/2489

Berler, A., Pavlopoulos, S., & Koutsouris, D. (2004). Design of an interoperability framework in a regional healthcare system. In *Proceedings of Engineering in Medicine and Biology Society* (*Vol. 2*, pp. 3093–3096). IEEE. doi:10.1109/IEMBS.2004.1403874.

Berler, A., Pavlopoulos, S., & Koutsouris, D. (2005). Using key performance indicators as knowledge-management tools at a regional health-care authority level. *IEEE Transactions on Information Technology in Biomedicine, 9*(2), 184–192. doi:10.1109/TITB.2005.847196 PMID:16138535.

Berler, A., Pavlopoulos, S., & Koutsouris, D. (2008). Key performance, indicators and information flow: The cornerstones of effective knowledge management for managed care. In Jennex, M. E. (Ed.), *Knowledge Management: Concepts, Methodologies, Tools, and Applications* (pp. 2808–2828). San Diego, CA: San Diego State University. doi:10.4018/978-1-60566-050-9.ch022.

Berlin, A., Sorani, M., & Sim, I. (2006). A taxonomic description of computer-based clinical decision support systems. *Journal of Biomedical Informatics, 39*(6), 565–667. doi:10.1016/j.jbi.2005.12.003 PMID:16442854.

Berner, E., & La Lande, T. (n.d.). Overview of clinical decision support systems. In Berner, E. (Ed.), *Clinical Decision Support Systems Theory and Practice*. Academic Press.

Biermann, J. S., Golladay, G. J., & Peterson, R. N. (2006). Using the internet to enhance physician-patient communication. *The Journal of the American Academy of Orthopaedic Surgeons, 14*, 136–144. PMID:16520364.

Birnbaum, M. (2012). A conversation with donald berwick on implementing national health reform. *Journal of Health Politics, Policy and Law, 37*(4), 709–727. doi:10.1215/03616878-1597511 PMID:22466046.

Black, A. D., Car, J., Pagliari, C., Anandan, C., & Cresswell, K. et al. (2011). The impact of ehealth on the quality and safety of health care: A systematic overview. *PLoS Medicine, 8*(1), e1000387. doi:10.1371/journal.pmed.1000387 PMID:21267058.

Blackwell, R. (2012, April 10). Toronto's economy marches on its stomach. *The Globe and Mail*.

Blank, T. O., & Adam-Blodnieks, M. (2007). The who and the what of usage of two cancer online communities. *Computers in Human Behavior, 23*, 1249–1257. doi:10.1016/j.chb.2004.12.003.

Bloom, D. E., Canning, D., & Fink, G. (2011). *Implications of population aging for economic growth* (Working Paper 64). Boston: Harvard. Retrieved 30 December 2012 from http://www.hsph.harvard.edu/pgda/WorkingPapers/2011/PGDA_WP_64.pdf

Blumenthal, D. (2009). Stimulating the adoption of health information technology. *The New England Journal of Medicine, 260*, 1477–1479. doi:10.1056/NEJMp0901592.

Blumenthal, D., & Glasor, J. (2007). Information technology comes to medicine. *The New England Journal of Medicine, 356*(24), 2527–2534. doi:10.1056/NEJMhpr066212 PMID:17568035.

Bodenheimer, T., & Fernandez, A. (2005). High and rising health care costs: Part 4: Can costs be controlled while preserving quality? *Annals of Internal Medicine, 143*(1), 26–31. doi:10.7326/0003-4819-143-1-200507050-00007 PMID:15998752.

Bond, S., & Cooper, S. (2006). Modelling emergency decisions: Recognition-primed decision making: The literature in relation to an opthalmic critical incident. *Journal of Clinical Nursing, 15*(8), 1023–1032. doi:10.1111/j.1365-2702.2006.01399.x PMID:16879547.

Booth, A., & Brice, A. (2004). Knowledge management. In Walton, G., & Andrew, B. (Eds.), *Exploiting knowledge in health services*. London, UK: Facet Publishing.

Bordage, G., & Lemieux, M. (1991). Semantic structures and diagnostic thinking of experts and novices. *Academic Medicine, 66*(Suppl), 70–72. doi:10.1097/00001888-199109000-00045 PMID:1930535.

Borlaug, B. A., Melenovsky, V., Russell, S. D., Kessler, K., Pacak, K., Becker, L. C., & Kass, D. A. (2006). Impaired chronotropic and vasodilator reserves limit exercise capacity in patients with heart failure and a preserved ejection fraction. *Circulation, 114*(20), 2138–2147. doi:10.1161/CIRCULATIONAHA.106.632745 PMID:17088459.

Boswell, R., & Boudreau, W. (2000). Employee satisfaction with performance appraisals and appraisers: The role of perceived appraisal use. *Human Resource Development Quarterly, 11*(3), 283–299. doi:10.1002/1532-1096(200023)11:3<283::AID-HRDQ6>3.0.CO;2-3.

Botsis, T., Demiris, G., Pedersen, S., & Hartvigsen, G. (2008). Home telecare technologies for the elderly. *Journal of Telemedicine and Telecare, 14*, 333–337. doi:10.1258/jtt.2008.007002 PMID:18852311.

Botsis, T., & Hartvigsen, G. (2008). Current status and future perspectives in telecare for elderly people suffering from chronic diseases. *Journal of Telemedicine and Telecare, 14*, 194–203. doi:10.1258/jtt.2008.070905 PMID:18534954.

Boulos, M. N. (2004). Towards evidence-based, GIS-driven national spatial health information infrastructure and surveillance services in the United Kingdom. *International Journal of Health Geographics, 3*(1). PMID:14748927.

Boulos, M., Roudsari, A., & Carson, E. (2001). Health geomatics: An enabling suite of technologies in health and healthcare. *Journal of Biomedical Informatics, 34*, 195–219. doi:10.1006/jbin.2001.1015 PMID:11723701.

Bourgeois, F., Taylor, P., Emans, S., Nigrin, D., & Mandl, K. (2008). Whose personal control? Creating private, personally controlled health records for pediatric and adolescent patients. *Journal of the American Medical Informatics Association, 15*(6), 737–743. doi:10.1197/jamia.M2865 PMID:18755989.

Bowles, K. H., & Baugh, A. C. (2007). Applying research evidence to optimize telehomecare. *The Journal of Cardiovascular Nursing, 22*(1), 5–15. PMID:17224692.

boyd, D.M., & Ellison, N.B. (2007). Social network sites: Definition, history, and scholarship. *Journal of Computer-Mediated Communication, 13*, 210-230.

Brandt, J. (2011). *The changing world of patient advocacy.* Retrieved 30 December 2012 from http://pixelsandpills.com/2011/04/04/changing-world-patient-advocacy/

Bressler, H., Keyes, J., Rochon, P., & Badley, E. (1999). The prevalence of low back pain in the elderly. *Spine, 24,* 1813–1819. doi:10.1097/00007632-199909010-00011 PMID:10488512.

Bright, T., Wong, A., Dhurjati, R., Bristow, E., Bastian, L., & Coeytaux, R. et al. (2012). Effect of clinical decision-support systems a systematic review. *Annals of Internal Medicine, 157*(1), 29–43. doi:10.7326/0003-4819-157-1-201207030-00450 PMID:22751758.

Britton, B. P., Engelke, M. K., Rains, D. B., & Mahmud, K. (2000). Measuring costs and quality of telehomecare. *Home Health Care Management & Practice, 12*(4), 27–32. doi:10.1177/108482230001200409.

Brown, S., Fischetti, L., Graham, G., Bates, J., Lancaster, A., McDaniel, D.,... Kolodner, R. (2007). Use of electronic health records in disaster response: The experience of department of veterans affairs after hurricaine Katrina. *American Journal of Public Health, 97*(S1), S136-S141. doi:102105/AJPH 2006.10494B

Brunenberg, D. E., van Styn, M. J., Sluimer, J. C., Bekebrede, L. L., Bulstra, S. K., & Joore, M. A. (2005). Joint recovery programme versus usual care: An economic evaluation of a clinical pathway for joint replacement surgery. *Medical Care, 43*(10), 1018–1026. doi:10.1097/01.mlr.0000178266.75744.35 PMID:16166871.

Buckley, B., Murphy, A., & MacFarlane, A. (2011). Public attitudes to the use in research of personal health information from general practitioners' records: a survey of the Irish general public. *Journal of Medical Ethics, 37*(1), 50–55. doi:10.1136/jme.2010.037903 PMID:21071570.

Bujnowska-Fedak, M.M., Puchala, E., & Steciwko, A. (2011). The impact of telehome care status and quality of life among patients with diabetes in primary care setting in Poland. *Telemedicine and e-Health Journal, 17*(3), 153-163.

Burr, L., & Dawson, S. (2003). Codification of interaction within a large scale online forum environment. In *Proceedings of Educause.* EDUCAUSE.

Burton, L. C., German, P., Gruber-Baldini, A., Hebel, R., Zimmerman, S., & Magaziner, J. (2001). Medical care for nursing home residents: Differences by dementia status. *Journal of the American Geriatrics Society, 49,* 142–147. doi:10.1046/j.1532-5415.2001.49034.x PMID:11207867.

Busse, R., & Wismar, M. (2002). Scenarios on the development of consumer choice for healthcare services. In Busse, R., Wismar, M., & Berman, P. C. (Eds.), *The European Union and Health Services* (pp. 249–258). Amsterdam: IOS Press.

Cadario, B. (2005). New appreciation of serious adverse drug reactions. *British Columbia Medical Journal, 47*(1), 14.

Caldwell, S. E., & Mays, N. (2012). Studying policy implementation using a macro, meso and micro frame analysis: The case of the collaboration for leadership in applied health research & care (CLAHRC) programme nationally and in North West London. *Health Research Policy and Systems, 10*(1), 32. doi:10.1186/1478-4505-10-32 PMID:23067208.

California Healthcare Foundation. (2008). *Report: Improving decision support tools for long term care.* Sacramento, CA: California Healthcare Foundation.

Calliope. (2010). *CALLIOPE D4.3 standardisation status report.* Retrieved 29 August 2012 from http://www.calliope-network.eu/Portals/11/assets/documents/CALLIOPE_D4_3_Standardisation_Status_ReportN.pdf

Calliope. (2010). *EU ehealth interoperability roadmap.* Retrieved 29 August 2012 from http://www.calliope-network.eu/Consultation/tabid/439/Default.aspx

Cambria, E., Hussain, A., Durrani, T., Havasi, C., Eckl, C., & Munro, J. (2010). Sentic computing for patient centered applications. In *Proceedings of the 2010 IEEE 10th International Conference on Signal Processing (ICSP),* (pp. 1279-1282). IEEE.

Campbell, E. M., Sittig, D. F., Ash, J. S., Guappone, K. P., & Dykstra, R. H. (2006). Types of unintended consequences related to computerized provider order entry. *Journal of the American Medical Informatics Association, 13*(5), 547–554. doi:10.1197/jamia.M2042 PMID:16799128.

Canadian Association for Health Services and Policy Research. (2012). *About CAHSPR.* Retrieved 12, 16, 2012, from https://cahspr.ca/en/about

Canadian Health Services Research Foundation. (2000). *Health services research and evidence-based decision-making.* Ottawa, Canada: Canadian Health Services Research Foundation.

Canadian Institute for Health Information Update. (2012). *National rehabilitation reporting system.* Ottawa, Canada: Canadian Institute for Health Information Update.

Canadian Institute for Health Information. (2006). *Discharge abstracts database 2005-2006: Executive summary: Data quality documentation.* Ottawa, Canada: Canadian Institute for Health Information.

Canadian Institute for Health Information. (2010). *Choice of a case mix system for use in acute care activity-based funding options and considerations* (Discussion Paper: Activity-Based Funding Unit). Ottawa, Canada: Canadian Institute for Health Information.

Canadian Institute for Health Information. (2010). *Healthcare in Canada 2010.* Ottawa, Canada: Canadian Institute for Health Information.

Canadian Institute for Health Information. (2011). [*A focus on seniors and aging.* Ottawa, Canada: CIHI.]. *Health Care in Canada,* 2011.

Canadian Institute for Health Information. (2011). *Funding models to support quality and sustainability: A pan Canadian dialogue summary report.* Ottawa, Canada: Canadian Institute for Health Information, Institute of Health Economics, & Canadian Health Services Research Foundation.

Canadian Institute for Health Information. (2011). *Case mix RPG grouping methodology and rehabilitation cost weights information sheet.* Ottawa, Canada: Canadian Institute of Health Information.

Canadian Policy and Procedure Network. (2010). *Canadian policy & procedure network.* Retrieved 12, 16, 2012, from http://ca.groups.yahoo.com/group/cppn/

Canadian, R. A. I. Conference. (2008). *Making the quality connection.* Slide presentation. Canadian RAI Conference.

Capital Health. (2011). *Health record forms management.* Retrieved from http://policy.nshealth.ca/Site_Published/DHA9/document_render.aspx?documentRender.IdType=6&documentRender.GenericField=&documentRender.Id=34962

Capital Health. (2012). *Policy development, implementation and evaluation.* Retrieved 12 16, 2012, from http://policy.nshealth.ca/Site_Published/DHA9/document_render.aspx?documentRender.IdType=6&documentRender.GenericField=&documentRender.Id=17121

Cardozo, L., & Steinberg, J. (2010). Telemedicine for recently discharged older patients. *Telemedicine and e-Health, 16*(1), 49-55.

Carter, M. (2003). Factors associated with ambulatory care-sensitive hospitalizations among nursing home residents. *Journal of Aging and Health, 15*(2), 295–329. doi:10.1177/0898264303015002001 PMID:12795274.

Casalino, L., Nicholson, S., Gans, D., Hammons, T., Morra, D., Karrison, T., & Levinson, W. (2009). What does it cost physician practices to interact with health insurance plans? *Health Affairs, 28*(4), w533–w543. doi:10.1377/hlthaff.28.4.w533 PMID:19443477.

Casey, M. M., Moscovice, I. S., & Davidson, G. (2006). Pharmacist staffing, technology use, and implementation of medication safety practices in rural hospitals. *Journal of National Rural Health Association, 22*(4), 321–330. doi:10.1111/j.1748-0361.2006.00053.x PMID:17010029.

Castellese, S. R. (2006). *Guatemala health care practitioners' leadership styles: Medical worker perception versus leader self-perception.* (Unpublished doctoral dissertation). Capella University, Minneapolis, MN.

Castillo-Salgado, C. (2010). Trends and directions of global public health surveillance. *Epidemiologic Reviews, 32*(1), 93–109. doi:10.1093/epirev/mxq008 PMID:20534776.

Celler, B. G., Lovell, N. H., & Basilakis, J. (2003). Using information technology to improve the management of chronic disease. *The Medical Journal of Australia, 179*(5), 242–246. PMID:12924970.

Center for Health Transformation. (2008). *Electronic prescribing: building, deploying and using e-prescribing to save lives and save money.* Retrieved 6 September 2012 from http://www.surescripts.com/media/660347/cht_eprescribing_paper_06.10.2008.pdf

Chang, Y., Ng, C., Wu, C., Li-Chin, C., Chen, C., & Kuang-Hung, H. (2012). Effectiveness of a five-level pediatric triage system: an analysis of resource utilization in the emergency department in Tawaan. *Emergency Medicine Journal.* doi:10.1136/emermed-2012-201362 PMID:22983978.

Charreire, H., Casey, R., Salze, P., Simon, C., Chaix, B., & Banos, A. et al. (2010). Measuring the food environment using geographical information systems: A methodological review. *Public Health Nutrition, 13*(11), 1773–1785. doi:10.1017/S1368980010000753 PMID:20409354.

Chaudhry, B., Wang, J., We, S., Maglione, M., Mojica, W., Roth, E., & Morton, S. (2006). Systematic review: Impact of health information technology on quality, efficiency, and costs of medical care. *Annals of Internal Medicine, 144*, 742–752. doi:10.7326/0003-4819-144-10-200605160-00125 PMID:16702590.

Chen, C., Garrido, T., Chock, D., Okawa, G., & Liang, L. (2009). The kaiser permanente electronic health record: Transforming and streamlining modalities of care. *Health Affairs, 28*(2), 323–333. doi:10.1377/hlthaff.28.2.323 PMID:19275987.

Chopra, A., Park, T., & Levin, P. L. (2010). *Blue button provides access to downloadable personal health data.* Retrieved 30 December 2012 from http://www.whitehouse.gov/blog/2010/10/07/blue-button-provides-access-downloadable-personal-health-data

Chou, W. S., Hunt, Y. M., Beckjord, E. B., Moser, R. P., & Hesse, B. W. (2009). Social media use in the United States: Implications for health communication. *Journal of Medical Internet Research, 11*(4). Retrieved 30 December 2012 from http://www.jmir.org/2009/4/e48/

Chou, S.-W., Min, H.-T., Chang, Y.-C., & Lin, C.-T. (2010). Understanding continuance intention of knowledge creation using extended expectation–confirmation theory: An empirical study of Taiwan and China online communities. *Behaviour & Information Technology, 29*(6), 557–570. doi:10.1080/01449290903401986.

Chuang, Y., Ginsburg, L., & Berta, W. B. (2007). Learning from preventable adverse events in health care organizations: Development of a multilevel model of learning and propositions. *Health Care Management Review, 32*(4), 330–340. doi:10.1097/01.HMR.0000296790.39128.20 PMID:18075442.

Chumbler, N., Haggstrom, D., & Saleem, J. (2011). Implementation of health information technology in veterans health administration to support transformational change: Telehealth and personal health records. *Medical Care, 49*(12), S36–S42. doi:10.1097/MLR.0b013e3181d558f9 PMID:20421829.

City of Toronto. (n.d.). *Key industry sector: Food & beverage.* Retrieved September 10, 2012, from http://www.toronto.ca/invest-in-toronto/food.htm

Civan, A., & Pratt, W. (2007). Threading together patient expertise. In *Proceedings of the AMIA Annual Symposium* (pp. 140-144). AMIA.

Civan, A., McDonald, D. W., Unruh, K. T., & Pratt, W. (2009). Locating patient expertise in everyday life. In *Proceedings of the International ACM SIGCHI Conference on Supporting Group Work* (pp. 291-300). ACM.

Clayton, P. D., & Hripcsak, G. (1995). Decision support in healthcare. *International Journal of Bio-Medical Computing*, *39*(1), 59–66. doi:10.1016/0020-7101(94)01080-K PMID:7601543.

Cleverley, O. W., & Cameron, A. E. (2007). *Essentials of health care finance*. New York: Jones & Bartlett Learning Ed.

COACH. (2001). *Guidelines for the protection of health information*. Edmonton, Canada: COACH - Canada's Health Informatics Association.

Coates, G. (1996). Image and identity: Performance appraisal in a trust hospital. *Health Manpower Management*, *22*(3), 16–22. doi:10.1108/09552069610125883 PMID:10161774.

Coburn, A., Keith, R., & Bolda, E. (2002). The impact of rural residence on multiple hospitalizations in nursing facility residents. *The Gerontologist*, *42*(5), 661–666. doi:10.1093/geront/42.5.661 PMID:12351801.

Coffield, R., DeLoss, G., & Mooty, G. (2008). The rise of the personal health record: panacea or pitfall of health information. *Health Law News. University of Houston. Health Law and Policy Institute*, *12*(10), 8–13.

Conference Board of Canada. (2011). *Elements of an effective innovation strategy for long term care in Ontario*. Ontario, Canada: Ontario Long Term Care Association.

Cornette, P., Swine, C., Malhomme, B., Gillet, J., Meert, P., & D'Hoore, W. (2005). Early evaluation of the risk of functional decline following hospitalization of older patients: Development of a predictive tool. *European Journal of Public Health*, *16*(2), 203–208. doi:10.1093/eurpub/cki054 PMID:16076854.

Coughlin, J. F., Pope, J. E., & Leedle, B. R. (2006). Old age, new technology, and future innovations in disease management and home health care. *Home Health Care Management & Practice*, *18*(3), 196–207. doi:10.1177/1084822305281955.

Coyte, P. C. (1998). The economic cost of musculoskeletal disorders in Canada. *Arthritis Care and Research*, *5*, 315–335. doi:10.1002/art.1790110503 PMID:9830876.

Croner, C. M. (2003). Public health, GIS, and the internet. *Annual Review of Public Health*, *24*, 57–82. PMID:12543872.

Croskerry, P. (2009). A universal model of diagnostic reasoning. *Academic Medicine*, *84*(8), 1022–1028. doi:10.1097/ACM.0b013e3181ace703 PMID:19638766.

Crowe, B., & Sim, L. (2005). An assessment of the effect of the introduction of a PACS and RIS on clinical decision making and patient management at Princess Alexandra Hospital Brisbane, Australia. *International Congress Series*, *1281*, 964–967. doi:10.1016/j.ics.2005.03.347.

Cryderman, P. (1987). *Developing policy and procedure manuals*. Ottawa, Canada: Canadian Hospital Association.

Cryderman, P. (1999). *Customized manuals for changing times*. Ottawa, Canada: CHA Press.

Curran-Smith, J., Abidi, S. S. R., & Forgeron, P. (2005). Towards a collaborative learning environment for children's pain management: Leveraging an online discussion forum. *Health Informatics Journal*, *11*(1), 19–31. doi:10.1177/1460458205050682.

Cusack, C. (2008). Electronic health records and electronic prescribing: Promise and pitfalls. *Obstetrics and Gynological Clinics of North America*, *35*, 63–79. doi:10.1016/j.ogc.2007.12.010 PMID:18319129.

Cushman, R., & Froomkin, A. (2010). Ethical, legal and social issues for personal health records and applications. *Journal of Biomedical Informatics*, *43*(5), S51–S55. doi:10.1016/j.jbi.2010.05.003 PMID:20937485.

Cutler, D. M., Feldman, N. E., & Horwitz, J. R. (2005). US adoption of computerized physician order entry system. *Journal of Health Affairs*, *24*(6), 1654–1664. doi:10.1377/hlthaff.24.6.1654.

Cypress, B. (1983). Characteristics of physician visits for back symptoms: A national perspective. *American Journal of Public Health*, *73*, 389–395. doi:10.2105/AJPH.73.4.389 PMID:6219588.

D'Astolfo, C., & Humphreys, B. K. (2006). *A record review of reported musculoskeletal pain in an Ontario long term care facility.* BMJ Geriatrics.

Daft, R., & Marcic, D. (2001). *Understanding management* (3rd ed.). Hercourt.

Dalkir, K. (2008). Computer-mediated knowledge sharing. In Bolisani, E. (Ed.), *Building the Knowledge Society on the Internet: Sharing and Exchanging Knowledge in Networked Environments* (pp. 89–109). New York: Information Science Reference. doi:10.4018/978-1-59904-816-1.ch005.

Danchev, S., Tsakanikas, A., & Ventouris, N. (2011). *Cloud computing: A driver for Greek economy.* Retrieved 14 September 2012 from http://www.iobe.gr/media/meletes/CloudComputing.pdf

Dansky, K. H., Palmer, L., Shea, D., & Bowles, K. H. (2001). Cost analysis of telehomecare. *Telemedicine Journal and e-Health*, *7*(3), 225–232. doi:10.1089/153056201316970920 PMID:11564358.

Datta, G. (2010). HL7 international health level seven introduction. *HL7 Ambassador Presentation.* Retrieved 31 December 2012 from http://www.phdsc.org/standards/pdfs/naphit-Webinar-phdsc-business-case-gora-datta.pdf

Dave, D., & Kaestner, R. (2009). Health insurance and ex ante moral hazard: Evidence from Medicare. *International Journal of Health Care Finance and Economics*, *9*(4), 367–390. doi:10.1007/s10754-009-9056-4 PMID:19277859.

Davies, H. (2006). Improving the relevance of management research: Evidence-based management: Design, science or both? *Business Leadership Review*, *3*(3), 1–6.

Davis, D. A., & Taylor-Vaisey, A. (1997). Translating guidelines into practice: A systematic review of theoretic concepts, practical experience, and research evidence in the adoption of clinical practice guidelines. *Canadian Medical Association Journal*, *157*, 408–416. PMID:9275952.

de Boer, M. J., Versteegen, G. J., & van Wijhe, M. (2007). Patients' use of the internet for pain-related medical information. *Patient Education and Counseling*, *68*(1), 86–97. doi:10.1016/j.pec.2007.05.012 PMID:17590563.

DeJong, G., Tian, W., Smout, R., Horn, S., Putman, K., & Hsieh, C. et al. (2009). Long-term outcomes of joint replacement rehabilitation patients discharged from skilled nursing and inpatient rehabilitation facilities. *Archives of Physical Medicine and Rehabilitation*, *90*. PMID:19651264.

Denton, I. (2001). Will patients use electronic personal health records? Responses from a real-life experience. *Journal of Healthcare Information Management*, *15*(3), 251–259. PMID:11642143.

Detmer, D., Raymond, B., Tang, P., & Bloomrosen, M. (2008). Integrated personal health records: transformative tools for consumer-centric care. *BMC Medical Informatics and Decision Making*, *8*(45). doi:doi:10.1186/1472-6947-8-45 PMID:18837999.

DeVries, P. (2012). Electronic social media in the healthcare industry. *International Journal of Electronic Finance*, *6*(1), 49–61. doi:10.1504/IJEF.2012.046593.

Diamond, C., Mostashari, F., & Shirky, C. (2009). Collecting and sharing data for population health: A new paradigm. *Health Affairs*, *28*(2), 454–466. doi:10.1377/hlthaff.28.2.454 PMID:19276005.

Djulbegovic, B., Hozo, I., Beckstead, J., Tsalatsanis, A., & Pauker, S. (2012). Dual processing model of medical decision-making. *BMC Medical Informatics and Decision Making*, *12*(1), 94. doi:10.1186/1472-6947-12-94 PMID:22943520.

Donabedian, A. (1980). Explorations in quality assessment and monitoring: *Vol. I. The definition of quality approaches to its measurement.* Ann Arbor, MI: Health Administration Press.

Donabedian, A. (1982). Explorations in quality assessment and monitoring: *Vol. II. The criteria and standards of quality.* Ann Arbor, MI: Health Administration Press.

Donabedian, A. (1985). Explorations in quality assessment and monitoring: *Vol. III. The methods and findings of quality assessment and monitoring – An illustrated analysis.* Ann Arbor, MI: Health Administration Press.

Donabedian, A. (1993). Continuity and change in the quest for quality. *Clinical Performance and Quality Health Care*, *1*, 9–16. PMID:10135611.

Donabedian, A., & Bashshur, R. (2003). *An introduction to quality assurance in health care.* Oxford, UK: Oxford University Press.

Dong, S., Bullard, M., Blitz, S., Ohinmaa, A., & Holroyd, B. et al. (2006). Reliability of computerized emergency triage. *Academic Emergency Medicine, 13*(3). doi:10.1111/j.1553-2712.2006.tb01691.x PMID:16495428.

Dong, S., Bullard, M., Meurer, D., Colman, I., Blitz, S., & Holroyd, B. et al. (2005). Emergency triage: comparing a novel computer triage program with standard triage. *Academic Emergency Medicine, 12*(6), 502–507. doi:10.1111/j.1553-2712.2005.tb00889.x PMID:15930400.

Donnelly, L. F., Gessner, K. E., Dickerson, J. M., Koch, B. L., Towbin, A. J., & Lehkamp, T. W. et al. (2010). Quality initiatives: Department scorecard: A tool to help drive imaging care delivery performance. *Radiographics, 30*(7), 2029–2038. doi:10.1148/rg.307105017 PMID:20801869.

Doolan, D. F., & Bates, D. W. (2002). Computerized physician order entry systems in hospitals: Mandates and incentives. *Journal of Health Affairs, 21*(4), 180–185. doi:10.1377/hlthaff.21.4.180 PMID:12117128.

Doupi, P., et al. (2010). *eHealth strategies country brief: Iceland.* Retrieved 9 September 2012 from http://ehealth-strategies.eu/database/documents/Iceland_CountryBrief_eHStrategies.pdf

Dove, N. (2009). Can international medical graduates help solve Canada's shortage of rural physicians? *Canadian Journal of Rural Medicine, 14*(3), 120–123. PMID:19594998.

Dowd, S. B., & Tilson, E. (1996). The benefits of using CQI/TQM data (continuous quality improvement/total quality management). *Radiologic Technology, 67*(6), 533–535. PMID:8827822.

Ducrou, A. J. (2009). *Complete interoperability in healthcare: Technical, semantic and process interoperability through ontology mapping and distributed enterprise integration techniques.* (Doctor of Philosophy Thesis). University of Wollongong, Wollongong, Australia. Retrieved 31 December 2012 from http://ro.uow.edu.au/theses/3048

Dunn, K., & Wynia, M. (2010). Dreams and nightmares:practical and ethical issues for patients and physicians using personal health records. *The Journal of Law, Medicine & Ethics, 38*(1), 64–73. doi:10.1111/j.1748-720X.2010.00467.x PMID:20446985.

Echeverri, M., & Abels, E. G. (2008). Opportunities and obstacles to narrow the digital divide: Sharing scientific knowledge on the internet. In Bolisani, E. (Ed.), *Building the Knowledge Society on the Internet: Sharing and Exchanging Knowledge in Networked Environments* (pp. 146–171). Hershey, PA: Information Science Publishing. doi:10.4018/978-1-59904-816-1.ch008.

Eckert, J., & Shetty, S. (2011). Food systems, planning and quantifying access: Using GIS to plan for food retailing. *Applied Geography (Sevenoaks, England), 31*(4), 1216–1223. doi:10.1016/j.apgeog.2011.01.011.

Economics, T. D. (2010). *Charting a path to sustainable healthcare in Ontario: 10 proposals to restrain cost growth without compromising quality of care.* Retrieved January 20, 2012, from http://www.td.com/document/PDF/economics/special/td-economics-special-db0510-health-care.pdf

Eder, L. (2000). *Managing healthcare information systems with web enabled technologies.* Hershey, PA: Idea Group Publishing.

Edmonstone, J. (1996). Appraising the state of performance appraisal. *Health Manpower Management, 22*(6), 9. doi:10.1108/09552069610153071 PMID:10164227.

Edwards, D. (1986). *Out of the crisis.* Cambridge, MA: MIT Center for Advanced Engineering Studies.

E-Health Governance Initiative. (2012). *Discussion paper on semantic and technical interoperability.* Retrieved 30 December 2012 from http://www.ehgi.eu/Download/eHealth%20Network%20-%20eHGI%20Discussion%20Paper%20Semantic%20and%20Technical%20Interoperability-2012-10-22.pdf

EHR4CR. (2011). *EHR4CR executive summary.* EHR4CR.

EIPA - European Institute of Public Administration. (2011). *European public sector award 2011, project catalogue, eprescribing in Estonia.* Retrieved 9 September 2012 from http://www.bka.gv.at/DocView.axd?CobId=45974

Ekberg, J., Ericson, L., Timpka, T., Eriksson, H., Nordfeldt, S., Hanberger, L., & Ludvigsson, J. (2008). Web 2.0 systems supporting childhood chronic disease management: Design guidelines based on information behaviour and social learning theories. *Journal of Medical Systems, 34*(2), 107–117. doi:10.1007/s10916-008-9222-0 PMID:20433049.

Elstein, A., Shulman, L., & Sprafka, S. (1978). *Medical problem solving: An analysis of clinical reasoning.* Cambridge, MA: Harvard University Press.

Elwyn, G., Légaré, F., van der Weijden, T., Edwards, A., & May, C. (2008). Arduous implementation: Does the normalisation process model explain why it's so difficult to embed decision support technologies for patients in routine clinical practice. *Implementation Science; IS, 3*(1), 57. doi:10.1186/1748-5908-3-57 PMID:19117509.

EpSOS. (2008). *epSOS home.* Retrieved from www.epsos.eu

EpSOS. (2009). *D2.1: Legal and regulatory constraints on epSOS, design- Participating member states T2.1.1: Analysis and comparison.* epSOS Project Deliverable. Retrieved September 14 2012 from http://www.epsos.eu/uploads/tx_epsosfileshare/D2.1.1_legal_requ_final_01.pdf

EpSOS. (2010). *D3.3.3 epSOS interoperability framework.* epSOS Project Deliverable. Retrieved September 14 2012 from http://www.epsos.eu/uploads/tx_epsosfileshare/D3.3.3_epSOS_Final_Interoperability_Framework_01.pdf

Ericsson. (2011). *More than 50 billion connected devices – Taking connected devices to mass market and profitability* (white paper). Retrieved September 14 2012 from http://www.ericsson.com/res/docs/whitepapers/wp-50-billions.pdf

Estabrooks, C. A., Hutchinson, A. M., Squires, J. E., Birdsell, J., Cummings, G. G., & Degner, L. et al. (2009). Translating research in elder care: An introduction to a study protocol series. *Implementation Science; IS, 4*(51). PMID:19664285.

Estabrooks, C. A., Squires, J. E., Cummings, G. G., Teare, G. F., & Norton, P. G. (2009). Study protocol for the translating research in elder care (TREC), building context - An organizational monitoring program in long-term care project (project one). *Implementation Science; IS, 4*(52). PMID:19671166.

European Commission. (2004). *Communication from the commission to the council: The European parliament, the European economic and social committee and the committee of the regions e-Health - Making healthcare better for European citizens: An action plan for a European e-Health area.* Retrieved 1 September 2012 from http://eur-lex.europa.eu/LexUriServ/LexUriServ.do?uri=COM:2004:0356:FIN:EN:PDF

European Commission. (2007). *eHealth priorities and strategies in European countries, eHealth ERA report, towards the establishment of a European eHealth research area.* Retrieved 8 September 2012 from http://www.ehealth-era.org/documents/2007ehealth-era-countries.pdf

European Commission. (2010). *Communication from the commission Europe 2020: A strategy for smart, sustainable and inclusive growth.* Retrieved 1 September 2012 from http://ec.europa.eu/research/era/docs/en/investing-in-research-european-commission-europe-2020-2010.pdf

European Commission. (2010). *Communication from the commission to the European parliament, the council, the European economic and social committee and the committee of the regions a digital agenda for Europe.* Retrieved 1 September 2012 from http://ec.europa.eu/information_society/digital-agenda/documents/digital-agenda-communication-en.pdf

Eysenbach, G. (2008). Medicine 2.0: Social networking, collaboration, participation, apomediation, and openness. *Journal of Medical Internet Research, 10*(3). Retrieved 30 December 2012 from http://www.ncbi.nlm.nih.gov/pmc/articles/PMC2626430/

Eysenbach, G., & Wyatt, J. (2002). Using the internet for surveys and health research. *Journal of Medical Internet Research, 4*(13). Retrieved 30 December 2012 from http://www.jmir.org/2002/2/e13/

Eysenbach, G. (2001). What is e-health? *Journal of Medical Internet Research, 3*(2), e20. doi:10.2196/jmir.3.2.e20 PMID:11720962.

Eyserbach, G. (2008). Medicine 2.0: Social networking, collaboration, participation, apomediation, and openness. *Journal of Medical Internet Research, 10*(3), e22. doi:10.2196/jmir.1030 PMID:18725354.

Falas, T., Papadopoulos, G., & Stafylopatis, A. (2003). A review of decision support systems in telecare. *Journal of Medical Systems*, 27(4), 347–356. doi:10.1023/A:1023705320471 PMID:12846466.

Fang, H., Peifer, K., Chan, J., & Rizzo, J. (2011). Health information technology and physicians' perceptions of healthcare quality. *The American Journal of Managed Care*, 17(3), e66–e70. PMID:21504261.

Fickenscher, K. (2005). The new frontier of data mining. *Health Management Technology*, 26(10), 26–30. PMID:16259138.

Finkelstein, J., Knight, A., Marinopoulos, S., Gibbons, M. C., & Berger, Z. … Bass, E.B. (2012). Enabling patient-centered care through health information technology. Rockville, MD: Agency for Healthcare Research and Quality.

Fisher, G., & Bibo, M. (2000). No leadership without representation. *International Journal of Organisational Behaviour*, 6(2), 307–319.

Fitzpatrick, M. (2006). Using data to drive performance improvement in hospitals. *Health Management Technology*, 27(12), 10–16. PMID:17256646.

Fletcher, C. (1993). Appraisal: An idea whose time has gone? *Personnel Management*, 25(9), 34.

Flim, C., et al. (2010). *eHealth strategies country brief: The Netherlands*. Retrieved 9 September 2012 from http://www.ehealth-strategies.eu/database/documents/Netherlands_CountryBrief_eHStrategies.pdf

Follen, M., Castaneda, R., Mikelson, M., Johnson, D., Wilson, A., & Higuchi, K. (2007). Implementing health information technology to improve the process of health care delivery: A case study. *Disease Management*, 10(4), 208–215. doi:10.1089/dis.2007.104706 PMID:17718659.

Food and Agriculture Organization of the United Nations. (2010). *Special programme for food security*. Retrieved October 9, 2010, from http://www.fao.org/spfs/en/

Forni, A., Chu, H. T., & Fanikos, J. (2010). Technology utilization to prevent medication errors. *Current Drug Safety*, 5(1), 13–18. doi:10.2174/157488610789869193 PMID:20210714.

Forsyth, R., Maddock, C., Iedema, R., & Lassere, M. (2010). Patient perceptions of carrying their own health information: Approaches towards responsibility and playing an active role in their own health--Implications for a patient-held health file. *Health Expectations*, 13(4), 416–426. doi:10.1111/j.1369-7625.2010.00593.x PMID:20629768.

Fraunhofer, I. S. S. T. (2009). *Study on multilingualism*. Semantic Interoperability Centre Europe. Retrieved 14 September 2012 from https://www.opengroup.org/projects/si/uploads/40/19571/multilingualism-study.pdf

Fulcher, C., & Kaukinen, C. (2005). Mapping and visualizing the location HIV service providers: An exploratory spatial analysis of Toronto neighborhoods. *AIDS Care*, 17(3), 386–396. doi:10.1080/09540120512331314312 PMID:15832887.

Gans, D. (2005). Medical groups' adoption of electronic health records and information systems. *Health Affairs*, 24(5), 1323–1333. doi:10.1377/hlthaff.24.5.1323 PMID:16162580.

Garde, S., Knaup, P., Hovenga, E., & Heard, S. (2007). Towards semantic interoperability for electronic health records: Domain knowledge governance for open EHR archetypes. *Methods of Information in Medicine*, 46(3), 332–343. PMID:17492120.

Garg, A. X., Adhikari, N. K. J., & McDonald, H. et al. (2005). *Effects of computerized clinical decision support systems on practitioner performance and patient outcomes*. Academic Press. doi:10.1001/jama.293.10.1223.

Gartner. (2009). *e-Health for a healthier Europe! Opportunities for a better use of healthcare resources*. Retrieved 20 September 2009 from http://www.se2009.eu/

Gaylin, D., Moiduddin, A., Mohamoud, S., Lundeen, K., & Kelly, J. (2011). Public attitudes about health information technology, and its relationship to health care quality, costs, and privacy. *Health Services Research*, 46(3), 920–934. doi:10.1111/j.1475-6773.2010.01233.x PMID:21275986.

Gellerman, S. W., & Hodgson, W. G. (1988). Cyanamid's new take on performance appraisal. *Harvard Business Review*, 66(3), 36.

Georgiou, A. (2002). Data, information and knowledge: The health informatics model and its role in evidence-based medicine. *Journal of Evaluation in Clinical Practice*, *8*(2), 127–130. doi:10.1046/j.1365-2753.2002.00345.x PMID:12180361.

Gibbons., et al. (2007). *Coming to terms: Scoping interoperability for health care.* Retrieved 31 December 2012 from http://www.hl7.org/documentcenter/public/wg/ehr/ComingtoTerms2007-03-22.zip

Gigerenzer, G. (2008). Fast and frugal heuristics. In *Rationality for Mortals: How People Cope with Uncertainty.* New York: Oxford University Press.

Gigerenzer, G., & Gaissmaier, W. (2011). Heuristic decision making. *Annual Review of Psychology*, *62*, 451–482. doi:10.1146/annurev-psych-120709-145346 PMID:21126183.

Glinos, I. (2012). Worrying about the wrong thing: Patient mobility versus mobility of health care professionals. *Journal of Health Services Research & Policy*, *17*, 254–256. doi:10.1258/jhsrp.2012.012018 PMID:22914545.

Glouberman, S., & Mintzberg, H. (2001). Managing the care of health and the cure of disease-Part II: Integration. *Health Care Management Review*, *26*(1), 70–84. doi:10.1097/00004010-200101000-00007 PMID:11233356.

Godfrey, C. M., Harrison, M. B., Friedberg, E., Medves, J. M., & Tranmer, J. E. (2007). The symptom of pain in individuals recently hospitalized for heart failure. *The Journal of Cardiovascular Nursing*, *22*(5), 368–374. PMID:17724418.

Goel, V. (1996). Indicators of health determinants and health status. In *Patterns of HealthCare in Ontario: The ICES Practice Atlas* (2nd ed., pp. 5–26). Ottawa, Canada: CMA.

Gold, M., McLaughlin, C., Devers, K., Berenson, R., & Bovbjerg, R. (2012). Obtaining providers' 'buy-in' and establishing effective means of information exchange will be critical to HITECH's success. *Health Affairs*, *31*(3), 514–526. doi:10.1377/hlthaff.2011.0753 PMID:22392662.

Goldzweig, C. L., Towfigh, A., Maglione, M., & Shekelle, P. G. (2009). Cost and benefit of health information technology: New trends from the literature. *Journal of Health Affairs*, *28*(2), 282–293. doi:10.1377/hlthaff.28.2.w282.

Government of Ontario. (2009). *Ontario population projections update 2009-2036.* Ontario, Canada: Government of Ontario.

Graber, M., & VanScoy, D. (2003). How well does decision support software perform in the emergency department? *Emergency Medicine Journal*, *20*(5), 426–428. doi:10.1136/emj.20.5.426 PMID:12954680.

Graffigna, G., Libreri, C., & Bosio, A. C. (2012). Online exchanges among cancer patients and caregivers: Constructing and sharing health knowledge about time. *Qualitative Research in Organizations and Management: An International Journal*, *7*(3). Retrieved September 10, 2012 from http://www.emeraldinsight.com/journals.htm?articleid=17053129

Grant, A. M., Moshyk, A. M., Kushniruk, A., & Moehr, J. R. (2003). Reflections on an arranged marriage between bioinformatics and health informatics. *Methods of Information in Medicine*, *42*(2), 116–120. PMID:12743646.

Gray, J. A. (2009). *Evidence-based healthcare and public health: How to make decisions about health services and public health.* London: Elsevier Health Sciences.

Green, C. (2012). *Geographic information systems and public health: Benefits and challenges.* Winnipeg, Canada: National Collaborating Centre for Infectious Diseases.

Greene, J. A., Choudhry, N. K., Kilabuk, E., & Shrank, W. H. (2010). Online social networking by patients with diabetes: A qualitative evaluation of communication with facebook. *Journal of General Internal Medicine*. doi: doi:10.1007/s11606-010-1526-3 PMID:20945113.

Greenhalgh, T., Hinder, S., Stramer, K., Bratan, T., & Russell, J. (2010). Adoption, non-adoption, and abandonment of a personal electronic health record: Case study of HealthSpace. *British Medical Journal*, *341*, c5814. doi:10.1136/bmj.c5814 PMID:21081595.

Grilo, A. (2010). *Interoperability frameworks, theories and models.* Retrieved 29 December from https://www.google.gr/url?sa=t&rct=j&q=&esrc=s&source=Web&cd=5&ved=0CEUQFjAE&url=http%3A%2F%2Fwww.fines-cluster.eu%2Ffines%2Fjm%2Fdocman%2FDownload-document%2F54-Interoperability-Frameworks-Theories-and-Models-Grilo.html&ei=nNDqUIfRB5T54QSoy4HYCg&usg=AFQjCNGUl_fR4QHqpkwH0n5p44nHBTBf_w&bvm=bv.1355534169,d.bGE

Grivet Foiaia, L. (2007). *Web 2.0: Guida al nuovo fenomeno della rete.* Milano, Italy: Ulrico Hoepli Editore.

Grote, D. (2000). Performance appraisal reappraised. *Harvard Business Review, 78*(1), 21.

Gwee, S. (2011). 6 P's of social health. *Social Media Club Reporter.* Retrieved 14 September 2012 from http://socialmediaclub.org/blogs/from-the-clubhouse/6-ps-health

Hackman, J. R., & Wageman, R. (1995). Total quality management: Empirical, conceptual, and practical issues. *Administrative Science Quarterly, 40*(2), 309. doi:10.2307/2393640.

Halamka, J., Mandl, K., & Tang, P. (2008). Early experiences with personal health records. *Journal of the American Medical Informatics Association, 15*(1), 1-7. doi:10.1197/jamia M2562

Hale, P. L. (2007). *Electronic prescribing for the medical practice: Everything you wanted to know but were afraid to ask.* Chicago: Healthcare Information Management Systems Society.

Hallett, L. F., & McDermott, D. (2011). Quantifying the extent and cost of food deserts in Lawrence, Kansas, USA. *Applied Geography (Sevenoaks, England), 31*(4), 1210–1215. doi:10.1016/j.apgeog.2010.09.006.

Hamilton, D., Dahlgren, E., Hult, A., Roos, B., & Söderström, T. (2004). When performance is the product: Problems in the analysis of online distance education. *British Educational Research Journal, 30*(6), 841–854. doi:10.1080/0141192042000279530.

Hammar, T., Nyström, S., Petersson, G., Åstrand, B., & Rydberg, T. (2011). Patients satisfied with e-prescribing in Sweden: A survey of a nationwide implementation. *Journal of Pharmaceutical Health Services Research, 2,* 97–105. doi:10.1111/j.1759-8893.2011.00040.x.

Handy, C. (1993). *Understanding organisation* (4th ed.). London: Penguin.

Harmoni, A. (2002). *Effective healthcare information systems.* Hershey, PA: IGI Global.

Hart, L., Deyo, R., & Cherkin, D. (1995). Physician office visits for low back pain: frequency, clinical evaluation and treatment patterns from a US National survey. *Spine, 20,* 11–19. doi:10.1097/00007632-199501000-00003 PMID:7709270.

Hartzema, A., Winterstein, A., Johns, T., De Leon, J., Bailey, W., McDonald, K., & Pannell, R. (2007). Planning for pharmacy health information technology in critical access hospitals. *American Journal of Health-System Pharmacists, 64,* 315–321. doi:10.2146/ajhp060134 PMID:17244881.

Harvey, G., Loftus-Hills, A., Rycroft-Malone, J., Titchen, A., Kitson, A., McCormack, B., & Seers, K. (2002). Getting evidence into practice: The role and function of facilitation. *Journal of Advanced Nursing, 37*(6), 577–588. doi:10.1046/j.1365-2648.2002.02126.x PMID:11879422.

Hashemi Beni, L., Villeneuve, S., LeBlanc, D. I., Côté, K., Fazil, A., & Otten, A. et al. (2012). Spatio-temporal assessment of food safety risks in Canadian food distribution systems using GIS. *Spatial and Spatia-temporal Epidemiology, 3,* 215–223. doi:10.1016/j.sste.2012.02.009 PMID:22749207.

Hatzakis, M., Allen, C., Haselkorn, M., Anderson, S., Nichol, P., Lai, C., & Haselkorn, J. (2006). Use of medical informatics for management of multiple sclerosis using a chronic-care model. *Journal of Rehabilitation Research and Development, 43*(1), 1–16. doi:10.1682/JRRD.2004.10.0135 PMID:16847767.

Hawkins, J., & Li, J. (2001). *A system for evaluating inpatient care cost-efficiency in hospital.* Retrieved December 18, 2012, 2012 from http://www.ncbi.nlm.nih.gov/pmc/articles/PMC2243448/pdf/procamiasymp00002-0408.pdf

Hay, D., Varga-Toth, J., & Hines, E. (2006). Frontline health care in Canada: Innovations in delivering services to vulnerable populations. *Canadian Policy Research Networks.* Retrieved from http://www.frontlinehealth.ca/pdfs/CPRNResearchReport.pdf

Haynes, B., & Haines, A. (1998). Barriers and bridges to evidence based clinical practice. *British Medical Journal*, *317*, 273. doi:10.1136/bmj.317.7153.273 PMID:9677226.

Haynes, R. B., Ackloo, E., Sahota, N., McDonald, H. P., & Yao, X. (2008). Interventions for enhancing medication adherence[review]. *Cochrane Database of Systematic Reviews*, *2*(2), 1–127.

Hayrinen, K., Saranto, K., & Nykanen, P. (2008). Definition, structure, content, use and impacts of electronic records: A review of the research literature. *International Journal of Medical Informatics*, *77*(5), 291–304. doi:10.1016/j.ijmedinf.2007.09.001 PMID:17951106.

Head, A. L. (1996). *An examination of the implications for NHS information providers of staff transferring from functional to managerial roles*. Aberystwyth, UK: University College of Wales.

Health Canada. (2012). *Household food insecurity in Canada in 2007-2008: Key statistics and graphics*. Retrieved September 10, 2012, from http://www.hc-sc.gc.ca/fn-an/surveill/nutrition/commun/insecurit/key-stats-cles-2007-2008-eng.php

Health Council of Canada. (2011). *Progress report 2011: Health care renewal in Canada*. Toronto, Canada: HCC.

Health Level 7. (2006). *Health level 7*. Retrieved June 28th 2007, from http://www.HL7.org

Hébert, M. A., Korabek, B., & Scott, R. E. (2006). Moving research into practice: A decision framework for integrating home telehealth into chronic illness care. *International Journal of Medical Informatics*, *75*, 786–794. doi:10.1016/j.ijmedinf.2006.05.041 PMID:16872892.

Hébert, R., Dubios, M., Wolfson, C., Chambers, L., & Cohen, C. (2001). Factors associated with long-term institutionalization of older people with dementia: Data from the Canadian study of health and aging. *Journal of Gerontology*, *56*(11), 693–699.

Heller, F. P., Drenth, P., Koopman, P., & Rus, V. (1988). *Decisions in organizations: A three county comparative study*. London: Sage.

Hellström, L., Waern, K., Montelius, E., Åstrand, B., Rydberg, T., & Petersson, G. (2009). Physicians' attitudes towards eprescribing – Evaluation of a Swedish full-scale implementation. *BMC Medical Informatics and Decision Making*, *9*, 37. doi:10.1186/1472-6947-9-37 PMID:19664219.

Hersh, W. (2004). Health care information technology: Progress and barriers. *Journal of the American Medical Association*, *292*(18), 2273–2274. doi:10.1001/jama.292.18.2273 PMID:15536117.

Hersh, W., Helfand, M., Wallace, J., Kraemer, D., Patterson, P., Shapiro, S., & Greenlick, M. (2002). A systematic review of the efficacy of telemedicine for making diagnostic and management decisions. *Journal of Telemedicine and Telecare*, *8*, 197–209. doi:10.1258/135763302320272167 PMID:12217102.

Heubusch, K. (2008). IT standards for PHRs: Are PHRs ready for standards? Are standards ready for PHRs? *Journal of American Health Information Management Association*, *79*(6), 31–36. PMID:18604973.

Hew, K. F., & Cheung, W. S. (2010). Higher-level knowledge construction in asynchronous online discussions: An analysis of group size, duration of online discussion, and student facilitation techniques. *Instructional Science*, *39*(3), 303–319. doi:10.1007/s11251-010-9129-2.

Hider, P. (2002). *Electronic prescribing, a critical appraisal of the literature*. Retrieved 29 December 2012 from http://www.otago.ac.nz/christchurch/otago014044.pdf

Higgs, G., & Gould, M. (2001). Is there a role for GIS in the 'new NHS'? *Health & Place*, *7*, 247–259. doi:10.1016/S1353-8292(01)00014-4 PMID:11439259.

Hillestad, R., Bigelow, J., & Bower, A. (2005). Can electronic medical record systems transform health care? Potential health benefits, savings, and costs. *Health Affairs*, *24*, 1103–1117. doi:10.1377/hlthaff.24.5.1103 PMID:16162551.

Hirzalla, F., van Zoonen, L., & de Ridder, J. (2011). Internet use and political participation: Reflections on the mobilization/normalization controversy. *The Information Society*, *27*, 1–15. doi:10.1080/01972243.2011.534360.

HL7. (2012), *Press release: HL7 standards soon to be free of charge.* Retrieved 14 September 2012 from http://www.hl7.org/documentcenter/public_temp_BAC62A60-1C23-BA17-0C72ECEC786D7A54/pressreleases/HL7_PRESS_20120904.pdf

Hogan, S., & Kissam, S. (2010). Measuring meaningful use. *Health Affairs, 29*(4), 601–606. doi:10.1377/hlthaff.2009.1023 PMID:20368588.

Holt, C. (2011). Emerging technologies: Web 2.0. *Health Information Management Journal, 40*(1), 33–35.

Honeyman, A., Cox, B., & Fisher, B. (2005). Potential impacts of patients access to their electronic records. *Informatics in Primary Care, 13,* 55–60. PMID:15949176.

Hsu, C., Tseng, K. C., & Chuang, Y. (2011). Predictors of future use of telehomecare health services by middle-aged people in Taiwan. *Journal of Social Behavior and Personality, 39*(9), 1252–1262. doi:10.2224/sbp.2011.39.9.1251.

Huczynski, A., & Buchanan, D. (2001). *Organizational behaviour: An introductory text* (4th ed.). Englewood Cliffs, NJ: Prentice Hall.

Hu, M., Pavlicek, W., Liu, P. T., Zhang, M., Langer, S. G., Wang, S., & Wu, T. T. (2011). Informatics in radiology: Efficiency metrics for imaging device productivity. *Radiographics, 31*(2), 603–616. doi:10.1148/rg.312105714 PMID:21257928.

Hunt, D., Haynes, R., Hanna, S., & Smith, K. (1998). Effects of computer-based clinical decision support systems on physician performance and patient outcome. *Journal of the American Medical Association, 280*(15), 1339–1346. doi:10.1001/jama.280.15.1339 PMID:9794315.

Hutt, E., Ecord, M., Eilertsen, T., Fredrickson, E., & Kramer, A. (2002). Precipitants of emergency room visits and acute hospitalization in short-stay medicare nursing home residents. *Journal of the American Geriatrics Society, 50,* 223–229. doi:10.1046/j.1532-5415.2002.50052.x PMID:12028202.

Iakovidis, I. (1998). Towards personal health record: Current situation, obstacles and trends in implementation of electronic healthcare records in Europe. *International Journal of Medical Informatics, 52*(123), 105–117. doi:10.1016/S1386-5056(98)00129-4 PMID:9848407.

Iakovidis, I. (2000). Towards a health telematics infrastructure in the European Union. In *Information technology strategies from US and the European Union: Transferring research to practice for healthcare improvement.* Amsterdam: IOS Press.

IDIKA. (2011). *Implementation and support of the national e-prescription system.* Retrieved 12 September 2012 from http://www.idika.gr/diabouleuseis/222-04-08-2011-26

IDIKA. (2012). *The Greek e-prescription system is the larger online system in Greece.* Retrieved 14 September 2012 from http://www.idika.gr/files/deltiatypou/deltio_typoy__31.08.12.pdf

IDIKA. (2012). *e-Prescription enterprise information bus presentation.* Retrieved 14 September 2012 from http://www.idika.gr/files/%20%CE%BC%CE%B7%CF%87%CE%B1%CE%BD%CE%B9%CF%83%CE%BC%CE%BF%CF%8D%20%CE%97%CE%9A%CE%95%CE%A3%2014-3-2012.pdf

IEEE-USA. (2009). *Interoperability for the national health information network.* Retrieved 30 December 2012 from http://www.ieeeusa.org/policy/positions/NHINInteroperability1109.pdf

Imhoff, M., Webb, A., & Goldschmidt, A. (2001). Health informatics. *Intensive Care Medicine, 27,* 179–186. PMID:11280631.

Innvær, S. (2009). The use of evidence in public governmental reports on health policy: An analysis of 17 Norwegian official reports (NOU). *BMC Health Services Research, 9*(1), 177. doi:10.1186/1472-6963-9-177 PMID:19785760.

Innvaer, S., Vist, G., Trommald, M., & Oxman, A. (2002). Health policy-makers' perceptions of their use of evidence: A systematic review. *Journal of Health Services Research & Policy*, *7*(4), 239–244. doi:10.1258/135581902320432778 PMID:12425783.

Institute of Electrical & Electronics Engineers. (1990). *IEEE standard computer dictionary: A compilation of IEEE standard computer glossaries*. New York: IEEE.

Institute of Medicine. (2000). *To err is human: Building a safer health system*. Washington, DC: National Academy Press.

Institute of Medicine. (2001). *Crossing the quality chasm: A new health system for the 21st century*. Retrieved 31 December 2012 from http://iom.edu/Reports/2001/Crossing-the-Quality-Chasm-A-New-Health-System-for-the-21st-Century.aspx

Interoperability Solutions for European Public Administrations – ISA. (2011). *European interoperability framework (EIF) towards interoperability for European public services*. Retrieved 10 September 2012 from http://ec.europa.eu/isa/documents/eif_brochure_2011.pdf

Intrator, O., Castle, N., & Mor, V. (1999). Facility characteristics associated with hospitalization of nursing home residents: Results of a national study. *Medical Care*, *37*(3), 228–237. doi:10.1097/00005650-199903000-00003 PMID:10098567.

Intrator, O., Zinn, J., & Mor, V. (2004). Nursing home characteristics and potentially preventable hospitalizations of long-stay residents. *Journal of the American Geriatrics Society*, *52*(10), 1–7. doi:10.1111/j.1532-5415.2004.52469.x PMID:14687307.

Isabel Health Care. (2012). *Home*. Retrieved 07 05, 2012, from www.isabelhealthcare.com/home/default

Jarvenpaa, S. L., & Majchrzak, A. (2010). Vigilant interaction in knowledge collaboration: Challenges of online user participation under ambivalence. *Information Systems Research*, *21*(4), 773–784. doi:10.1287/isre.1100.0320.

Jensen, P., Jensen, L., & Brunak, S. (2012). Mining electronic health records: Towards better research applications and clinical care. *National Review*, *13*, 395–405. doi:10.1038/nrg3208 PMID:22549152.

Johnson, J. R. (1991). No excuses performance appraisals. *Harvard Business Review*, *69*(1), 188.

Johnson, L. M., Richards, J., Pink, G. H., & Campbell, L. (1998). *Case mix tools for decision making in healthcare*. Ottawa, Canada: Canadian Institute for Health Information.

Joseph, D., Griffin, M., Hall, R., & Sullivan, E. (2001). Peer coaching: An intervention for individuals struggling with diabetes. *The Diabetes Educator*, *27*, 703–710. doi:10.1177/014572170102700511 PMID:12212020.

Joyce, K. (2009). To me it's just another tool to help understand the evidence: Public health decision-makers' perceptions of the value of geographical information systems (GIS). *Health & Place*, *15*, 831–840. doi:10.1016/j.healthplace.2009.01.004.

Kadane, J. B. (2005). Bayesian methods for health-related decision making. *Statistics in Medicine*, *24*(4), 563–567. doi:10.1002/sim.2036 PMID:15678444.

Kaelber, D., & Pan, E. (2008). The value of personal health record (PHR) systems. In *Proceedings of AMIA Annual Symposium* (pp. 343-347). AMIA.

Kaelber, D., Jha, A., Johnston, D., Middleton, B., & Bates, D. (2008). A research agenda for personal health records. *Journal of the American Informatics Association, 15*(6), 729-736. doi:10.1197/jamia. M2547

Kahn, J., Aulakh, V., & Bosworth, A. (2009). What it takes: Characteristics of the ideal personal health record. *Health Affairs*, *28*(2), 369–376. doi:10.1377/hlthaff.28.2.369 PMID:19275992.

Kaiser, H. J. (2012). Family foundation. In *Health Care Costs: A Primer Key Information on Health Care Costs and their Impact*. The Henry J. Kaiser Family Foundation. Retrieved 31 December 2012 from http://www.kff.org/insurance/upload/7670-03.pdf

Karsh, B., Weinger, M., Abbott, P., & Wears, R. (2010). Health information technology: Fallacies and sober realities. *Journal of the American Medical Informatics Association*, *17*, 617–623. doi:10.1136/jamia.2010.005637 PMID:20962121.

Kaufman, D. R., Patel, V. L., Hilliman, C., Morin, P. C., Pevzner, J., Weinstock, R. S., & Starren, J. (2003). Usability in the real world: Assessing medical information technologies in patients' homes. *Journal of Biomedical Informatics*, *36*(1-2), 45–60. doi:10.1016/S1532-0464(03)00056-X PMID:14552846.

Kaushal, R., Jha, A. K., Franz, C., Glaser, J., Shetty, K. D., & Jaggi, T. et al. (2006). Return on investment for a computerized physician order entry system. *Journal of the American Medical Informatics Association*, *13*(3), 261–266. doi:10.1197/jamia.M1984 PMID:16501178.

Kearns, R. A., & Barnett, J. R. (1999). Auckland's starship enterprise: Placing metaphor in a children's hospital. In Williams, A. (Ed.), *Therapeutic landscapes: The dynamic between place and wellness* (pp. 169–200). Lanham, MD: University Press of America Inc..

Kerr, K. (2008). Metadata repositories in health care. *Health Care and Informatics Review Online*, *12*(3), 37–44.

Keshavjee, K., Manji, A., Singh, B., & Pairaudeau, N. (2009). Failure of electronic medical records in Canada: A failure of policy or a failure of technology? In McDaniel, J. G. (Ed.), *Advances in Information Technology and Communication in Health* (pp. 107–114). Amsterdam: IOS Press BV.

Keyhani, S., Wang, S., Hebert, P., Carpenter, D., & Anderson, G. (2010). US pharmaceutical innovation in an international context. *American Journal of Public Health*, *100*(6), 1075–1080. doi:10.2105/AJPH.2009.178491 PMID:20403883.

Kharrazi, H., Chisholm, R., VanNasdale, D., & Thompson, B. (2012). Mobile personal health records: An evaluation of features and functionality. *International Journal of Medical Informatics*, *81*(9), 579–593. doi:10.1016/j.ijmedinf.2012.04.007 PMID:22809779.

Kim, M., & Johnson, K. (2002). Personal health records: evaluation of functionality and utility. *Journal of the American Medical Informatics Association*, *9*(2), 171–180. doi:10.1197/jamia.M0978 PMID:11861632.

Kimura, M. (1991). *PACS, RIS, HIS - Each as a part of allied healthcare information system*.

Kissick, W. L. (1994). *Medicine's dilemmas: Infinite needs versus finite resources*. New Haven, CT: Yale University Press.

Kitson, A., Harvey, G., & McCormack, B. (1998). Enabling the implementation of evidence based practice: A conceptual framework. *Quality in Health Care*, *7*, 149–158. doi:10.1136/qshc.7.3.149 PMID:10185141.

Klein, G., & Klinger, D. (1991). Naturalistic decision making. *Human Systems IAC Gateway*, *11*(3), 16–19.

Kleinke, J. (2005). Dot-gov: Market failure and the creation of a national health information technology system. *Health Affairs*, *24*(5), 1246–1262. doi:10.1377/hlthaff.24.5.1246 PMID:16162569.

Klonoff, D. C., & True, M. W. (2009). The missing element of telemedicine for diabetes: Decision support software. *Journal of Diabetes Science and Technology*, *3*(5), 996–1001. PMID:20144411.

Knaus, W., & Draper, E. D. (1986). An evaluation of outcome from intensive care in major medical centers. *Annals of Internal Medicine*, *104*, 410–418. doi:10.7326/0003-4819-104-3-410 PMID:3946981.

Kneck, A., Klang, B., & Fagerberg, I. (2011). Learning to live with illness: experiences of persons with recent diagnoses of diabetes mellitus. *Scandinavian Journal of Caring Sciences*, *12*. doi: doi:10.1111/j.1471-6712.2010.00864.x PMID:21244458.

Kobb, R., Chumber, N.R., Brennan, D.M., & Robinowitz, T. (2008). Home telehealth: Mainstreaming what we do well. *Telemedicine and e-Health Journal*, *14*(90), 977-981.

Koch, S. (2006). Home telehealth–Current state and future trends. *International Journal of Medical Informatics*, *75*(8), 565–576. doi:10.1016/j.ijmedinf.2005.09.002 PMID:16298545.

Kohn, L. T., Corrigan, J. M., & Donaldson, M. S. (2000). *To err is human, building a safer health system*. Washington, DC: National Academy Press.

Kolbitsch, J., & Maurer, H. (2006). The transformation of the web: How emerging communities shape the information we consume. *Journal of Universal Computer Science*, *12*(2), 187–213.

Koppel, R., Metlay, J., & Cohen, A. (2005). Role of computerized physician order entry systems in facilitating medical errors. *Journal of the American Medical Association, 293*, 1197–1203. doi:10.1001/jama.293.10.1197 PMID:15755942.

Korica, P., Maurer, H., & Schinagl, W. (2006). *The growing importance of e-communities on the web*. Paper presented at IADIS International Conference on Web Based Communities. San Sebastian, Spain.

Kovner, A. R., & Rundall, T. G. (2006). Evidence-based management reconsidered. *Frontiers of Health Services Management, 22*(3), 3–22. PMID:16604900.

KPMG International Cooperative. (2012). *Accelerating innovation: The power of the crowd*. KPMG.

Kremer, P., & DeLiberty, T. L. (2011). Local food practices and growing potential: Mapping the case of Philadelphia. *Applied Geography (Sevenoaks, England), 31*(4), 1252–1261. doi:10.1016/j.apgeog.2011.01.007.

Krugman, P. (2011, April 22). Patients are not consumers. *New York Times*, p. A23.

Kruskal, J. B., Anderson, S., Yam, C. S., & Sosna, J. (2009). Strategies for establishing a comprehensive quality and performance improvement program in a radiology department. *Radiographics, 29*(2), 315–329. doi:10.1148/rg.292085090 PMID:19168762.

Kukafka, R., & Yasnoff, W. A. (2007). Public health informatics. *Journal of Biomedical Informatics, 40*, 365–369. doi:10.1016/j.jbi.2007.07.005 PMID:17656158.

Kulkarni, G. (2005). Diagnostic decision support in the ED: Practical considerations. *Emergency Medicine Journal, 22*(6), 462. PMID:15911967.

Kwon, Y.-S., Kim, S.-W., & Park, S. (2009). An analysis of information diffusion in the blogworld. In J. Wang & S. Zhou (Eds.), *CNIKM '09 Proceedings of the 1st ACM International Workshop on Complex Networks meet Information and Knowledge Management* (pp. 27-30). New York: ACM.

Labadie, J.-F. (2005). Inter-regional front-line services knowledge brokering alliance. In *Proceedings of the Fourth Annual National Knowledge Brokering Workhop* (p. 8). Retrieved from http://www.cfhi-fcass.ca/migrated/pdf/event_reports/National_Workshop_Report_2005_e.pdf

Lahey, W. (2012, November 29). Collaboration vital to better health care, improved regulation. *The Chronicle Herald*.

Lahey, W., & Currie, R. (2005). Regulatory and medico-legal barriers to interprofessional practice. *Journal of Interprofessional Care, 19*(S1), 197–223. doi:10.1080/13561820500083188 PMID:16096156.

Lau, F., Kuziemsky, C., Price, M., & Gardner, J. (2010). A review on systematic reviews of health information system studies. *Journal of the American Medical Informatics Association, 17*(6), 637–645. doi:10.1136/jamia.2010.004838 PMID:20962125.

Laurent, S. (2002). Rural Canada: Access to health care. *Government of Canada Economics Division*. Retrieved from http://dsp-psd.pwgsc.gc.ca/Collection-R/LoPBdP/BP/prb0245-e.htm#2Age

Lawrence, P. (2005). Preparing a cultural strategy for PACS. *Radiology Management, 27*(1), 21–29. PMID:15794374.

Lee, R., & Garvin, T. (2003). Moving from information transfer to information exchange in health and health care. *Social Science & Medicine, 56*, 449–464. doi:10.1016/S0277-9536(02)00045-X PMID:12570966.

Lehrer, J. (2009). The Predictions of Dopamine. In *How We Decide* (pp. 28–56). New York: Houghton Mifflin Harcourt Publishing Co..

Leon, D. A. (2011). Trends in European life expectancy: A salutary view. *International Journal of Epidemiology, 40*, 271–277. Retrieved 31 December 2012 from http://ije.oxfordjournals.org/content/early/2011/03/16/ije.dyr061.full

Lewis, S., Barer, M. L., Sanmartin, C., Sheps, S., Shortt, S. E., & McDonald, P. W. (2000). Ending waiting-list mismanagement: Principles and practice. *Canadian Medical Association Journal, 162*, 1297–1300. PMID:10813011.

Liddy, C., Dusseault, J. J., Dahrouge, S., Hogg, W., Lemelin, J., & Humbert, J. (2008). Telehomecare for patients with multiple chronic illnesses. *Canadian Family Physician Medecin de Famille Canadien, 54*, 58–65. PMID:18208957.

Liederman, E., & Morefield, C. (2003). Web messaging: a new tool for patient-physician communication. *Journal of the American Medical Informatics Association, 10*, 260–270. doi:10.1197/jamia.M1259 PMID:12626378.

Lin, C., Lin, I., & Roan, J. (2012). Barriers to physicians' adoption of healthcare information technology: An empirical study on multiple hospitals. *Journal of Medical Systems*, *36*(3), 1965–1977. doi:10.1007/s10916-011-9656-7 PMID:21336605.

Liu, P., Arnold, M., Belenkie, I., Howlett, J., Huckell, V., & Ignazewski, A. et al. (2001). The 2001 Canadian cardiovascular society consensus guideline update for the management and prevention of heart failure. *The Canadian Journal of Cardiology*, *17*(Suppl E), 5E–25E. PMID:11773943.

Loh, C., Cobb, S., & Johnson, C. (2009). Potential and actual accessibility to hospital and hospital services in northeast Florida. *Southeastern Geographer*, *49*(2), 171–184. doi:10.1353/sgo.0.0043.

London Development Agency. (2006). *Healthy and sustainable food for London: The mayor's food strategy*. London: London Development Agency.

Longhurst, C., & Hahn, J. (2005). Clinical decision-support systems in pediatrics. *COCIT Newsletter, 10*.

Lorenzo, V., Giesen, D., Jansen, P., & Klokgieters, K. (2010). *Business models for ehealth final report*. Retrieved 5 September 2012 from http://ec.europa.eu/information_society/activities/health/docs/studies/business_model/business_models_eHealth_report.pdf

Lown, B., Rosen, J., & Marttila, J. (2011). An agenda for improving compassionate care: A survey shows about half of patients say such care is missing. *Health Affairs*, *30*(9), 1772–1778. doi:10.1377/hlthaff.2011.0539 PMID:21900669.

Lumpkin, J. (2007). Archimedes: A bold step into the future. *Health Affairs*, *26*(2), w137–w139. doi:10.1377/hlthaff.26.2.w137 PMID:17259195.

MacDonald, J. M. (2011). *The information sharing behaviour of health service managers: A three-part study*. (Unpublished PhD Dissertation). Sheffield, UK: University of Sheffield Information School.

MacDonald, J., Bath, P., & Booth, A. (2008). Healthcare services managers: What information do they need and use? *Evidence Based Library and Information Practice*, *3*(3), 18–38.

MacPherson, S. L., Joseph, D., & Sullivan, E. (2004). The benefits of peer support with diabetes. *Nursing Forum*, *39*(4), 5-12. Retrieved September 10, 2012, from http://www.ncbi.nlm.nih.gov/pubmed/15700481

Magnusson, L., Hanson, E., & Borg, M. (2004). A literature review study of information and communication technology as a support for frail older people living at home and their family carers. *Technology and Disability*, *16*(4), 223–235.

Magrabi, F., Lovell, N. H., Huynh, K., & Celler, B. G. (2001). *Home telecare: System architecture to support chronic disease management*. Paper presented at the 23rd Annual International Conference of the IEEE Engineering in Medicine and Biology Society. Istanbul, Turkey.

Maloney, F., & Wright, A. (2010). USB-based personal health records: an analysis of features and functionality. *International Journal of Medical Informatics*, *79*, 97–111. doi:10.1016/j.ijmedinf.2009.11.005 PMID:20053582.

Mandl, K., Kohame, I., & Brandt, A. (1998). Electronic patient-physician communication: problems and promise. *Annals of Internal Medicine*, *129*, 495–500. doi:10.7326/0003-4819-129-6-199809150-00012 PMID:9735088.

Mandl, K., Szolovits, P., & Kohane, I. (2001). Public standards and patients' control: how to keep electronic medical records accessible but private. *British Medical Journal*, *322*(7281), 283–287. doi:10.1136/bmj.322.7281.283 PMID:11157533.

Man, E. (2005). A functional approach to appraisal and retention scheduling. *Records Management Journal*, *15*(1), 21–33. doi:10.1108/09565690510585402.

March, J., & Olsen, J. (1986). Garbage can models of decision making in organizations. In March, K., & Weissinger-Baylon, R. (Eds.), *Ambiguity and Command* (pp. 11–35). New York: Longman Inc..

Markle Connecting for Health. (2003). *Americans want benefits of personal health records.* New York: Markle Foundation.

Markle Connecting for Health. (2004). *Connecting Americans to their healthcaare: Final report of the working group on policies for electronic information sharing between doctors and patients.* New York: Markle Foundation.

Markle Connecting for Health. (2006). *Survey finds Americans want electronic personal health information to improve own health care.* New York: Markle Foundation.

Martz, B., Zhang, X., & Ozanich, G. (2007). Information systems and healthcare XIV: Developing an integrative health informatics. *Communications of AIS, 19.*

Matern, R., & Kim, S. (2012). *Who's hungry faces of hunger: 2012 profile of hunger in the GTA.* Toronto, Canada: Daily Bread Food Bank.

Mawani, A. (2011). *Can we get better for less: Value for money in Canadian health care.* Retrieved December 2, 2011 from http://www.cga-canada.org/en-ca/ResearchReports/ca_rep_2011-04_healthcare.pdf

Mayan, M. (2009). *Essential of qualitative inquiry.* Walnut Creek, CA: Left Coast Press.

Mbananga, N., & Sekokotla, D. (2002). *The utilisation of health management information in Mpumalanga Province.* Retrieved from http://www. hst. org. za/research

McCally, M., Haines, A., Fein, O., Addington, W., Lawrence, R., & Cassel, C. (1998). Poverty and ill health: Physicians can and should make a difference. *Annals of Internal Medicine, 129*(9), 726–733. doi:10.7326/0003-4819-129-9-199811010-00009 PMID:9841606.

McClure, M., & Hinshaw, A. S. (Eds.). (2002). *Magnet hospitals revisited: Attraction and retention of professional nurses.* Washington, DC: American Nurses Publishing.

McCormack, B., Kitson, A., Harvey, G., Rycroft-Malone, J., Titchen, A., & Seers, K. (2002). Getting evidence into practice: The meaning of 'context'. *Journal of Advanced Nursing, 38*(1), 94–104. doi:10.1046/j.1365-2648.2002.02150.x PMID:11895535.

McCray, A. (2005). Promoting health literacy. *Journal of the American Medical Informatics Association, 12,* 153–163. PMID:15561782.

McGregor, D. (1972). An uneasy look at performance appraisal. *Harvard Business Review, 50*(5), 133.

McPake, B., Kumaranayake, L., & Normand, C. (2006). *Health economics: An international perspective.* New York, NY: Routledge Publishing.

McShane, S. L. (2006). *Canadian organizational behaviour* (6th ed.). New York: McGraw-Hill Ryerson.

MEDCOM. (2012). *eHealth in Denmark eHealth as a part of a coherent Danish health care system.* Retrieved 9 September 2012 from http://www.medcom.dk/dwn5350

Menachemi, N., & Collum, T. (2011). Benefits and drawbacks of electronic health record systems. *Risk Management and Healthcare Policy, 4,* 47–55. doi:10.2147/RMHP.S12985 PMID:22312227.

Mendes, W. (2008). Implementing social and environmental policies in cities: The case of food policy in Vancouver, Canada. *International Journal of Urban and Regional Research, 32*(4), 942–967. doi:10.1111/j.1468-2427.2008.00814.x.

Mensink, N. M. (2004). *Facilitating the development of a graduate-level university program using processes and principles of adult education.* (Unpublished MAdEd thesis). St. Francis Xavier University, Antigonish, Canada.

Mensink, N., & Paterson, G. (2010). The evolution and uptake of a drug information system: The case of a small Canadian province. *Studies in Health Technology and Informatics, 160*(Pt 1), 141–145. PMID:20841666.

Menzies, D., Lewis, M., & Oxlade, O. (2008). Cost for tuberculosis care in Canada. *Canadian Journal of Public Health, 5*(99), 391–396.

Mettler, T., & Vimarlund, V. (2009). Understanding business intelligence in the context of health care. *Health Informatics Journal, 15,* 254–264. doi:10.1177/1460458209337446 PMID:19713399.

Metzger, J., & Turisco, F. (2001). Computerized physician order entry: A look at the vendor marketplace and getting started. *The Leapfrog Group*. Retrieved from http://www.leapfroggroup.org/media/file/Leapfrog-CPO_Guide.pdf

Meyer, E. T., & Schroeder, R. (2009). The world wide web of research and access to knowledge. *Knowledge Management Research & Practice*, 7(3), 218–233. doi:10.1057/kmrp.2009.13.

Meyer, H. H., Kay, E., & French, J. R. P. (1989). Split roles in performance appraisal. *Harvard Business Review*, 67(1), 26.

Middleton, B., Hammond, W., Brennan, P., & Cooper, G. (2005). Accelerating U.S. EHR adoption: How to get there from here: Recommendations based on the 2004 ACMI retreat. *Journal of the American Medical Informatics Association*, 12, 13–19. doi:10.1197/jamia.M1669 PMID:15492028.

Milenković, A., Otto, C., & Jovanov, E. (2006). Wireless sensor network for personal health monitoring: Issues and implementation. *Computer Communications*, 29, 2521–2533. doi:10.1016/j.comcom.2006.02.011.

Miles, A. (2009). Of butterflies and wolves: enacting lupus transformations on the internet. *Anthropology & Medicine*, 16(1), 1–12. doi:10.1080/13648470802425906.

Miller, R. (2009). Computer-assisted diagnostic decision support: History, challenges and possible paths forward. *Advances in Health Science Education*, 14(Suppl 1), 89–106. doi:10.1007/s10459-009-9186-y PMID:19672686.

Miller, R., West, C., Brown, T., Sim, I., & Ganchoff, C. (2005). The value of electronic health records in solo or small group practices. *Health Affairs*, 24, 1127–1137. doi:10.1377/hlthaff.24.5.1127 PMID:16162555.

Ministry of Health and Long Term Care. (1998). *Access to quality health care in rural and northern Ontario*. Retrieved from https://ospace.scholarsportal.info/bitstream/1873/7175/1/10276872.pdf

Ministry of Health and Long Term Care. (2010, July 1). *LTCH level-of-care per diem funding policy*. Ottawa, Canada: Ministry of Health and Long Term Care.

Ministry of Health and Long Term Care. (2012, March). *Long term care home financial policy*. Ottawa, Canada: Ministry of Health and Long Term Care.

Ministry of Health and Long-Term Care (MOHLTC). (2012). *Health analyst's toolkit*. December 18, 2012 from http://www.health.gov.on.ca/english/providers/pub/healthanalytics/health_toolkit/health_toolkit.pdf

Ministry of Health and Long-Term Care (MOHLTC). (2012). *Ontario case costing guide. Data Standards Unit, Health Data Branch*. MOHLTC.

Mirkin, B., & Weinberger, M. B. (2001). *The demography of population ageing, population ageing and living arrangements of, older persons: Critical issues and policy responses*. Retrieved 31 December 2012 from http://www.un.org/esa/population/publications/bulletin42_43/weinbergermirkin.pdf

Mitchell, R. (2010). *Patient-centred e-health: Helping to improve quality of care through e-health*. Retrieved 30 December 2012 from http://www.healthfirsteurope.org/uploads/Modules/Newsroom/HFE-EqualityInE-health_BROCH_LayA_V23_spreads-2.pdf

Moahi, K. H. (2000). *A study of the information behavior of health care planners, managers and administrators in Botswana and implications for the design of a national health information system(NHIS)*. (Unpublished PhD dissertation). University of Pittsburgh, Pittsburgh, PA.

Mohaghan, V., & Cooke, J. (2004). The health and social care context. In Walton, G., & Andrew, B. (Eds.), *Exploiting knowledge in health services* (p. 16). London: Facet Publishing.

MOHLTC. (2006). *Ontario guide to case costing*. MOHLTC.

MOHLTC. (2010). *Externally-informed annual health systems trends report* (3rd ed.). Academic Press.

Mo, P. K. H., & Coulson, N. S. (2010). Empowering processes in online support groups among people living with HIV/AIDS: A comparative analysis of 'lurkers' and 'posters'. *Computers in Human Behavior*, 26, 1183–1193. doi:10.1016/j.chb.2010.03.028.

Morrison, K. T., Nelson, T. A., & Ostry, A. S. (2011). Mapping spatial variation in food consumption. *Applied Geography (Sevenoaks, England), 31*, 1262–1267. doi:10.1016/j.apgeog.2010.11.020.

Moss, L. J. (2000). *Perceptions of meeting effectiveness in the capital health region.* (Unpublished MA thesis). Royal Roads University, Victoria, Canada.

MoU. (2010). *Memorandum of understanding between the European Union and the United States related to information and communication technologies for health activities.* Retrieved 14 September 2012 from http://ec.europa.eu/information_society/newsroom/cf/document.cfm?action=display&doc_id=751

Mullner, R. M., Chung, K., Croke, K. G., & Mensah, E. K. (2004). Geographic information systems in public health and medicine. *Journal of Medical Systems, 28*(3), 215–221. doi:10.1023/B:JOMS.0000032972.29060.dd PMID:15446613.

Mulvaney, J. (2002). The case for RIS/PACS integration. *Radiology Management, 24*(3), 24–29. PMID:12080929.

Murray, G., Hannam, R., & Wong, J. (2004). *Case costing in Ontario hospitals: What makes for success.* Toronto, Canada: The Change Foundation.

Mykkänen, J. A., & Tuomainen, M. P. (2006). An evaluation and selection framework for interoperability standards. *Information and Software Technology, 50*(3), 176–197. doi:10.1016/j.infsof.2006.12.001.

Nagy, P. G., Warnock, M. J., Daly, M., Toland, C., Meenan, C. D., & Mezrich, R. S. (2009). Informatics in radiology: Automated web-based graphical dashboard for radiology operational business intelligence. *Radiographics, 29*(7), 1897–1906. doi:10.1148/rg.297095701 PMID:19734469.

Nambisan, P., & Nambisan, S. (2009). Models of consumer value cocreation in health care. *Health Care Management Review, 34*(4), 344–354. doi:10.1097/HMR.0b013e3181abd528 PMID:19858919.

National Institutes of Health National Center for Research Resources. (2006). *Electronic health records overview.* Retrieved April 10, 2010, from http://www.ncrr.nih.gov/publications/informatics/ehr.pdf

Nettleton, S., Burrows, R., & O'Malley, L. (2005). The mundane realities of the everyday lay use of the Internet for health, and their consequences for media convergence. *Sociology of Health & Illness, 27*(7), 972–992. doi:10.1111/j.1467-9566.2005.00466.x PMID:16313525.

Neuhauser, L., & Kreps, G. L. (2003). Rethinking communication in the e-health era. *Journal of Health Psychology, 8*(1), 7–23. Retrieved 30 December 2012 from http://www.uk.sagepub.com/ciel/study/articles/Ch10_Article.pdf

Newhouse, I., Heckman, G., Harrison, D., D'Elia, T., Kaasalainen, S., Strachan, P., & Demers, C. (2012). Barriers to the management of heart failure in Ontario long term care homes: An interprofessional perspective. *Journal of Research in Interprofessional Practice and Education, 2*(3).

Newman, M. W., Lauterbach, D., Munson, S. A., Resnick, P., & Morris, M. E. (2011). It's not that I don't have problems, I'm just not putting them on Facebook: Challenges and opportunities in using online social networks for health. In *Proceedings of the ACM 2011 Conference on Computer Supported Cooperative Work* (pp. 341-350). Hangzhou, China: ACM.

NHMRC. (2010). *Australian guidelines for the prevention and control of infection in healthcare.* Commonwealth of Australia. Retrieved 30 December 2012 from http://www.nhmrc.gov.au/_files_nhmrc/publications/attachments/cd33_complete.pdf

NHS Connecting for Health. (2012). *HealthSpace.* Retrieved 12, 16, 2012, from http://www.connecting-forhealth.nhs.uk/systemsandservices/healthspace

Niedźwiedzka, B. (2003). A proposed general model of information behaviour. *Information Research, 9*(1), Paper 164.

Nor, F. M., Razak, N. A., & Aziz, J. (2010). E-learning: Analysis of online discussion forums in promoting knowledge construction through collaborative learning. *WSEAS Transactions on Communications, 9*(1), 53–62.

Norman, G. (2009). Dual processing and diagnostic error. *Advances in Health Science Education, 14*(Suppl 1), 37–39. doi:10.1007/s10459-009-9179-x.

Norman, G., & Eva, K. (2010). Diagnostic error and reasoning. *Medical Education, 44*(1), 94–100. doi:10.1111/j.1365-2923.2009.03507.x PMID:20078760.

Norman, G., Young, M., & Brooks, L. (2007). Non-analytical models of clinical reasoning: The role of experience. *Medical Education, 41*(12), 1140–1145. doi:doi:10.1111/j.1365-2923.2007.02914.x PMID:18004990.

Norris, A. C. (2002). Current trends and challenges in health informatics. *Health Informatics Journal, 8*, 205–213. doi:10.1177/146045820200800407.

Norris, D., Mason, J., & Lefrere, P. (2003). *Transforming e-knowledge: A revolution in the sharing of knowledge.* Ann Arbor, MI: Society for College and University Planning.

Nourizadeh, S., Deroussent, C., Song, Y. Q., & Thomesse, J. P. (2009). A distributed elderly healthcare system. *Inria.* Retrieved from http://hal.inria.fr/docs/00/43/12/02/PDF/A_Distributed_Elderly_healthcare_System.pdf

Nova Scotia Department of Health and Wellness. (2012). *Personal health information act.* Retrieved 12, 16, 2012, from https://www.gov.ns.ca/dhw/phia/

Nova Scotia Department of Health and Wellness. (2012,). *Overview and discussion paper, health services and insurance act.* Retrieved 12, 16, 2012, from http://www.gov.ns.ca/health/hsil/doc/OverviewDiscussionDocument.pdf

Nykiforuk, C. I., & Flaman, L. M. (2008). *Exploring the utilization of geographic information systems in health promotion and public health.* Edmonton, Canada: Centre for Health Promotion Studies, School of Public Health, University of Alberta.

O'Brien-Pallas, L. (2002). Where to from here? *Canadian Journal of Nursing Research, 33*(4), 3–14. PMID:11998195.

O'Grady, L. A., Witteman, H., & Wathen, C. N. (2008). The experiential health information processing model: Supporting collaborative web-based patient education. *BMC Medical Informatics and Decision Making, 8*, 58. doi:10.1186/1472-6947-8-58 PMID:19087353.

OASIS. (2005). *XACML - eXtensible access control markup language v2.0 normative XACML 2.0 documents.* Retrieved 30 December 2012 from http://docs.oasis-open.org/xacml/2.0/XACML-2.0-OS-NORMATIVE.zip

OASIS. (2005). *SAML - Security assertion markup language v2.0, the complete SAML v2.0 OASIS standard set.* Organization for the Advancement of Structured Information Standards – OASIS.

O'Connor, A. M., Stacey, D., & Jacobsen, M. J. (2011). *Ottawa decision support tutorial: Improving practitioners' decision support skills Ottawa hospital research institute: Patient decision aids.* Academic Press.

OECD Health Data. (2010). Retrieved from www.oecd.org/health/healthdata

OECD. (2010). *OECD health policy studies improving health sector efficiency: The role of information and communication technologies.* Paris: Organisation for Economic Co-operation and Development. Retrieved 1 September 2012 from http://www.oecd.org/els/health-policiesanddata/improvinghealthsectorefficiency.htm

OECD. (2011). *Help wanted? Providing and paying for long-term care.* Paris, France: OECD. Retrieved from www.oecd.org/health/longtermcare

OECD. (2011). *OECD-NSF workshop building a smarter health and wellness.* Retrieved 14 September from http://www.oecd.org/Internet/Interneteconomy/47039222.pdf

Office of the Auditor General of Ontario. (2009). *Ontario's electronic health records initiative, special report.* Toronto, Canada: Office of the Auditor General of Ontario.

Official Journal of the European Union. (2006). *Directive 2006/123/EC of the European parliament and of the council of 12 December 2006 on services in the internal market* (L 376, 27/12/2006 P. 0036 - 0068). Retrieved 29 August 2012 from http://eur-lex.europa.eu/JOHtml.do?uri=OJ:L:2011:088:SOM:en:HTML

Official Journal of the European Union. (2011). *Directive 2011/24/EU of the European parliament and of the council of 9 March 2011 on the application of patients' rights in cross-border healthcare.* Retrieved 22 August 2012 from http://eur-lex.europa.eu/JOHtml.do?uri=OJ:L:2011:088:SOM:en:HTML

Oliver, A. (2008). Public-sector health-care reforms that work? A case study of the US veterans health administration. *Lancet, 371*(9619), 1211–1213. doi:10.1016/S0140-6736(08)60528-0 PMID:18395583.

Ontario Case Costing Initiative (OCCI). (2012). *About the OCCI.* Retrieved on December 18, 2012 from http://www.occp.com

Ontario Case Costing Initiative (OCCI). (2012). *OCCI costing analysis tool (CAT).* Retrieved December 18, 2012 from http://www.occp.com

Ontario Case Costing Initiative (OCCI). (2012). *Ontario case costing facilities.* Retrieved December 18, 2012 from http://www.occp.com

Ontario Health Association (OHA). (2009). *Supporting transformation: A vision for e-health human resources for Ontario.* Retrieved December 18, 2012 from http://www.oha.com/KnowledgeCentre/Library/Documents/Supporting_Transformation_FINAL.pdf

Ontario Hospital Association (OHA). (2010). *Ideas and opportunities for bending the health care cost curve: Advice for the government of Ontario.* Retrieved December 2, 2011 from http://www.ccac-ont.ca/Upload/on/General/Bending%20the%20Health%20Care%20Cost%20Curve%20(Final%20Report%20-%20April%2013,%202010).pdf

Ontario Institute for Cancer Research (OICR). (2012). *Ontario institute for cancer research.* Retrieved December 18, 2012, 2012 from http://oicr.on.ca/files/public/OICR%20Slidedeck%2010Feb12%20revised%207%20August%202012.pdf

Ontario Joint Policy and Planning Committee. (2006). *Evaluation and selection of a group and weighting methodology for adult inpatient rehabilitation care.* Reference Document RD10-10.

Ontario Ministry of Agriculture & City of Toronto Economic Development. (2002). *Food industry outlook: A study of food industry growth trends in Toronto.* Toronto, Canada: City of Toronto.

Ontario Ministry of Health and Long-Term Care. (2012). *Ontario's action plan for health care.* Retrieved from http://www.health.gov.on.ca/en/ms/ecfa/healthy_change/docs/rep_healthychange.pdf

Ontario Professional Planners Institute. (2011). *Planning for food systems in Ontario: A call to action.* Retrieved June 27, 2011, from http://www.ontarioplanners.on.ca/pdf/a_call_to_action_from_oppi_june_24_2011.pdf

OP3: One Province, One Process, One Policy. (2011). *Style guide for writers and developers of NS DHA and IWK policy documents.* Retrieved 12 16, 2012, from http://policy.nshealth.ca/Site_Published/dha9/document_render.aspx?documentRender.IdType=5&documentRender.Id=29030

Orizio, G., Schulz, P., Gasparotti, C., Caimi, L., & Gelatti, U. (2010). The world of e-patients: A content analysis of online social networks focusing on diseases. *Telemedicine and e-Health, 16*(10), 1060-1066.

Osheroff, J. A., Teich, J. M., & Middleton, B. F. et al. (2006). *A roadmap for national action on clinical decision support.* Washington, DC: American Medical Informatics Association.

Osman, M. (2004). An evaluation of the dual-process theories of reasoning. *Psychonomic Bulletin & Review, 11*(6), 988–1010. doi:10.3758/BF03196730 PMID:15875969.

Page, D. (2010, September). The two paths to PHRs. *Hospital and Health Networks Magazine.*

Pagliari, C., Detmer, D., & Singleton, P. (2007). Potential of electronic personal health records. *British Medical Journal, 335*(7615), 330–333. doi:10.1136/bmj.39279.482963.AD PMID:17703042.

Palmer, K. T., McElearney, N., & Harrington, M. (2004). Appraisal standards in occupational medicine. *Occupational Medicine, 54*(4), 218–226. doi:10.1093/occmed/kqh068 PMID:15190157.

Papp, J. (2006). *Quality management in the imaging sciences* (3rd ed.). MOSBY.

Parente, S., & McCullough, J. (2009). Health information technology and patient safety: Evidence from panel data. *Health Affairs, 28*(2), 357–360. doi:10.1377/hlthaff.28.2.357 PMID:19275990.

Park, W., Kim, J. S., Chae, Y. M., Yu, S., Kim, C., Kim, S., & Jung, S. H. (2003). Does the physician order-entry system increase the revenue of a general hospital? *Journal of Medical Informatics, 71,* 25–32. doi:10.1016/S1386-5056(03)00056-X PMID:12909155.

Paterson, G. I. (2008). *Boundary infostructures for chronic disease: Constructing infostructures to bridge communities of practice.* Saarbrücken, Germany: VDM Verlag Dr. Muller.

Pauly, M. (2011). The trade-off among quality, quantity, and cost: How to make it-if we must. *Health Affairs*, *30*(4), 574–580. doi:10.1377/hlthaff.2011.0081 PMID:21471475.

Pauly, M., Herring, B., & Song, D. (2006). Information technology and consumer search for health insurance. *International Journal of the Economics of Business*, *13*(1), 45–63. doi:10.1080/13571510500519970.

Pauly, M., & Satterthwaite, M. (1981). The pricing of primary care physicians services: A test of the role of consumer information. *The Bell Journal of Economics*, *12*(2), 488–506. doi:10.2307/3003568.

Pear, R. (2011, December 3). Health official takes parting shot at 'waste'. *New York Times*, p. A23.

Percival, J., & Hanson, J. (2006). Big brother or brave new world? Telecare and its implications for older people's independence and social inclusion. *Critical Social Policy*, *26*(4), 888–909. doi:10.1177/0261018306068480.

Perry, L., Bellchambers, H., Howie, A., Moxey, A., Parkinson, L., Capra, S., & Byles, J. (2011). Examination of the utility of the promoting action on research in health services framework for implementation of evidence based practice in residential aged care setting. *Journal of Advanced Nursing*, *67*(10), 2139–2150. doi:10.1111/j.1365-2648.2011.05655.x PMID:21535089.

Peters, C. J., Bills, N. L., Lembo, A. J., Wilkins, J. L., & Fick, G. W. (2009). Mapping potential foodsheds in New York state: A spatial model for evaluating the capacity to localize food production. *Renewable Agriculture and Food Systems*, *24*(1), 72–84. doi:10.1017/S1742170508002457.

Phinney, J., MacDonald, J. M., & Spiteri, L. (2012). *A health policy language for Nova Scotia: A Dalhousie school of information management reading course project*. Paper presented at APLA 2012: Discovering Hidden Treasures. Wolfville, Canada.

Pirtle, B., & Chandra, A. (2011). An overview of consumer perceptions and acceptance as well as barriers and potential of electronic personal health records. *American Journal of Health Sciences*.

PointClickCare. (2011). Retrieved from http://www.pointclickcare.com/solutions/solutions.php

Poley, M., Edelenbos, K., Mosseveld, M., van Wijk, M., Bakker, D., & van der Lei, J. et al. (2007). Cost consequences of implementing an electronic decision support system for ordering laboratory tests in primary care: Evidence from a controlled prospective study in The Netherlands. *Clinical Chemistry*, *53*(2), 213–219. doi:10.1373/clinchem.2006.073908 PMID:17185371.

Poon, E. G., Blumenthal, D., Jaggi, T., & Honour, M. M. (2004). Overcoming barriers to adopting and implementing computerized physician order entry systems in U.S. hospitals. *Journal of Health Affairs*, *23*(4), 184–190. doi:10.1377/hlthaff.23.4.184 PMID:15318579.

Poon, E., Blumenthal, D., Jaggi, T. H. M., Bates, D., & Kaushal, R. (2004). Overcoming bariers to adopting and impementing computerized physician order entry systems in U.S. Hospitals. *Health Affairs*, *23*(4), 184–190. doi:10.1377/hlthaff.23.4.184 PMID:15318579.

Poon, E., Jha, A., Christino, M., Honour, M., Fernandopulle, R., Middleton, B., & Kaushal, R. (2006). Assessing the level of healthcare information technology adoption in the United States: A snapshot. *BMC Medical Informatics and Decision Making*, *6*(1). doi:10.1186/1472-6947-6-1 PMID:16396679.

Pothukuchi, K., & Kaufman, J. L. (1999). Placing the food system on the urban agenda: The role of municipal institutions in food systems planning. *Agriculture and Human Values*, *16*, 213–224. doi:10.1023/A:1007558805953.

Pothukuchi, K., & Kaufman, J. L. (2000). The food system: A stranger to the planning field. *Journal of the American Planning Association. American Planning Association*, *66*(2), 113–124. doi:10.1080/01944360008976093.

Powell, J., Fitton, R., & Fitton, C. (2006). Sharing electronic health records: the patient view. *Informatics in Primary Care*, *14*, 55–57. PMID:16848967.

Proulx, M.-J., Bernier, E., & Bédard, Y. (2007). *Environmental health systemic review: How the new analytical geomatics technologies can help environmental health professionals and decision-makers to make further use of mapping than what is offered traditionally by geographic information systems (GIS) a*. Quebec City, Canada: Centre de recherche en géomatique, Université Laval.

Public Health Agency of Canada. (2012, February 1). *Disease surveillance on-line - Surveillance des maladies en direct.* Retrieved September 11, 2012, from http://dsol-smed.hc-sc.gc.ca/dsol-smed/

Purves, I., & Scholte, N. (2002). *The Danish ETP model.* Newcastle, UK: Sowerby Centre for Health Informatics at Newcastle, University of Newcastle.

Pyper, C., Amery, J., Watson, M., & Crook, C. (2004). Patients' experiences when accessing their on-line electronic patient records in primary care. *The British Journal of General Practice, 54,* 38–43. PMID:14965405.

Quintero, J., Abraham, M., Aguilera, A., Villegas, H., Montilla, G., & Solaiman, B. (2001, October). *Collaborative medical reasoning in telemedicine.* Paper presented at the 23rd Annual International Conference of the IEEE Engineering in Medicine and Biology Society. Istanbul, Turkey.

Rahimpour, M., Lovell, N. H., Celler, B. G., & McCormick, J. (2008). Patients' perceptions of a home telecare system. *International Journal of Medical Informatics, 77,* 486–498. doi:10.1016/j.ijmedinf.2007.10.006 PMID:18023610.

Ramnarayan, P., & Britto, J. (2002). Pediatric decision support systems. *Archives of Disease in Childhood, 87*(5), 361–362. doi:10.1136/adc.87.5.361 PMID:12390900.

Raphael, D. (2007). Canadian public policy and poverty in international perspective. In Raphael, D. (Ed.), *Poverty and Policy in Canada: Implications for Health and Quality of Life* (pp. 335–364). Toronto, Canada: Canadian Scholars' Press.

Raskovic, D., Martin, T., & Jovanov, E. (2004). Medical monitoring applications for wearable computing. *The Computer Journal, 47*(4), 495–504. doi:10.1093/comjnl/47.4.495.

Registered Nurses' Association of Ontario. (2005). *Risk assessment and prevention of pressure ulcers (revised).* Toronto, Canada: Registered Nurses' Association of Ontario.

Reuben, D. B., & Tinetti, M. E. (2012). Goal-oriented patient care — An alternative health outcomes paradigm. *The New England Journal of Medicine, 366,* 777–779. doi:10.1056/NEJMp1113631 PMID:22375966.

Riches, G. (1997). Hunger in Canada: Abandoning the right to food. In Riches, G. (Ed.), *First world hunger: Food security and welfare politics* (pp. 46–77). Toronto, Canada: Garamond Press.

Riva, G., Milani, L., & Gaggioli, A. (2010). Networked flow. In *Comprendere e sviluppare la creatività in rete.* Milan, Italy: LED.

Roback, K., & Herzog, A. (2003). Home informatics in healthcare: Assessment guidelines to keep up quality of care and avoid adverse effects. *Technology and Health Care, 11,* 195–206. PMID:12775936.

Rogers, E. M. (1983). *Diffusion of innovations* (3rd ed.). New York: Free Press.

Rogoski, R. R. (2003). PACS as an enterprise resource: Digital imaging comes of age, as improved web, storage, network and EMR technologies support its extended reach throughout the healthcare enterprise. *Health Management Technology, 24*(11), 14–16, 20. PMID:14608707.

Rosenmöller, M., McKee, M., & Baeten, R. (2012). *Patient mobility in the European Union learning from experience.* Retrieved 31 December 2012 from http://www.euro.who.int/__data/assets/pdf_file/0005/98420/Patient_Mobility.pdf

Rosenstein, A. (1999). Measuring the benefits of clinical decision support: Return on investment. *Health Care Management Review, 24*(2), 32–43. PMID:10358805.

Rosser, W. W. (1993). Dissemination of guidelines on cholesterol: Effects on patterns of practice of general practitioners and family physicians in Ontario. *Canadian Family Physician Medecin de Famille Canadien, 39,* 280–284. PMID:8495119.

Ross, J., Normand, S., Wang, Y., Nallamothu, B., & Lichtman, J. (2008). Hospital remoteness and thirty-day mortality from three serious conditions. *Health Affairs, 27*(6), 1707–1717. doi:10.1377/hlthaff.27.6.1707 PMID:18997230.

Roukema, J., Steyerberg, E., van der Lei, J., & Moll, H. (2008). Randomized trial of a clinical decision support system: Impact on the management of children with fever without apparent source. *Journal of the American Medical Informatics Association, 15*(1), 107–113. doi:10.1197/jamia.M2164 PMID:17947627.

Routledge, P. A., Mahony, M. S., & Woodhouse, K. W. (2003). Adverse drug reactions in elderly patients. *British Journal of Clinical Pharmacology*, *57*(2), 121–126. doi:10.1046/j.1365-2125.2003.01875.x PMID:14748810.

Rubin, D. L. (2011). Informatics in radiology: Measuring and improving quality in radiology: Meeting the challenge with informatics. *Radiographics*, *31*(6), 1511–1527. doi:10.1148/rg.316105207 PMID:21997979.

Rubin, I., & Beckhard, R. (1972). Factors influencing the effectiveness of health teams. *The Milbank Memorial Fund Quarterly*, *50*(3), 317–335. doi:10.2307/3349352 PMID:5043085.

Ruchlin, H. S., Dubbs, N. L., Callahan, M. A., & Fosina, M. J. (2004). The role of leadership in instilling a culture of safety: Lessons from literature. *Journal of Healthcare Management*, *49*(1), 47–59. PMID:14768428.

Rull, R. P., Ritz, B., & Shaw, G. M. (2006). Neural tube defects and maternal residential proximity to agricultural pesticide applications. *American Journal of Epidemiology*, *163*(8), 743–753. doi:10.1093/aje/kwj101 PMID:16495467.

Rushton, G. (1998). Improving the geographic basis of health surveillance using GIS. In Gatrell, A., & Loytonen, M. (Eds.), *GIS and Health* (pp. 63–80). Philadelphia: Taylor and Francis.

Russell, S. E., & Keidkamp, P. (2011). Food desertification: The loss of a major supermarket in New Haven, Connecticut. *Applied Geography (Sevenoaks, England)*, *31*(4), 1197–1209. doi:10.1016/j.apgeog.2011.01.010.

Ryan, C. (2003). Understanding performance appraisal. *Journal of Community Nursing*, *17*(8), 9–14.

Rycroft-Malone, J. (2004). The PARIHS framework - A framework for guiding the implementation of evidence-based practice. *Journal of Nursing Care Quality*, *19*(4), 297–304. doi:10.1097/00001786-200410000-00002 PMID:15535533.

Rycroft-Malone, J., Dopson, S., Degner, L., Hutchinson, A. M., Morgan, D., Stewart, N., & Estabrooks, C. A. (2009). Study protocol for the translating research in elder care (TREC), building context through case studies in long-term care project (project two). *Implementation Science; IS*, *4*, 53. doi:10.1186/1748-5908-4-53 PMID:19671167.

Rycroft-Malone, J., Kitson, A., Harvey, G., McCormack, B., Seers, K., Titchen, C., & Estabrooks, C. (2002). Ingredients for change: Revisiting a conceptual framework. *Quality & Safety in Health Care*, *11*, 174–180. doi:10.1136/qhc.11.2.174 PMID:12448812.

Rycroft-Malone, J., Seers, K., Titchen, A., Harvey, G., Kitson, A., & McCormack, B. (2004). What counts as evidence in evidence-based practice. *Journal of Advanced Nursing*, *47*(1), 81–90. doi:10.1111/j.1365-2648.2004.03068.x PMID:15186471.

Ryerson University. (2010). *Food security defined*. Retrieved October 9, 2010, from http://www.ryerson.ca/foodsecurity/definition/

Saha, A., Grabowski, H., Birnbaum, H., Greenberg, P., & Bizan, O. (2005). Generic competition in the US pharmaceutical industry. *International Journal of the Economics of Business*, *13*(1), 15–38. doi:10.1080/13571510500519905.

Sahota, N., Lloyd, R., Ramakrishna, A., Mackay, J., Prorok, J., & Weise-Kelly, L. et al. (2011). Computerized clinical decision support systems for acute care management: A decision-maker-researcher partnership systematic review of effects on process of care and patient outcomes. *Implementation Science; IS*, *6*(91). PMID:21824385.

Samb, B., Evans, T., & Dybul, M. (2009). An assessment of interactions between global health initiatives and country health systems. *Lancet*, *373*(9681), 2137–2169. doi:10.1016/S0140-6736(09)60919-3 PMID:19541040.

Schiff, G. D., Fung, S., Speroff, T., & McNutt, R. A. (2003). Decompensated heart failure: Symptoms, patterns of onset, and contributing factors. *The American Journal of Medicine*, *114*(8), 625–630. doi:10.1016/S0002-9343(03)00132-3 PMID:12798449.

Schmidt, H., & Boshuizen, H. (1993). On the origin of intermediate effects in clinical case recall. *Memory & Cognition*, *21*(3), 338–351. doi:10.3758/BF03208266 PMID:8316096.

Scotch, M., & Parmanto, B. (2006). Development of SOVAT: A numerical-spatial decision support system for community health assessment research. *International Journal of Medical Informatics*, *75*, 771–784. doi:10.1016/j.ijmedinf.2005.10.008 PMID:16359916.

Seggewiss, K. (2009). Variations in home care programs across Canada demonstrate need for national standards and pan-Canadian program. *Canadian Medical Association Journal, 180*(2), E90–E92. doi:10.1503/cmaj.090819 PMID:19506265.

Shapiro, J., Mostashari, F., Hripcsak, G., Soulakis, N., & Kuperman, G. (2011). Using health information exchange to improve public health. *American Journal of Public Health, 101*(4), 616–623. doi:10.2105/AJPH.2008.158980 PMID:21330598.

Shekelle, P., Morton, S., & Keeler, E. (2006). *Costs and benefits of health information technology.* Rockville, MD: Agency for Healthcare Research and Quality.

Sherer, J. L. (1994). Retooling leaders: Facilitative leadership helps clarify process and underpin culture change. *Hospitals & Health Networks, 68*(1), 42–44. PMID:8269006.

Shortliffe, E. H., Perreault, L. E., Wiederhold, G., & Fagan, L. M. (2001). *Medical informatics, computer applications, healthcare and biomedicine* (2nd ed.). London: Springer Ed.

Sibbald, B. (2001). Use computerized systems to cut adverse drug events: Report. *Canadian Medical Association Journal, 164*(13), 1878.

Siliquini, R., Ceruti, M., Lovato, E., Bert, F., Bruno, S., & De Vito, E. … La Torre, G. (2011). Surfing the Internet for health information: An Italian survey on use and population choices. *BMC Medical Informatics and Decision Making, 11*(21). Retrieved September 10, 2012, from http://www.biomedcentral.com/1472-6947/11/21

Silvestre, A., Sue, V., & Allen, J. (2009). If you build it, will they come? The Kaiser Permanente model of online health care. *Health Affairs, 28*(2), 334–344. doi:10.1377/hlthaff.28.2.334 PMID:19275988.

Simmons, R., & Shiffman, J. (2007). Scaling up health service inovations: A framework for action. In Simmons, R., Fajans, P., & Ghiron, L. (Eds.), *Scaling up health services delivery from pilot innovations to policies and programmes* (pp. 1–30). Geneva, Switzerland: World Health Organization.

Sketris, I., Ingram, E. L., & Lummis, H. (2007). *Optimal prescribing and medication use in Canada: Challenges and opportunities.* Ottawa, Canada: Health Council of Canada.

Smith, P. (2003). Implementing an EMR system: One clinic's experience. *Family Practice Management, 10*(5), 37–42. PMID:12776405.

Smith, R. (1996). What clinical information do doctors need? *British Medical Journal, 313*(7064), 1062–1068. doi:10.1136/bmj.313.7064.1062 PMID:8898602.

Sommers, L., Marton, K., & Barbaccia, J. C. (2000). Physician, nurse, and social worker collaboration in primary care for chronically ill seniors. *Archives of Internal Medicine, 160*, 1825–1833. doi:10.1001/archinte.160.12.1825 PMID:10871977.

Sonnino, R. (2009). Feeding the city: Towards a new research and planning agenda. *International Planning Studies, 14*(4), 425–435. doi:10.1080/13563471003642795.

Speedie, S.M., Ferguson, A.S., Sanders, J., & Doarn, C.R. (2008). Telehealth: The promise of new care delivery models. *Telemedicine and e-Health Journal, 14*(9), 964-967.

Stanciole, A. (2008). Health insurance and lifestyle choices: Identifying ex ante moral hazard in the US market. *The Geneva Papers on Risk and Insurance, 33*, 627–644. doi:10.1057/gpp.2008.27.

Statistics Canada. (2009). *Human activity and the environment: Annual statistics.* Ottawa, Canada: Statistics Canada.

StatsCan. (2007). *Residential care facilities (2006/2007).* StatsCan.

Stegwee, R., & Spil, T. (2001). *Strategies for healthcare information systems.* Hershey, PA: Idea Group Publishing.

Steinbrook, R. (2008). Personally controlled online health data--The next big thing in medical care. *The New England Journal of Medicine, 358*(16), 1653–1656. doi:10.1056/NEJMp0801736 PMID:18420496.

Stephanovich, P. L., & Uhrig, J. D. (1999). Decision making in high-velocity environments: Implications for healthcare. *Journal of Healthcare Management, 44*(3), 195–205.

Stineman, M. G., Escarce, J. J., Tassoni, C. J., Goin, J. E., Granger, C. V., & Williams, S. V. (1998). Diagnostic coding and medical rehabilitation length of stay: Their relationship. *Archives of Physical Medicine and Rehabilitation*, 79. PMID:9523773.

Straus, S. E., & McAlister, F. A. (2000). Evidence-based medicine: A commentary on common criticisms. *Canadian Medical Association Journal*, *163*(7), 837–841. PMID:11033714.

Stroetmann, K. A., Artmann, J., & Stroetmann, V. N. (2011). *European countries on their journey towards national eHealth infrastructures final European progress report*. Retrieved 5 September 2012 from www.ehealthstrategies.eu/report/report.html

Stroetmann, V. N., Kalra, D., Lewalle, P., Rector, A., Rodrigues, J. M., & Stroetmann, K. A. ... Zanstra, P. E. (2009). *Semantic interoperability for better health and safer healthcare research and deployment roadmap for Europe*. Retrieved 30 December 2012 from http://ec.europa.eu/information_society/activities/health/docs/publications/2009/2009semantic-health-report.pdf

Stuckler, D., Feigl, B. A., & Basu, S. (2010). *The political economy of universal health coverage*. Retrieved 30 December from http://www.hsr-symposium.org/images/stories/8political_economy.pdf

Studer, M. (2005). The effect of organizational factors on the effectiveness of EMR system implementation--What have we learned? *Electronic Healthcare*, *4*(2), 92–97.

Subramanian, S., Hoover, S., Gilman, B., Field, T. S., Mutter, R., & Gurwitz, J. H. (2007). Computerized physician order entry with clinical decision support in long-term care facilities: Costs and benefits to stakeholders. *Journal of the American Geriatrics Society*, *55*(9), 1451–1457. doi:10.1111/j.1532-5415.2007.01304.x PMID:17915344.

Surescripts. (2011). *The national progress report on e-prescribing and interoperable health care, year 2011*. Retrieved 6 September 2012 from http://www.surescripts.com/downloads/npr/National%20Progress%20Report%20on%20E%20Prescribing%20Year%202011.pdf

Sutherland, J. (2011). *Hospital payment mechanisms: An overview and options for Canada*. Ottawa, Canada: Canadian Health Services Research Foundation Series of Reports on Cost Drivers and Health System Efficiency.

Sutherland, J., & Walker, J. (2006). *Technical report: Development of the rehabilitation patient group (RPG) case mix classification methodology and weighting system for adult inpatient rehabilitation*. Toronto, Canada: Ontario Joint Policy and Planning Committee.

Tamber, P. (2012). *Doctors only trust doctors*. Retrieved 09 01, 2012, from http://blogs.bmj.com/bmj/2012/07/09/pritpal-s-tambar-doctors-only-trust-doctors/

Tang, P., Ash, J., Bates, D., Overhage, J., & Sands, D. (2006). Personal health records: Definitions, benefits, and strategies for overcomming barriers to adoption. *Journal of the American Medical Informatics Association*, *13*(2), 121–126. doi:10.1197/jamia.M2025 PMID:16357345.

Tang, P., & Lansky, D. (2005). The missing link: Bridging the patient-provider health information gap. *Health Affairs*, *24*, 1290–1295. doi:10.1377/hlthaff.24.5.1290 PMID:16162575.

Tang, P., & Lee, T. (2009). Your doctor's office or the internet? Two paths to personal health records. *The New England Journal of Medicine*, *360*(13), 1276–1278. doi:10.1056/NEJMp0810264 PMID:19321866.

Tan, R., McClure, T., Lin, C. K., Jea, D., Dabiri, F., & Massey, T. et al. (2009). Development of a fully implantable wireless pressure monitoring system. *Biomedical Microdevices*, *11*, 259–264. doi:10.1007/s10544-008-9232-1 PMID:18836836.

Tarasuk, V. (2001). A critical examination of community-based responses to household food insecurity in Canada. *Health Education & Behavior*, *28*(4), 487–499. doi:10.1177/109019810102800408 PMID:11465158.

Tarasuk, V. (2003). Low income, welfare and nutritional vulnerability. *Canadian Medical Association Journal*, *168*(6), 709–710. PMID:12642427.

Tarasuk, V. (2009). Health implications of food insecurity. In Raphael, D. (Ed.), *Social Determinants of Health* (2nd ed., pp. 205–220). Toronto, Canada: Canadian Scholars Press.

Taylor, R., Bower, A., Frederico, G., & Bigelow, J. (2005). Promoting health information technology: Is there a case for more-aggressive government action? *Health Affairs*, *24*(5), 1234–1245. doi:10.1377/hlthaff.24.5.1234 PMID:16162568.

Teich, J., Bordenick, J., et al. (2004). *Electronic pre-scribing: Toward maximum value and rapid adoption recommendations for optimal design and implementation to improve care, increase efficiency and reduce costs in ambulatory care a report of the electronic prescribing initiative ehealth initiative*. Washington, DC: Foundation for eHealth Initiative. Retrieved 6 September 2012 from http://c.ymcdn.com/sites/www.azhec.org/resource/resmgr/files/erx_toward_maximum_value_and.pdf

Tengelin, E., Arman, R., Wikström, E., & Delive, L. (2011). Regulating time commitments in healthcare organizations: Managers' boundary approaches at work and in life. *Journal of Health Organization and Management*, *25*(5), 578–599. PMID:22043654.

Teufel, R. J., Kazley, A. S., & Basco, W. T. Jr. (2009). Early adopters of computerized physician order entry in hospitals that care for children: A picture of US health care shortly after the institute of medicine reports on quality. *Journal of Clinical Pediatrics*, *48*(4), 389–396. doi:10.1177/0009922809331801 PMID:19224864.

The Scarborough Hospital (TSH). (2012). *Key facts and figures*. Retrieved December 18, 2012 from http://www.tsh.to/pages/Key-Facts--Figures

Thornett, A. M. (2001). Computer decision support systems in general practice. *International Journal of Information Management*, *21*, 39–47. doi:10.1016/S0268-4012(00)00049-9.

Tong, H., Tong, L., & Tong, J. (2009). The Vioxx recall case and comments. *International Business Journal*, *29*(2), 114–118.

Toronto Public Health. (2008). *The state of Toronto's food*. Toronto, Canada: Toronto Public Health.

Toronto Public Health. (2010). *Cultivating food connections: Towards a healthy and sustainable food system for Toronto*. Toronto, Canada: Toronto Public Health.

Torres, L. S., Dutton, A. G., & Norcutt, T. A. L. (2003). *Basic medical techniques and patient care in imaging technology* (6th ed.). Philadelphia: Lippincott, Williams and Wilkins.

Trainor, J., & Stamos, J. (2011). Fever without a localizing source. *Pediatric Annals*, *40*(1), 21–25. doi:10.3928/00904481-20101214-06 PMID:21210596.

Translating Research in Elder Care: TREC Overview. (2012). Retrieved March 18, 2012, from http://www.trec.ualberta.ca/TRECOverview.aspx

Tukker, A., Huppes, G., Guinée, J., Heijungs, R., de Koning, A., & van Oers, L. et al. (2006). *Environmental impact of products (EIPRO): Analysis of the life-cycle environmental impacts related to the final consumption of the EU-25*. Seville, Spain: European Commission.

Turner, A., Kabashi, A., Guthrie, H., Burket, R., & Turner, P. (2011). Use and value of information sources by parents of child psychiatric patients. *Health Information and Libraries Journal*, *28*(2), 101–109. doi:10.1111/j.1471-1842.2011.00935.x PMID:21564493.

U.S. National Library of Medicine. (2012). *Unified medical language system (UMLS®)*. Retrieved 12, 16, 2012, from http://www.nlm.nih.gov/research/umls/

United States Department of Agriculture. (2012, December 11). *Food environment atlas*. Retrieved December 28, 2012, from http://www.ers.usda.gov/data-products/food-environment-atlas.aspx

United States Executive Office of the President. President's Council of Advisors on Science and Technology. (2010). *Report to the President realizing the full potential of health information technology to improve healthcare for Americans: The path forward*. Retrieved August 20, 2012, from http://www.whitehouse.gov/sites/default/files/microsites/ostp/pcast-health-it-report.pdf

United States Government Accountability Office. (2003). *Medical malpractice insurance: Multiple factors have contributed to increased premium rates* (GAO Publication No. GAO-03-702). Retrieved August 20, 2012, from http://www.gao.gov/new.items/d03702.pdf

University of Arizona. (2011). *Administrative policy formulation*. Retrieved 12, 16, 2012, from http://policy.arizona.edu/policy-formulation

University of Manitoba. (2009, December 18). *Population health research data repository*. Retrieved September 13, 2012, from http://umanitoba.ca/faculties/medicine/units/community_health_sciences/departmental_units/mchp/resources/repository/index.html

Vaitheeswaran, V. (2011, March 31). A very big HIT. *The Economist: The World in 2011, 133.*

Valeri, L., Giesen, D., Jansen, P., & Klokgieters, K. (2010). *Business models for ehealth, final report*. Retrieved 30 December 2012 from http://ec.europa.eu/information_society/activities/health/docs/studies/business_model/business_models_eHealth_report.pdf

van Aalst, J. (2009). Distinguishing knowledge-sharing, knowledge- construction, and knowledge-creation discourses. *Computer-Supported Collaborative Learning, 4,* 259–287. doi:10.1007/s11412-009-9069-5.

van den Hooff, B., Elving, W., Meeuwsen, J. M., & Dumoulin, C. (2003). Knowledge sharing in knowledge communities. In Huysman, M., Wenger, E., & Wulf, V. (Eds.), *Communities and Technologies* (pp. 119–141). Dordrecht, The Netherlands: Kluwer Academic Publishers. doi:10.1007/978-94-017-0115-0_7.

Van Dijk, L. Villalba, De Vries, H., & Bell, D.S. (2011). Electronic prescribing in the United Kingdom and in The Netherlands. Rockville, MD: Agency for Healthcare Research and Quality.

Venkatraman, S., Bala, H., Venkatesh, V., & Bates, J. (2008). Six strategies for electronic medical records systems. *Communications of the ACM, 51*(11), 140–144. doi:10.1145/1400214.1400243.

Vitacca, M., Assoni, G., Pizzocaro, P., Guerra, A., Marchina, L., & Scalvini, S. et al. (2006). A pilot study of nurse-led, home monitoring for patients with chronic respiratory failure and with mechanical ventilation assistance. *Journal of Telemedicine and Telecare, 12*(7), 337–342. doi:10.1258/135763306778682404 PMID:17059649.

Waegemann, C. (2005). Closer to reality: Personal health records represent a step in the right direction for interoperability of healthcare IT systems and accessibility of patient data. *Health Management Technology, 26,* 16–18. PMID:15932068.

Wagner, E. H. (1998). Chronic disease management: What will it take to improve care for chronic illness? *Efficient Clinical Practice, 1*(1), 2–4. PMID:10345255.

Wagstaff, A. (2002). Poverty and health sector inequalities. *Bulletin of the World Health Organization,* 97–105. PMID:11953787.

Wakefield, D., Ward, M., Loes, J., O'Brien, J., & Speery, L. (2010). Implementation of a telepharmacy service to provide round-the-clock medication order review by pharmacists. *American Journal of Health-System Pharmacists, 67,* 2052–2057. doi:10.2146/ajhp090643 PMID:21098378.

Wald, J., & McCormack, L. (2012). *Patient empowerment and health information technology* (White Paper). Retrieved 30 December 2012 from http://www.himss.org/content/files/RTI_WhitePaper_patientEmpowerment.pdf

Walker, J., & Carayon, P. (2009). From tasks to processes: The case for changing health information technology to improve health care. *Health Affairs, 28*(2), 467–477. doi:10.1377/hlthaff.28.2.467 PMID:19276006.

Walton, G., & Booth, A. (2004). *Exploiting knowledge in health services*. London: Facet Publishing.

Wang, B., Wan, T., Burke, D., Bazzoli, G., & Lin, B. (2005). Factors influencing health information system adoption in American hospitals. *Health Care Management Review, 30*(1), 44–51. doi:10.1097/00004010-200501000-00007 PMID:15773253.

Wang, S., Middleton, B., & Prosser, L. (2003). A cost-benefit analysis of electyronic medical records in primary care. *The American Journal of Medicine, 114,* 397–403. doi:10.1016/S0002-9343(03)00057-3 PMID:12714130.

Warden, G., et al. (2012). *Health IT and patient safety: Building safer systems for better care*. Washington, DC: The National Academy Press. Retrieved 5 September 2012 from http://www.iom.edu/Reports/2011/Health-IT-and-Patient-Safety-Building-Safer-Systems-for-Better-Care.aspx

Ware, C. (2004). Foundation for a Science of data visualization. In Ware, C. (Ed.), *Information Visualization Perception for Design* (pp. 1–27). San Francisco, CA: Morgan Kaufman Publishers. doi:10.1016/B978-155860819-1/50004-2.

Webster, P. (2010). United States to compel physicians to make meaningful use' of electronic health records. *Canadian Medical Association Journal*, *182*(14), 1500–1502. doi:10.1503/cmaj.109-3361 PMID:20837690.

Wedlake, S. (2012). *Law amendments bill 147 - An act respecting the Nova Scotia regulated health professions network*. Retrieved 12, 16, 2012, from http://nslegislature.ca/pdfs/committees/61_4_LACSubmissions/20121129/20121129-147-03.pdf

Wei, L., & Yan, Y. (2010). Knowledge production and political participation: Reconsidering the knowledge gap theory in the web 2.0 environment. In D. Wen & J. Zhu (Eds.), *The 2nd IEEE International Conference on Information Management and Engineering (ICIME)* (pp. 239-243). Los Alamitos, CA: IEEE Computer Society.

Weitzman, E., Kaci, L., & Mandl, K. (2010). Sharing medical data for health research: The early personal health record experience. *Journal of Medical Internet Research*, *12*(2), e14. doi:10.2196/jmir.1356 PMID:20501431.

Weitzman, E., Kelemen, S., Kaci, L., & Mandl, K. (2012). Willigness to share personal health record data for care improvement and public health: A survey of experienced personal health record users. *BMC Medical Informatics and Decision Making*, *12*(39). PMID:22616619.

Wenger, E., White, N., & Smith, J. D. (2009). Digital habitats stewarding technology for communities. Portland, OR: CPsquare.

Wenger, E. (1998). *Communities of practice, learning, meaning and identity*. Cambridge, UK: Cambridge University Press.

Wenger, E., McDermott, R., & Snyder, W. R. (2002). *Cultivating communities of practice*. Boston: Harvard Business School Press.

West, S., Blake, C., Liu, Z., McKoy, J., Oertel, M., & Carey, T. (2009). Reflections on the use of electronic health record data for clinical research. *Health Informatics Journal*, *15*(2), 106–121. doi:10.1177/1460458209102972 PMID:19474224.

Wilkinson, A., Papaioannou, D., Keen, C., & Booth, A. (2009). The role of the information specialist in supporting knowledge transfer: A public health information case study. *Health Information and Libraries Journal*, *26*(2), 118–125. doi:10.1111/j.1471-1842.2008.00790.x PMID:19490150.

Williams, C., Mostashari, F., Mertz, K., Hogin, E., & Atwal, P. (2012). From the office of the national coordinator: The strategy for advancing the exchange of health information. *Health Affairs*, *31*(3), 527–536. doi:10.1377/hlthaff.2011.1314 PMID:22392663.

Willis, C. D., Mitton, C., Gordon, J., & Best, A. (2012). System tools for system change. *BMJ Quality & Safety*, *21*(3), 250–262. doi:10.1136/bmjqs-2011-000482 PMID:22129934.

Wilson, J., & Cole, G. (1990). A healthy approach to performance appraisal. *Personnel Management*, *22*(6), 46.

Winstanley, N. B. (1980). Legal and ethical issues in performance appraisals. *Harvard Business Review*, *58*(6), 186–192.

Wismar, M., Palm, W., Figueras, J., Ernst, K., & van Ginneken, E. (2011). *Cross-border health care in the European Union: Mapping and analysing practices and policies*. Retrieved 21 August 2012 from http://www.euro.who.int/__data/assets/pdf_file/0004/135994/e94875.pdf

Witry, M., Doucette, W., Daly, J., Levy, B., & Chrischilles, E. (2010). Family physician perceptions of personal health records. *Perspectives in Health Information Management*, *7*(Winter), 1–12. PMID:20697465.

Wolter, J., & Friedman, B. (2005). Health records for the people: Touting the benefits of the consumer-based personal health record. *Journal of American Health Information Management Association*, *76*(10), 28–32. PMID:16333941.

World Bank. (2011, April 14). *High and volatile food prices continue to threaten the world's poor*. Retrieved April 20, 2011, from http://go.worldbank.org/DGNYAFM0Y0

World Health Organization. (2002). *The world health report 2002, reducing risks, promoting healthy life*. Geneva, Switzerland: WHO. Retrieved 21 August 2012 from http://www.who.int/entity/whr/2002/en/index.html

World Health Organization. (2002). *WHO global burden of disease (GBD) 2002 estimates (revised)*. Retrieved 30 December 2012 from http://www.who.int/healthinfo/bodestimates/en/

World Health Organization. (2005). *International health regulations (2005)* (2nd Ed.). Geneva, Switzerland: WHO. Retrieved 31 December 2012 from http://whqlibdoc.who.int/publications/2008/9789241580410_eng.pdf

World Health Organization. (2006). *Active aging – A policy framework*. Retrieved September 3, 2012, from http://whqlibdoc.who.int/hq/2002/who_nmh_nph_02.8.pdf

World Health Organization. (2008). *The world health report 2008 - Primary health care (now more than ever)*. Geneva, Switzerland: WHO. Retrieved 21 August 2012 from http://www.who.int/whr/2008/en/index.html

World Health Organization. (2008). *Global burden of disease*. Retrieved 30 December 2012 from http://www.who.int/healthinfo/global_burden_disease/en/index.html

World Health Organization. (2010). *The world health report - Health systems financing: The path to universal coverage*. Geneva, Switzerland: WHO. Retrieved 21 August 2012 from http://www.who.int/whr/2010/en/index.html

Worthy, S., Rounds, K. C., & Soloway, C. B. (2003). Strengthening your ties to referring physicians through RIS/PACS integration. *Radiology Management, 25*(2), 18–22. PMID:12800559.

WP 29. (2004). *Strategy document*. Retrieved 12 September 2012 from http://ec.europa.eu/justice/policies/privacy/docs/wpdocs/ 2004/wp98_en.pdf

Yamin, C., Emani, S., Williams, D., Lipsitz, S., Karson, A., Wald, J., & Bates, D. (2011). The digital divide in adoption and use of a personal health record. *Archives of Internal Medicine, 171*(6), 568–574. doi:10.1001/archinternmed.2011.34 PMID:21444847.

Yan, P., & Yang, X. (2009). To trade or to teach: Modeling tacit knowledge diffusion in complex social networks. In Q. Luo & J. Zhu (Eds.), *Second International Conference on Future Information Technology and Management Engineering* (pp. 151-154). Los Alamitos, CA: IEEE Computer Society.

Yasnoff, W. A., Humphreys, B. L., & Overhage, J. M. et al. (2004). A consensus action agenda for achieving the national health information infrastructure. *Journal of the American Medical Informatics Association, 11*(4), 332–338. doi:10.1197/jamia.M1616 PMID:15187075.

Yasnoff, W. A., O'Carroll, P. W., Koo, D., Linkins, R. W., & Kilbourne, E. M. (2000). Public health informatics: Improving and transforming public health in the information age. *Journal of Public Health Management and Practice, 6*(6), 67–75. PMID:18019962.

Yau, G., Williams, A., & Brown, J. (2011). Family physicians' perspectives on personal health records. *Canadian Family Physician Medecin de Famille Canadien, 57*(5), e178–e184. PMID:21642732.

Zeckhauser, R. (1970). Medical insurance: A case study of the tradeoff between risk spreading and appropriate incentives. *Journal of Economic Theory, 2*(1), 10–26. doi:10.1016/0022-0531(70)90010-4.

Zenios, M. (2011). Epistemic activities and collaborative learning: Towards an analytical model for studying knowledge construction in networked learning settings. *Journal of Computer Assisted Learning, 27*(3), 259–268. doi:10.1111/j.1365-2729.2010.00394.x.

Zhen, B., Li, H., & Kohno, R. (2009). Networking issues in medical implant communications. *International Journal of Multimedia and Ubiquitous Engineering, 4*(1), 23–37.

Zitner, D., Paterson, G. I., & Fay, D. F. (1998). Methods for identifying pertinent and superfluous activity. In Tan, J. (Ed.), *Health Decision Support Systems* (pp. 177–197). New York: Aspen Publishers, Inc..

About the Contributors

Christo El Morr (PhD Biomedical Engineering, Compiègne University of Technology-France, 1997) is an Assistant Professor of Health Informatics and the Undergraduate Program Director at the School of Health Policy and Management, York University, Canada. His cross-disciplinary research covers healthcare informatics, computer science, and computer engineering. His research interests focus on Health Virtual Communities and Mobile Communities; he also has research interests in Software Accessibility for people with Visual Disability, PACS, and Electronic Health Records. He has published books, chapters, and articles in these areas. He consulted for international organizations and was an Expert Reviewer for the Ministry of Research and Innovation, Ontario.

* * *

Valentina Al Hamouche received her diploma in Radiologic Technology from the American University of Beirut Medical Center (Lebanon) in 1989, and her BSc. in Radiologic Technology from Anglia Polytechnic University Cambridge (UK) in 1996; she has also received a Masters degree in Health Systems Management from University of London (UK) in 2006. She has a multinational teaching experience in Lebanon, United Kingdom, United Arab Emirates, and Canada. She conducted research in Radiography and Health Management, presented her findings in international conferences. Her research interests are in the domain of health management, medical imaging integration, and radiation protection. She joined the faculty of medical radiation science program (radiologic technology) at the Michener Institute for Applied Health Sciences/University of Toronto in December 2008. She enjoys both the patient care and the evolving technology aspects of her profession.

Sama Al Khudairy, a York graduate, enrolled at the university with determination and strong interests in healthcare Policy and Management. Her drive and perseverance allowed her to not only enjoy, but also excel in her coursework. She particularly enjoyed the Health Ethics and Law courses, which proved to be an aid in establishing a clear and honest motif. Sama's philosophy in and of her achievements is as simple as wanting to make a difference and create a positive and lasting impression. Her belief is that all individuals deserve the chance of attaining optimal health, and she continues working towards the achievement of this goal. Sama graduated with honors in 2009. She then found her place as a student representative on the Faculty of Graduate Studies and went on to graduate with high standings in 2011, obtaining her Masters in Health Policy and Equity. Today, Sama lives in Toronto and is a research assistant with experience in health management and is currently working towards a certification in project management.

Ioannis Apostolakis studied Mathematics in the University of Athens. He has an MSc in Informatics, Operational Research, and Education issues and also a PhD in Health Informatics. He has also Post Doctoral studies in Medical Informatics. He had been for several years scientific researcher in the Department of Clinical Therapeutics in the University of Athens. He has research and educational activities in issues of Health Informatics and Education. He is working as Professor at National School of Public Health. He has also taught in undergraduate and postgraduate level a wide range of courses: Health Informatics, Information Systems, Computational Statistics I, II, eGovernment, eDemocracy, Management and Operation of Virtual Communities, Research Methodology and the Internet, Teaching of Computer Science, Electronic Trade, Data Analysis Using Statistical Techniques. He has worked at the Therapeutic Clinic of National University of Athens as a Research Fellow, at the Ministry of Interior as an Informatics Specialist and at the National School of Public Administration as the Head of the Computer Studies Program. He has been also serving as a program committee member of many international conferences and as a reviewer of several journals in the area of E-Learning and Healthcare Service Management. More information is available at http://www.iapostolakis.gr.

Alexander Berler has an MSc in Biomedical Engineering and a PhD in Medical Informatics. He was affiliated with the Electrical Engineering Department, National Technical University of Athens, Greece, as a Postgraduate Student and Research Associate in the areas of healthcare information systems interoperability, medical informatics, and telemedicine since 1996. He has worked at Information Society SA, the official governmental information technology project office, as a project director responsible for the large healthcare informatics projects of the Greek government until 2006. He is currently employed as the Director of consulting services department at Gnomon Informatics with an expertise in international projects related to e-health, e-procurement and e-government. On behalf of Gnomon Informatics, he is a member of the epSOS Industry Team Steering Committee and participates in the development of the openNCP software components. He is currently a member of several societies, institutes, and organizations (IEEE, ACM, HIMSS, PMI, IHE), an external tutor to the National School of Public Health and the Chair of HL7 Hellas, the Greek HL7 Affiliate. More information available at http://gr.linkedin.com/in/aberler/.

Edward J. Cherian is Professor of Information Systems & Technology Management in the School of Business at George Washington University where he has been since 1985. For many years, he was responsible for the graduate MIS Degree Program, and served as Chair of the Department of Management Science. Dr. Cherian has developed and teaches courses in The Healthcare MBA Program, as well as the HITECH Certificate Program in the School of Public Health and Health Services. Some of his recent publications include; "A Health Information Technology System of Systems Architecture," under review. "Electronic Health Records and Electronic Medical Records: Using Information Technology for Healthcare Reform," 2012, International Technology, Education and Development Conference, Valencia, Spain. "Can Distance Education Equal Classroom Learning?" International Conference on Education, Research and Innovation, Madrid, Spain 2010, "Mobile Learning: The Beginning of the End of Classroom Learning," World Congress on Engineering and Computer Science, Berkeley, CA, October 2008. Professor Cherian holds BEE, MS, and PhD degrees from Rensselaer Polytechnic Institute.

Connie D'Astolfo is the President and Clinical Director of SPINEgroup. Dr. D'Astolfo is both a practicing clinician and consultant. Dr. D'Astolfo is currently completing a PhD in Health Management, Policy, and Informatics at York University. She has been registered with the College of Chiropractors of Ontario since 2001. She has consulted with the Ontario government and other health organizations on health-related policy and management projects and initiatives. Early in her career, Dr. D'Astolfo pioneered and led an inter-disciplinary pain management team for several Long-Term Care (LTC) homes and was the first chiropractor to be fully integrated in the LTC sector in Ontario. Her expertise lies in rehabilitation, performance management, and program evaluation.

Guendalina Graffigna received a PhD in Social Psychology at Università Cattolica del Sacro Cuore di Milano (Italy) where she is Assistant Professor. At the same university, she teaches "Qualitative Methodology," and she is vice-director for the II level Master Degree in "Qualitative Research for Marketing and Society" and member of the coordinating committee for the PhD School in Psychology. Guendalina is also editorial manager for the *Journal Micro & Macro Marketing*. Before her appointments, Guendalina was a Post Doc fellow and visiting professor in Qualitative Methods at the International Institute for Qualitative Methodology, University of Alberta, with which she still collaborates for several research and teaching initiatives as a scholar member. From January 2012, Guendalina is Associate Director for the Study and Training Centre of ASSIRM and Co-Chair for Education of MMRA. In June 2012, she received the award for International Leadership for Qualitative Health Research 2012. Her main areas of interests are consumer engagement, social media communication, online communities, qualitative methods applied to the study of consumption, and health.

Thuy Hoang is a performance and decision support consultant for a hospital in Ontario, Canada. She earned her Bachelor of Health Studies from York University. In addition, she holds a Master of Health Studies from Athabasca University. Thuy is currently a member of the Canadian College of Health Leaders (CCHL) and a member of the Utilization Managers' Network of Ontario (UMNO). Thuy possesses an extensive background in health care management. She supports the hospital's information and analysis needs by analyzing, interpreting, and reporting clinical and management information. She manages government and external agencies reporting requirements. In addition, Thuy provides information for the purposes of planning, evaluating performance, and improving patient safety and outcomes.

Chiara Libreri has a Master's Degree in "Organizational and Marketing Psychology" and an executive Master's Degree in "Qualitative methods applied to social and marketing research." Now she is a Ph.D candidate at the Faculty of Psychology at the Università Cattolica del Sacro Cuore di Milano. She mainly works on online exchanges and online knowledge processes between chronic patients. She spent part of her Ph.D. at the Faculty of Extension – University of Alberta, studying and working on knowledge transfer and qualitative methods. She is also didactic coordinator for the executive Master's degree in "Qualitative Research for Marketing and Society" and teaching assistant for the "Consumer Psychology and Marketing Research" course at the Faculty of Psychology at the Università Cattolica del Sacro Cuore. Her research interests and topics revolve around qualitative and online research applied to health promotion and communication, and consumer and marketing psychology. More specifically on the following keywords: online communities, online lay exchanges, online knowledge construction, and Web ethnography.

Grace Liu has worked as a Physiotherapist in the health industry in Ontario for 20 years. She has worked in a variety of settings, including acute care, rehabilitation, and home care, and has held the positions of Professional Practice Leader, Project Manager, Case Manager, and Research Analyst. Grace has achieved a Bachelor's degree in Physiotherapy, a Master's degree in Business Administration, and Case Management Certification. Currently, she is pursuing her Doctoral degree in Health Policy and Equity at York University. Her research interest is in health policy research at the systems level, particularly with funding and patient flow from emergency, acute care to rehabilitation or home care. In the future, Grace is interested in developing strategic health policies and transforming the health care delivery system focusing on quality and best practice standards with stakeholders to ensure sustainability.

Jacqueline MacDonald is a full-time health services manager in rural Nova Scotia, Canada. She is a part-time instructor at Dalhousie School of Information Management (SIM), and is an adjunct faculty at SIM and in Medical Informatics, Dalhousie Faculty of Medicine. Jackie's research interests include the health services research-practice gap and health services decision-making and related information, information behaviours, and information management practices. She has been a member of OP3, Nova Scotia's DHA/IWK policy working group since 2007.

Naomi Nonnekes Mensink is a Lecturer in Medical Informatics at Dalhousie University and a member of the Dalhousie faculty team delivering the Master of Health Informatics and Bachelor of Informatics programs. In addition to academic program development, teaching, strategic planning and program support, she has conducted evaluation studies on initiatives related to health-care and health informatics. Naomi has a Master of Adult Education degree from St. Francis Xavier University and has partially completed the requirements for a Doctor of Philosophy in Interdisciplinary Studies: Health Informatics. As an evaluator, Naomi has observed how the policies embedded in a provincial drug information system have impacted pharmacists' work, both positively and negatively.

Vishaya Naidoo is a doctoral candidate in the Health Policy and Equity program at York University. She holds an undergraduate degree in Political Science and a master's degree in Critical Disability Studies from York University. Her research seeks to understand the ways in which disability and later life intersect; including ageism and ableism, feminist perspectives of aging and the gendered body, and the medicalization of the aged body. Her doctoral research continues in this vein, exploring disability and age discrimination experienced by older adults in acute health care settings. From 2008-2011, she worked as a researcher with Disability Rights Promotion International (DRPI), and subsequently DRPI – Canada, a research project that explores a number of rights issues facing people with disabilities in both a Canadian and global context.

Yedishtra Naidoo completed his undergraduate degree in life sciences and psychology at the University of Toronto, where he assisted in research on Rett's syndrome and glycogen storage diseases at The Hospital for Sick Children in Toronto. He then went on to graduate with honors from Ross University medical school. While completing clinical rotations in California, he conducted conferences on prostate disease and cardiac arrhythmias. He subsequently went on to a psychiatry residency at Detroit Medical Center and Wayne State University, where he is currently in his second year. He has presented case reports on neuroleptic malignant syndrome and synthetic illicit drugs, and has research interests in posttraumatic stress disorder, from a behavioral and physiological perspective. He enjoys reading, various athletics, and travel in his leisure time.

Grace Paterson holds appointments as Associate Professor, Medical Informatics/Division of Medical Education in the Faculties of Medicine and Graduate Studies, Dalhousie University. Her research interests include semantic interoperability, ethnographic analysis of health information systems in the work setting, and clinical statements expressed using HL7 and SNOMED CT. As an investigator with the CMA EMR Case Studies and Canadian e-Pharmacy Task Force projects, she recognized the need to deal with clinical pragmatic issues to help ensure that systems are usable and useful in the work setting. She teaches in the Master in Health Informatics program and serves as a board member of Canada's National Institutes of Health Informatics (NIHI).

Nelson Ravka graduated with a DDS degree from the University of Toronto in 1971. Throughout his career in dentistry, he had the opportunity to work within and critically assess the three modalities of compensation: fee-for-service, salary, and capitation. He is currently in the master's program of Health Policy and Equity at York University. His area of interest is end of life health care and the political, legal, and social ramifications of medicalized dying. This includes the issues and conflicts that play a role in defining the rights of patients, surrogates, and health care professionals in determining the nature of the care received by the terminally ill.

Tom Ryan, originally from Littleton, Colorado, graduated from The George Washington University School of Business in 2011 with a Bachelor of Business Administration in Business Economics and Public Policy and a minor in Political Science. He spent a year working in healthcare as a Federal Analyst with Deloitte Consulting, LLP. There he worked with the United States Department of Defense, Navy Bureau of Medicine and Surgery on long-term strategic planning, project management, and organizational development. Currently, Mr. Ryan is pursuing his Juris Doctor at Harvard Law School in Cambridge, Massachusetts.

Brett W. Taylor is an academic emergency pediatrician and health informatician with the Department of Emergency Medicine at Dalhousie University and the IWK Health Centre Emergency Department in Halifax Nova Scotia Canada. Currently, his administrative and academic duties include Director, Centre for Therapeutic Technology at the IWK, Director Informatics for the Department of Emergency Medicine at Dalhousie, and Lead Physician, Informatics for the IWK Health Centre. Research interests include decision support in the acute care environment, decision-making theory, the e-therapeutics of minor traumatic brain injury, mobile applications for health, and information visualization. Dr. Taylor has been the director of two emergency pediatric programs and is a member of national pediatric research consortiums. He lives, works, and surfs in Halifax, Nova Scotia.

Julie Yang is a Project Manager at the Institute for Clinical Evaluative Sciences. She received her undergraduate degree in Health Studies from the University of Waterloo with a minor in Gerontology and her Master of Arts in Health Policy and Equity from York University. Her research interests include health and food policies, the impact of neoliberal discourse on food security, diaspora and food security, food systems analysis, and the intersection of place and space with food security.

Shahram Zaheer is currently enrolled in Health Policy and Management PhD program at York University. He is being supervised in his academic and research activities for the past four years by Dr. Liane Ginsburg. His area of interest includes patient safety, organizational culture, high reliability organizations, medical errors, and knowledge translation. Shahram has completed Masters of Science (MSc) degree in Kinesiology and Health Science from York University. His Master's Thesis examined the role of ease of reporting, group norms of openness, and participative leadership on frontline staff perceptions of patient safety culture. Shahram completed his undergraduate degree in Psychology (BSc). During this time period, he worked in a Psychology Assessment Laboratory under the supervision of Dr. Krista Trobst at York University. His undergraduate Thesis examined the effects of gender and emotions on social support provisions.

Index

CPSIA information can be obtained at www.ICGtesting.com
Printed in the USA
BVOW05*1204210713

326451BV00007B/114/P